Forensic Learning Series

Introduction to
Forensic Nursing
Principles and Practice
Forensic Learning Series

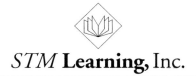

STM **Learning,** Inc.

Leading Publisher of Scientific, Technical, and Medical Educational Resources
Saint Louis
www.stmlearning.com

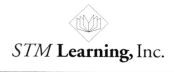

STM **Learning,** Inc.

We've partnered with Copyright Clearance Center to make it easy for you to request permissions to reuse content from STM Learning, Inc.

With copyright.com, you can quickly and easily secure the permissions you want.

Simply follow these steps to get started:

— Visit **copyright.com** and enter the title, ISBN, or ISSN number of the publication you'd like to reuse and hit "Go."
— After finding the title you'd like, choose "Pay-Per-Use Options."
— Enter the publication year of the content you'd like to reuse.
— Scroll down the list to find the type of reuse you want to request.
— Select the corresponding bubble and click "Price & Order."
— Fill out any required information and follow the prompts to acquire the proper permissions to reuse the content that you'd like.

For questions about using the service on **copyright.com**, please contact:

Copyright Clearance Center
222 Rosewood Drive
Danvers, MA 01923
Phone: +1-(978) 750-8400
Fax: +1-(978) 750-4470

Additional requests can be sent directly to **info@copyright.com**.

Introduction to
Forensic Nursing
Principles and Practice
Forensic Learning Series

Diana K. Faugno, MSN, RN, CPN, AFN-C, SANE-A, SANE-P, FAAFS, DF-IAFN, DF-AFN
Forensic Nurse
Dallas, Georgia
End Violence Against Women International
Former Board Director and Founding Member
Academy of Forensic Nursing
Former President and Founding Member
International Association of Forensic Nurses
Founding Member

Stacey A. Mitchell, DNP, MBA, MEd, RN, AFN-C, SANE-A, SANE-P, DF-AFN, FAAN
Clinical Professor and Director
Center of Excellence in Forensic Nursing
Texas A&M University School of Nursing
College Station, Texas
Forensic Nursing Certification Board
Former President and Founding Member
International Association of Forensic Nurses
Former President
Academy of Forensic Nursing
Founding Member

Valerie Sievers, MSN, RN, CNS, AFN-C, SANE-A, SANE-P, DF-AFN
Principal, Med Law Consultants LLC.
Peyton, Colorado
Care Team Consultant, Leda Health
Brooklyn, New York
Academy of Forensic Nursing
Founding Member

Sarah L. Pederson, BSN, RN, AFN-C, SANE-A, SANE-P
Georgia Statewide SANE Coordinator
Criminal Justice Coordinating Council
Atlanta, Georgia

Jessica M. Volz, DNP, CRNP, FNE A/P, FNP-BC, AFN-C, NE-BC, SANE-A, SANE-P, DM-AFN
Clinical Director of Forensics, Forensic Medical Unit
Adventist HealthCare Shady Grove Medical Center
Rockville, Maryland

Patricia M. Speck, DNSc, CRNP, FNP-BC, AFN-C, DF-IAFN, FAAFS, DF-AFN, FAAN
Professor; Coordinator Advanced Forensic Nursing
Department of Family, Community, & Health Systems
The University of Alabama at Birmingham School of Nursing
Birmingham, Alabama
Forensic Nursing Certification Board
President and Founding Member
International Association of Forensic Nurses Former President and
Founding Member Academy of Forensic Nursing Founding Member

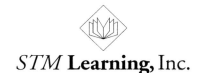

STM Learning, Inc.

Leading Publisher of Scientific, Technical, and Medical Educational Resources
Saint Louis
www.stmlearning.com

Publishers: Glenn E. Whaley and Marianne V. Whaley
Managing Editor: Olivia Sigmund
Graphic Design Director: Glenn E. Whaley
Graphic Designer: Connie H. C. Wang
Curriculum Developer: Olivia Sigmund
Associate Editor: Samantha Koester
Developmental Editor: Eleanor Stamer

Printed in the United States of America.

Publisher:
STM Learning, Inc.
Saint Louis, Missouri 63033
Phone: (314) 434-2424
http://www.stmlearning.com orders@stmlearning.com

Library of Congress Control Number: 2022912200

Print ISBN: 978-1-953119-07-0
eBook ISBN: 978-1-953119-08-7

CONTRIBUTORS

Sherry Arndt, BSN, MPA
Forensic Nursing Services
Comfrey, Minnesota

Molly V. Cooper, MSN, RN
AdventHealth Murray
Registered Nurse
Emergency Department
Chatsworth, Georgia

Callie Mersbergen, BSN, RN
Registered Nurse, Pediatric Intensive Care Unit
Phoenix Children's Hospital
Phoenix, Arizona

Varsha N., JD
Mayo Clinic Trained and Certified Wellness Coach
Certificate Harvard Program Refugee Trauma
Harvard Medical School of Continuing Education,
Founder & Consultant
ROAR Training & Consulting, LLC

Michelle M Tepper, DNP, MS, AGNP-C, SANE-A, SANE-P
Forensic Nurse Examiner
Suffolk County, New York
Clinical Instructor Emergency Medicine
Stony Brook Medicine
Stony Brook, New York

Elizabeth Burgess Dowdell, PhD, RN, AFN-C, FAAN
Professor
M. Louise Fitzpatrick College of Nursing
Villanova University
Villanova, Pennsylvania

Alexis Del Grosso, BSN, RNC-MNN
Registered Nurse
Summerlin Hospital Medical Center
Las Vegas, Nevada

Laquadria S. Robinson, MSN, APRN, PMHNP-BC
Quality of Life Health Service, Mental Health NP,
Substance Abuse Department, Alabama

Lauren C. Skinner, BSN, RN
University of Alabama at Birmingham, School of Nursing,
Birmingham, Alabama

Lynn Ellen Shay, DNP, FNP-C, CPM
Assistant Professor Assistant Dean of Faculty/Course
Leader MSN NP Track Chamberlain University
Downers Grove, Illinois

Steadman L. McPeters, DNP, CPNP-AC, CRNP, RNFA
Assistant Dean of Faculty
Chamberlain University College of Nursing
Chicago, Illinois

Tanja Gavrilovic, DNP, PMHNP
Doctor of Nursing Practice
Psychiatric Mental Health Nurse Practitioner
University of Alabama at Birmingham School of Nursing

Catherine Carter-Snell, PhD, RN, SANE-A
Professor
School of Nursing and Midwifery
Mount Royal University, Calgary
Alberta, Canada

Kathryn A. Swift, MSN, CRNP, FNE A/P, FNP-BC, CMSRN, SANE-A, SANE-P
Adventist Healthcare Shady Grove Medical Center
Forensic Nurse Practitioner, Forensic Medical Unit
Rockville, Maryland

Christine Foote-Lucero, MSN, RN, CEN, SANE-A, SANE-P, AFN-C
Forensic Nurse Examiner Program Manager Emergency
Department University of Colorado Hospital
Aurora, Colorado

Theresa Fay-Hillier, DrPH, MSN, PMHCNS-BC
Associate Clinical Professor
Distinguished Fellow- Academy of Forensic Nurses
(Inducted 2021)
Drexel University College of Nursing and Health Professions

Melanie Alexander, RN, MSN
Psychiatric Registered Nurse
Behavioral Health Ireland Center
Children's of Alabama
Birmingham, Alabama

Jennifer L. Johnson, DNP, APRN, WHNP-BC, AFN-BC, SANE-A, SANE-P, AFN-C, DF-AFN
Johnson Legal Nurse Consulting, Owner
Mission, Kansas
Adjunct Professor, Maryville University
St. Louis, Missouri

Joyce P. Williams, DNP, MFSA, RN, FAAFS, DF-IAFN, FAAN
Stevenson University
Randallstown, Maryland
AAFS Chair, Forensic Nursing Science Section

Laura Zimm, JD
Assistant Public Defender Sixth Judicial District Public
Defender's Office
Duluth, Minnesota

Alex L. Classen, MPS-HLS, BSN, RN, FNE-A/P, CPN, GFN-C
Forensic Nurse Examiner
Forensic Medical Unit
Adventist Healthcare Shady Grove Medical Center
Rockville, Maryland
Senior Clinical Research Nurse
The NIH Clinical Center
The National Institutes of Health
Bethesda, Maryland

Angela Morris, BSN, RN, CEN, SANE-A, SANE-P, EMT
Project Coordinator
Indiana SANE Training Project
University of Southern Indiana
Evansville, Indiana

Maud D'Arcy, BSN, RN
Pediatric Psychiatry Registered Nurse
Grace Grego Maxwell Mental Health Unit
Dell Children's Medical Center
Austin, Texas

Max Veltman, PhD, RN, CPNP-PC, AFN-C
Associate Professor
School of Nursing, Boise State University
Boise, Idaho

Pamela Harris Bryant, DNP, CRNP, PNP, AC/PC
Assistant Professor
The University of Alabama at Birmingham School of
Nursing
Birmingham, Alabama

Deborah L. St. Germain, DNP, RN, CEN, SANE-A, AFN-C
Clinical Assistant Professor (Retired)
LSU Health Sciences Center
School of Nursing
New Orleans, Louisiana

Heather J. Hayes, DNP, FNP-C, AFN-C
Executive Director/Director of Forensic Medical Services
Edmondson Telford Center for Children
Nurse Practitioner, Adolescent Medicine
Gynocology Services
The Longstreet Clinic, OBGYN Deptartment
Assistant Professor, Inez School of Nursing
Brenau University
Gainesville, Georgia

Jaclyn Rodriguez, BSN, BS, RN, SANE-A
SANE Coordinator
Crime Victims Services Division
Office of the Illinois Attorney General
Chicago, Illinois

Kimberly A. Foster, MBA, BSN, RN
Forensic Nurse
Douglas County Task Force on Family Violence, Inc.
Director of Health and Safety
KIPP Metro Atlanta Schools
Douglasville, Georgia

Amy Carney, PhD, NP, FAAFS
Professor
School Of Nursing
California State University San Marcos
San Marcos, California

Debra S. Holbrook, MSN, RN, SANE A, FNE A/P, AFN-C, DF-AFN, FAAN
Director - Forensic Nursing
Mercy Medical Center
Baltimore, Maryland
Executive Board - President Elect Academy of Forensic
Nursing
Adjunct Faculty Johns Hopkins School of Nursing
Baltimore, Maryland
Owner - Holbrook Forensic Consultants

Annette Cannon, PhD, MA, RN, MSN, D-ABMDI
Jefferson County Coroner
Golden, Colorado

Stacy A. Drake, PhD, MPH, RN, AFN-BC, D-ABMDI, FAAN
Associate Professor
Texas A&M University, School of Nursing
College Station, Texas

Kathy Bell, MS, RN, AFN-C, SANE-A, SANE-P, DF-AFN
Forensic Nursing Administrator
Tulsa Police Department
Tulsa, Oklahoma

Loretta Tsu, MA, BSN, RN, SANE-A, SCRN
University of Colorado Hospital
Aurora, Colorado

Michelle Patch, PhD, MSN, APRN-CNS, ACNS-BC, AFN-C
Assistant Professor
Johns Hopkins University School of Nursing
Baltimore, Maryland
Medical Advisory Board Member
Training Institute on Strangulation Prevention
San Diego, California

Barb Blackdeer-Mackenzie (Ho-Chunk), MEPD
Tribal Coordinator
Wisconsin Coalition Against Sexual Assault
Madison, Wisconsin
Student Retention Specialist
National Tribal Trial College, Southwest Law and Policy Center
Tucson, Arizona

Jeneile Luebke, PhD, RN (Bad River Band)
Post-Doctoral Nurse Research Fellow
University of Wisconsin-Madison, School of Nursing
Madison, Wisconsin

Ecoee Rooney, DNP, RN, AFN-C, SANE-A, DF-AFN
Director of Nursing Leadership Professional Development
Ochsner Health System Nursing Professional Development
New Orleans, Louisiana

Laura Kaiser, MBA, BSN, RN, SANE-A
Executive Director
Forensic Nursing Network, Inc.
Delaware, Ohio

Ruth Downing, MSN, RN, CNP, SANE-A
Director of Project Development
Forensic Nursing Network, Inc.
Delaware, Ohio
Family Nurse Practitioner
Immediate Health Associates, LLC
Westerville, Ohio
Founder and President
Forensic Nurse Consulting, LLC
Delaware, Ohio

Karen B. Silva, PhD, MSN, MFN, PMHRN-BC
Behavioral Health Nurse
Instructor of Psychiatry
Human Trafficking Response Team
West Hollywood, California

Laurie Charles, MSN, RN, CA-CPSANE, SANE-A, SANE-P, CHSE, AFN-C
Clinical Assistant Professor
Center of Excellence in Forensic Nursing
Texas A&M University, School of Nursing
Bryan, Texas

Rosario V. Sanchez, PhD, MSN, RN, CCRN (Alumnus), SANE-A
Comprehensive Community Case Manager - Toledo Gracehaven
Sylvania, Ohio
University of Toledo, College of Nursing
Toledo, Ohio

Heather Quaile, DNP, WHNP-BC, AFN-C, CSC, IF, FAANP
CEO/Founder
The SHOW Center
Nurse Practitioner/Medical Admin Wellspring Living
Adjunct Faculty
Vanderbilt University

Anita G Hufft, PHD, RN, FAAN
Dean and Professor of Nursing (retired)
Texas Woman's University
Denton, Texas

David A. Williams, DDS, MS, MPH.
Consultant
Trojan Horse Consulting
Randallstown, Maryland

Gordon Lee Gillespie, PhD, DNP, RN, CEN, CNE, CPEN, PHCNS-BC, FAEN, FAAN
Professor & Associate Dean for Research
Institute for Nursing Research and Scholarship
University of Cincinnati College of Nursing
Cincinnati, Ohio

Steven J. Palazzo, PhD, MN, RN, CNE
Associate Professor & Associate Dean for Academic Affairs
School of Nursing
University of Nevada, Las Vegas
Las Vegas, Nevada

Pamela Tabor, DNP, AFN-BC, DF-AFN, DF-IAFN
Consultant, Expert Witness, and Trainer
Little Rock, Arkansas

Sean P. Dugan, MD, FAAP, SAFE
Medical Director
California Clinical Forensic Medical Training Center
Sacramento, California
Director of Forensic Services
Shasta Community Health Center
Children's Legacy Center
Redding, California

Andrea B. Ward-Wiley, MS, BSN, RN, SANE-A, GFN-C
Owner
Cardinal Forensic Healthcare, LLC
Hanford, California
Forensic Nurse
Central Valley Forensic Nursing Specialists, Inc.
Fresno, California
Care Team Member
Leda Health
Brooklyn, New York

Teresa Devitt-Lynch, MSN, RN, AFN-C, AFN-BC, SANE-A
Forensic/Legal Nurse Consultant & Owner INTREPID
Forensic Healthcare Consulting
Fargo, North Dakota

Shelli A. Larkin, MSN, WHNP-BC, NE-BC, SANE-A
Associate Director & Chief Clinical Officer
Student Health Services
Adjunct Faculty, Department of Biobehavioral Nursing
Augusta University
Augusta, Georgia

Victoria A. Franz, DNP, APRN, FNP-C, AFN-BC, SANE-A, SANE-P, SAMFE
Family Nurse Practitioner
Forensic Healthcare Program Medical Director
SAMFE Program Manager
DDEAMC
Fort Gordon, Georgia

Josie Doss, PhD, RNC-OB, AFN-C, SANE-A
Director (Interim) and Associate Professor
Georgia College & State University
College of Health Sciences, School of Nursing
Program Director
HRSA ANE- Sexual Assault Nurse Examiner Grant
Milledgeville, Georgia

Shantee Henry, DNP, RN, SANE-A
ANE-SANE Clinical Coordinator
Georgia College & State University Assistant Professor
College of Health Sciences, School of Nursing
Milledgeville, Georgia

Deborah Pierce, RN, BSN, CEN, TNCC, TECC, ATCN, Sworn Law Enforcement Officer
SWAT Team Nurse
Fulton County Police Department
PRN ER Nurse
Emory Johns Creek Hospital
Johns Creek, Georgia

Jeremy Ackerman, MD, PhD, FACEP
Associate Professor
Department of Emergency Medicine
Emory University School of Medicine
Associate Professor
Wallace H. Coulter Department of Biomedical Engineering
Emory University and the Georgia Institute of Technology
Tactical Physician
Fulton County Police Department SWAT Team
Atlanta, Georgia

Our Mission

To become the world leader in publishing and

information services on child abuse,

maltreatment, diseases, and domestic violence.

We seek to heighten awareness of these issues

and provide relevant information to

professionals and consumers.

FOREWORD

As nurses, we recognize that violence is a health care issue. It does not discriminate against gender, race, age, geographic region, economic boundaries, or religion. For those who are intrigued by science, the law, and the ability to aid in the judicial process, there lies an opportunity to work at the intersection of them all. This intersection is forensic nursing. Forensic nurses provide and implement patient-centered and trauma-informed care to persons who have suffered the unimaginable. *Introduction to Forensic Nursing: Principles and Practice* offers insight into this care. It illuminates the vast and ever-changing practice environment of forensic nursing and arms nurses with the knowledge to provide care to those experiencing violence and trauma.

Through the exploration of this text, present and future forensic nurses will strengthen their inner passion for providing medical forensic care to the patient populations they serve. Forensic nurses choose to be a voice for the voiceless and to provide evidence-based, compassionate care in cases of violence. As you embark on your forensic adventure, realize that, going forward, you have the opportunity to be an advocate for science. As you work with patients, be authentic, speak the truth, earn their trust, be supportive, and be unafraid to ask the tough questions. You are capable of changing the landscape of the health care setting. Remember that though your patients may be in their darkest hour, you can be the light for all the days ahead.

Dr. Jennifer L. Johnson, DNP, MSN, APRN, WHNP-BC, AFN-BC, SANE-A, SANE-P, AFN-C, DF-AFN
President
Academy of Forensic Nursing

Preface

"As is often the case, when a radical improvement in health care takes place, one visionary emerges." —Virginia A. Lynch.

Virginia Lynch conceptualized nurses as the torchbearers and promoted improvement of medical-forensic practices, defined the practice of forensic nursing, and took the role to a global level. Over the past 3 decades, forensic nursing has emerged as a health care discipline that provides and improves the quality of care for society's most vulnerable populations. Forensic nurses combine compassionate trauma-informed care with the latest scientific practices to bring safety, medical treatment, and justice to patients who experience trauma in all its forms.

Introduction to Forensic Nursing: Principles and Practice provides a pathway into many different areas of forensic nursing with a focus on trauma-informed care. Forensic nurses play a key role in the identification, collection, and preservation of evidence that may otherwise be lost during a patient's hospital visit. They are specially educated to provide holistic, trauma-informed care to patients who have been victims of sexual assault, intimate partner violence, neglect, and/or physical assault. Their education includes training in the legal and forensic science aspects of the role. Forensic nurses work with those affected by many forms of maltreatment, including elder and child abuse and human trafficking.

Many of the chapters herein contain case studies designed to walk readers through scenarios encountered by forensic nurses, allowing readers to develop an understanding of the complexities of patients and the problems they face following violence. Both the experienced and novice health care provider will benefit from this new text.

Diana K. Faugno, MSN, RN, CPN, AFN-C, SANE-A, SANE-P, FAAFS, DF-IAFN, DF-AFN

Stacey A. Mitchell, DNP, MBA, MEd, RN, AFN-C, SANE-A, SANE-P, DF-AFN, FAAN

Valerie Sievers, MSN, RN, CNS, AFN-C, SANE-A, SANE-P, DF-AFN

Sarah L. Pederson, BSN, RN, AFN-C, SANE-A, SANE-P

Jessica M. Volz, DNP, CRNP, FNE A/P, FNP-BC, AFN-C, NE-BC, SANE-A, SANE-P, DM-AFN

Patricia M. Speck, DNSc, CRNP, FNP-BC, AFN-C, DF-IAFN, FAAFS, DF-AFN, FAAN

REVIEWS

Introduction to Forensic Nursing: Principles and Practice is an excellent resource for professionals that work at the intersection between the criminal justice system, forensic evidence collection, and medical care. Each chapter includes key points and case studies that enable the reader to easily digest the information and apply the lessons to their day to day work. Those who seek to understand the vital role that forensic nurses play in criminal investigations and the search for the truth should read this book.

Debbie Feinstein
Chief, Special Victims Division
State's Attorney's Office
Montgomery County, Maryland

Forensic nursing is a specialized field that not only requires general nursing knowledge and skills but also knowledge of the inner workings of the vast criminal system. The textbook, Introduction to Forensic Nursing: Principles and Practice *dives into the nuances necessary for nursing consideration when caring for assault victims. From the patient interview and evidence collection to the victim aftercare and legal proceedings,* Introduction to Forensic Nursing: Principles and Practice *succinctly details the current practices forensic nurses can incorporate to ensure victims of assault are cared for in a patient-centered environment and evidence is secured to strengthen the prosecution of the alleged perpetrator. Current and future forensic nurses will benefit greatly from the use of this textbook.*

Jennifer D. Bankston, DNP, MSN, BSN, WHNP-BC
Nursing Instructor
Hillsborough Community College
Tampa, Florida
Adjunct Lecturer
Regis College
Department of Nursing
Weston, Massachusetts

Introduction to Forensic Nursing: Principles and Practice is a comprehensive textbook for those interested in the dynamic field of forensic nursing. This long-awaited textbook includes descriptions of the many roles of the forensic nurse along with tools and information for successful practice. The organization of the textbook allows easy access to the content, including an overview and historical perspective of forensic nursing, as well as sections with specific content related to borrowed science, violence across the lifespan, special populations, and special crimes. The chapters detail the role of forensic nursing in various fields, and many include case studies with enlightening discussion on how the concepts of forensic nursing would be applied to the scenario. The concept of trauma-informed care is pervasive and emphasized throughout the text. Applying the principles of trauma-informed care reaches far beyond the forensic nurse practice and is a skill that can be utilized by all nurses.

Introduction to Forensic Nursing: Principles and Practice fills a void for a complete evidence-based practice resource about forensic nursing all in one place. This scholarly resource will be an asset for nursing curriculums.

Vicki J. Vawter, DNP, APRN, WHNP-BC
Professor of Nursing
Health Science Division Chair
Hillsborough Community College

The authors of Introduction to Forensic Nursing: Principles and Practice *have built a robust foundation of knowledge on forensic nursing, equally palatable to those already in the medical field as well as prospective practitioners. One aspect of forensic nursing that makes it so special is the sheer number of disciplines routinely engaged in the work. From biology to psychology to law and beyond,* Introduction to Forensic Nursing *gives each one its due. With this book, the authors successfully lay the groundwork for a future with knowledgeable, well-rounded, trauma-informed forensic nurses leading the charge to serve the medical needs of victims of abuse and violence in tandem with the justice system.*

Thomas Manion, Director
Director, Family Justice Center
Montgomery County Office of the Sheriff
Rockville, MD 20852

INSTRUCTIONS

OVERVIEW

Introduction to Forensic Nursing: Principles and Practice was developed in conjunction with the Academy of Forensic Nursing (AFN) to provide current and future forensic nurses with the opportunity to learn and grow within the field. Candidates who complete the book may register to take the posttest through AFN Learn to earn 13.0 contact hours. AFN is an approved provider of continuing education (CE) credits through the American Nurses Credentialing Center (ANCC).

EDUCATIONAL OBJECTIVES

Introduction to Forensic Nursing: Principles and Practice serves as an introduction to the broad field of forensic nursing and the care of patients whose cases intersect with legal systems. Upon completion of this text, the reader will have a strong understanding of forensic nursing, current best practices within subspecialties, and the possibilities for the forensic nurse of the future.

After reviewing this text, readers will be able to:

— Understand the history of the field of forensic nursing

— Describe the intersection of health care and the legal system in forensic nursing practice

— Identify the scientific fields that inform forensic nursing practice

— Describe the effects of violence across the lifespan

— Identify best practices when working with special populations

— Describe the role of the forensic nurse in cases of special crimes

— Delineate the steps of assessment and evidence collection

— Implement trauma-informed care in their own practice

COURSE FORMAT AND IMPLEMENTATION

For optimal results, the authors suggest reading the text in its entirety and completing the assessment in the back of the book.

If you are interested in receiving CE credits for the completion of this workbook, the posttest can be accessed on the AFN learning management system (LMS) at **www.goafn.thinkific.com**. Readers must purchase the CE for *Introduction to Forensic Nursing: Principles and Practice* and complete the available assessment. After registering and successfully completing the posttest with a score of 80% or higher, registrants will receive confirmation of earned credits from AFN and will be able to download their certificate for 13.0 contact hours immediately.

Registrants will be able to complete this process at their own pace. All fees related to receiving credit are determined by AFN and are the sole responsibility of the student.

CONTENTS IN BRIEF

CONTENTS IN DETAIL

Introduction to
Forensic Nursing

Principles and Practice

Forensic Learning Series

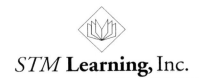

STM Learning, Inc.

Leading Publisher of Scientific, Technical, and Medical Educational Resources
Saint Louis
www.stmlearning.com

DEFINITIONS

OBJECTIVES
After reviewing this section, the reader will be able to:

1. *Clearly identify and define key terms related to forensic nursing.*

2. *Accurately apply terms when analyzing cases of forensic nursing.*

INSTRUCTIONS
The following terms are found throughout the text. This section should serve as a convenient reference for readers as they move through the chapters.

— **Adaptive Techniques:** Used by people with disabilities to provide developmentally specific care or assistance, such as wheelchairs, lifts, standing frames, gait trainers, augmentative communication devices, bath chairs, and recreational items (eg, swings or tricycles).

— **Actus Reus:** The guilty act (ie, the physical component of a crime).

— **Adolescent:** People between 10 and 19 years of age.

— **Adversarial Growth:** A phenomenon of acceptance of a traumatic event (or events), which includes positive psychological changes after the stages of recovery occur.

— **Adverse Childhood Experiences (ACEs):** Traumatic events that occur during childhood (eg, unstable housing; abandonment; domestic, sexual, physical, and emotional violence; and neglect) including witnessing violence and natural disasters.

— **Affiliated Volunteers:** Members of a recognized volunteer agency.

— **Alcohol-Enabled Sexual Assault (AESA):** Crime of sexual assault during which the perpetrator utilizes alcohol (either previously consumed by victim or provided by perpetrator) to incapacitate their victim.

— **All Hazards Approach:** Maximizes available resources to address the overall scope of emergency preparedness and planning, incorporating vulnerabilities and potential threats to the community.

— **Allostasis:** The process of the body responding to stressors in order to return to homeostasis.

— **Americans with Disabilities Act (ADA):** A civil rights act that came into effect in 1990 to prohibit discrimination against individuals with disabilities in all areas of public life, including jobs, schools, transportation, and all public and private places.

— **Anogenital Examination:** An examination of external genital organs.

— **Anoxia:** The absence of oxygen. During strangulation, the brain suffers an anoxic injury when the blood supply is completely obstructed.

— ***Anoxic Brain Injury:*** Caused by a complete lack of oxygen to the brain.

— ***Arraignment:*** An initial step in the criminal justice process, where a defendant is charged and informed of their constitutional rights.

— ***Asphyxia:*** A general term indicating the body is deprived of oxygen. Causes of asphyxia are divided into 4 primary categories: suffocation, strangulation, mechanical asphyxia, and drowning.

— ***BALD Step:*** A mnemonic that acts as a checklist for forensic nurses while they look for specific physical findings; it allows for a comprehensive testimony about all characteristics of a patient's wounds.

— ***Barriers to Reporting:*** Real or imagined ideas, beliefs, and stereotypes that can prevent a victim from coming forward about an assault.

— ***Biological Evidence:*** Body fluids such as saliva, breast or vaginal fluids, ear wax, and sweat.

— ***Bookend Cards:*** The initial and concluding images in a photodocumentation series that include identifiable information such as the patient's hospital wristband, a computer-generated identification label, or a commercially prepared label containing the name of the patient, their date of birth, the date and time of the examination, the health care provider's name and credentials, and the patient's case number.

— ***Bruise:*** Also known as "contusion;" an area of hemorrhage of soft tissue caused by the rupture of blood vessels from blunt trauma. Contusions may be present in skin and internal organs.

— ***Buccal Swab:*** Collected from the inside of the cheek as a reference sample.

— ***Bullying:*** Unwelcome verbal, visual, nonverbal, or physical conduct.

— ***Burnout:*** The result of persistent stress caused by the work environment; it includes fatigue, energy depletion, and reduction of professional productivity.

— ***Careful Nursing:*** A nursing model that focuses on the relational aspects of the nurse and their patients with the aim of providing excellent care.

— ***CATCH Program:*** Gives people making a restricted report the opportunity to anonymously disclose suspect information to help the Department of Defense identify serial offenders.

— ***Cause of Death:*** The condition, disease, or trauma that led to a death.

— ***Chain of Custody:*** The tracking of evidence from identification through maintenance and disposal.

— ***Child Maltreatment:*** An action or failure to act that results in harm (or the potential for harm) to a child (ie, anyone under the age of 18).

— ***Child Neglect:*** A form of child maltreatment that occurs when a caregiver fails to act on behalf of the child, resulting in harm or potential harm to the child. It includes failing to meet a child's basic physical, emotional, medical, or educational needs, as well as failure to provide adequate supervision.

— ***Chin Abrasion:*** Incurred when, in an effort to protect the neck, the victim instinctively lowers the head and creates a compression, sliding the chin against whatever is applying external pressure to the neck.

— ***Choking:*** Occurs when a foreign object lodges in the throat or windpipe, blocking airflow.

— *Civil Cases:* Lawsuits filed on behalf of 1 private party (eg, an individual) against another.

— *Cognitive Distortions:* Personal interpretations about what happened during an adverse event.

— *Compassion Fatigue:* The stress resulting from professionals continuously working with patients/clients who experience trauma.

— *Computed Tomography (CT):* A quick imaging technique that provides a detailed view of the internal organs and structures. CT imaging will identify injuries to neck structures (ie, bones and cartilage); however, it fails to evaluate injuries to the vasculature of the neck. A CT is *not* recommended to determine if there are injuries to the carotid or vertebral arteries.

— *Computed Tomographic Angiography (CTA):* Used to evaluate the arterial vessels. CTA is the gold standard for the evaluation of the carotid and vertebral arteries for a strangulation-induced dissection. CTA is sensitive for bony, cartilaginous, and soft tissue trauma as well as vascular injuries.

— *Contact Wound:* A wound resulting from the muzzle of a weapon being held against the skin.

— *Coroner:* An elected or appointed official whose duties include the oversight of medicolegal death investigations for a given geographical jurisdiction.

— *Correctional Facilities:* Places where people are kept when they have been arrested and are being punished for a crime.

— *Course of Conduct:* A pattern of multiple acts, serving as evidence of criminal purpose in a legal case.

— *Court Trial:* A type of trial in which attorneys present their cases to the judge, who serves as the "fact finder" and determines the outcome of a civil claim or criminal charges.

— *Coworker Workplace Violence:* Coworkers making derogatory comments about or threatening/committing physical harm against another coworker.

— *Crime Scene Investigation (CSI):* Use of physical evidence and deductive reasoning to gain knowledge about a crime.

— *Criminal Cases:* Cases that require probable cause in order to criminally charge a party with a crime.

— *Criminal Offenses:* Can include homicide, murder, sexual assault, robbery, aggravated assault, burglary, motor vehicle theft, and arson.

— *Criminal-Intent Workplace Violence:* An outside person entering a place of work and intentionally causing harm to employees and patrons.

— *Criminology:* The study of crime, what drives it, who perpetrates it and why, its interactions with society, and how to prevent it.

— *Cross Examination:* The questioning of a witness by the opposing attorney. The purpose is to discredit the witness or testimony provided on direct examination.

— *Customer/Client Workplace Violence:* A customer or patient intentionally causing harm to employees in a place of work.

— *Defense Health Agency (DHA):* An integrated combat support agency that enables the US Armed Forces medical services to have a medically ready force available.

— **Department of Defense (DOD):** The executive department of the federal government charged with coordinating and supervising all agencies and functions of the government directly related to national security and the US Armed Forces.

— **Dermis:** Includes the hair roots, sensory nerve fibers, sweat glands, sebaceous (ie, oil) glands, and capillaries.

— **Desistance:** The process by which gang members grow out of gang life or abstain from crime.

— **Developmental Disability:** A severe, chronic disability that is attributable to a mental or physical impairment or a combination of mental and physical impairments of an individual 5 years of age or older.

— **Digital Evidence:** Electronic devices, photography, and electronic records (eg, pornography).

— **Digital Immigrants:** Persons who were not born into the digital age but were typically born before the year 1990.

— **Digital Natives:** Persons born into and raised in a society with digital technology (ie, Generation Z and future generations).

— **Direct Examination:** The initial questioning of a witness by the attorney who called the witness with the intent to present testimony supporting a factual argument.

— **Disaster Cycle:** Comprised of 4 distinct phases for communities that wish to proactively address disasters; it includes preparedness, response, recovery, and mitigation.

— **Disparate Treatment/Impact:** Discriminatory practices in health care; may be intentional or unintentional.

— **Distance Wounds:** Occur when the distance to the weapon exceeds that of an intermediate wound and is far enough that there is no soot deposition or tattooing.

— **Domestic Violence (DV):** Physical, sexual, emotional, economic, psychological, spiritual, and financial abuse; may occur in any familial relationship between current or former intimate partners, married or unmarried couples, persons in heterosexual or same-sex relationships, parents or stepparents and their children, or persons with disabilities and their caregivers.

— **Drug-Facilitated Sexual Assault (DFSA):** Crime of sexual assault during which the perpetrator utilizes drugs (either previously consumed or provided by perpetrator) to incapacitate their victim.

— **Ecchymosis:** Discoloration caused by bleeding under the skin as a result of trauma.

— **Epidermis:** The outermost layer of the skin; it contains several layers of different types of cells, namely keratin, which provides structure and protection, and melanocytes, which produce the chemical melanin to create skin pigment.

— **Erotomania:** A person's delusional belief that someone is in love with them, and if not for an external barrier, they would be together; may lead a stalker to blame others for standing in the way of their "relationship."

— **Eustress:** Beneficial stress.

— *Evidence:* Available information/facts to prove an incident occurred (eg, photos, documentation).

— *Expert Witness:* In court, someone who is called upon to give their educated opinion on a topic.

— *Fact Witness:* In court, someone who was involved in the incident.

— *False Victimization Syndrome:* This type of stalker consciously or unconsciously believes that they are the victim and creates a fabricated claim; in these cases, the supposed "victim" is really the stalker; a rare motivation.

— *Family Advocacy Program (FAP):* The DOD's program designated to address domestic abuse, child abuse and neglect, and problematic sexual behavior in children and youth.

— *Financial Abuse:* Controlling the victim's ability to obtain, use, and maintain financial resources.

— *Forensic Anthropologists:* Typically specialize in physical anthropology and archeology (ie, the study of human osteology and skeleton interpretation).

— *Forensic Diagram:* A tool used in addition to forensic photography that supports descriptions of injury and findings; contributes to visual record of assessment findings.

— *Forensic Health Examiner (FHE):* Medical professional that has standardized training, maintains annual clinical competencies, and completes annual abuse/trauma-related continuing education.

— *Forensic Health Care Program (FHP):* A program that trains providers in forensic medical examinations, evidence collection techniques, and coordinated community response to violence.

— *Forensic Nursing:* The intersection of nursing and legal systems using borrowed elements of forensic science to assist patients.

— *Forensic Odontologist:* Identifies human remains by using the maxillofacial remains; has expertise in bite mark analysis through analysis of dentition impressions.

— *Forensic Pathologists:* Physicians who are board-certified in anatomic pathology and/or clinical pathology as well as forensic pathology; often serve as medical examiners.

— *Forensic Photography:* Also known as "photodocumentation;" a tool that supports descriptions of injury or normal findings and provides an authentic visual record of assessment findings at the time of the medical forensic examination.

— *Forensic Science:* The application of scientific methods to matters of criminal and civil law.

— *Gang:* An organized group commonly structured by racial, ethnic, or political lines that promotes permanent membership, engages in criminal activity, and employs threats, intimidation, or violence.

— *Gender Identity:* The personal conception one has of their gender (eg, male, female, nonbinary, etc.).

— *Gender-Based Crimes:* Violence committed against persons specifically due to their gender or gender role; may include domestic violence, dating violence, and stalking.

— *General Adaptation Syndrome (GAS):* Explains how the response to stress occurs and how chronic stress leads to physiological change and significant health problems.

— *Genital Swabs:* Includes samples from the penis, scrotum, vulva, vagina, and possibly the perineum/perianal area.

— *Gunshot Wounds (GSW):* Complex, penetrating injuries that are often encountered by health care professionals that work in the emergency department and other acute care and forensic settings.

— *Hate Crimes:* Can include larceny-theft; simple assault; intimidation; and destruction, damage, or vandalism of property.

— *Health Disparity:* A health difference that adversely affects disadvantaged populations based on a variety of health outcomes.

— *Hearsay:* Evidence based not on a witness's personal knowledge but on another's statement not made under oath.

— *Hemostasis:* Characterized by the constriction of blood vessels and capillaries where coagulation occurs.

— *Homeostasis:* The body's natural state of equilibrium.

— *Human Trafficking:* The recruitment, harboring, transportation, provision, obtaining, soliciting, or patronizing of a person for the purpose of sex exploitation, forced labor, and/or debt bondage.

— *Hybrid Disaster:* Caused by a combination of natural events and human actions.

— *Hypodermis:* The innermost layers of skin before the facia separation for underlying adipose, muscle, and bone.

— *Hypoxia:* The deficiency of sufficient oxygen in the blood, tissues, or cells to maintain normal physiological function.

— *Hypoxic Brain Injury:* Caused by a restriction of oxygen to the brain.

— *Impression Mark Abrasion:* Occurs when fingernails abrade the skin, leaving a curvilinear (ie, semicircular) mark.

— *Infiltrated Labor Unions:* Labor unions controlled or strongly influenced by crime organizations through fear and intimidation tactics.

— *Inflammatory Phase:* When damaged cells and pathogens are removed from the wound area via bleeding; the body's immediate response to trauma.

— *Integument:* The skin, the largest organ in the body. The integumentary system is composed of 3 layers: the epidermis, dermis, and hypodermis.

— *Intellectual Disability:* A condition that starts prior to adulthood and significantly decreases the ability to comprehend new or complex information, with reduced ability to learn or apply skills.

— *Interference:* Disruption of the victim's life personally, professionally, and/or socially.

— *International Organized Crime:* Groups of people who work together to gain power, influence, and money through illegal means; can vary from strict hierarchies to blood clans and networks.

— *Intimate Partner Violence (IPV):* Also known as "dating violence;" IPV occurs during the continuum of a romantic relationship, taking place anywhere from the introductory phase to its ending.

— ***Intimate Stalking:*** When a prior relationship exists between the stalker and victim, and the stalker is trying to reestablish that relationship; increased likelihood of prior history of abuse and domestic violence perpetrated by the stalker.

— ***Jail:*** Facilities for short-term confinement of people accused or convicted of crimes.

— ***Jury Trial:*** A type of trial in which attorneys present their cases to a panel of jurors. The jury then assesses the facts and evidence presented and makes the final decision regarding the civil claim or the criminal charges.

— ***Labor Trafficking:*** The recruitment, harboring, transportation, provision, or obtaining of a person for labor or services, through the use of force, fraud, or coercion for the purpose of subjection to involuntary servitude, peonage, debt bondage, or slavery.

— ***Life Invasion:*** When a stalker continually inserts themselves into the victim's life.

— ***Ligature Mark Abrasions:*** Typically horizontal abrasions on the neck that follow a predictable pattern; distinguishable from suicidal hanging marks because the suicidal suspension ligature mark rises diagonally toward the ear. However, if pressure is applied with a ligature at an upward angle, the mark may be indistinguishable from suicidal hanging marks.

— ***Magnetic Resonance Angiography (MRA):*** Used to evaluate the carotid and vertebral arteries for a possible dissection after strangulation. MRA is equally as sensitive as CTA for arterial dissection and does not involve ionizing radiation.

— ***Magnetic Resonance Imaging (MRI):*** A technique that uses a magnetic field and radio waves to create detailed images of the organs and tissues within the body. An MRI machine also produces 3-dimensional images that can be viewed from many different angles.

— ***Manmade Disaster:*** A disaster resulting directly from human actions.

— ***Manner of Death:*** A description of how the death occurred. There are 5 classifications: natural, accidental, homicidal, suicidal, and undetermined.

— ***MARCH:*** The acronym used in tactical combat or tactical emergency care situations. It stands for massive bleeding, airway, respiration, circulation, head and hypothermia.

— ***Maturation:*** The final stage in healing where the wound closes and is thick and the building blocks of collagen and fibrinogen are aligned with Langer's lines (ie, tension lines).

— ***Mechanism of Death:*** What occurred physiologically to cause a person to die.

— ***Medical Examiner (ME):*** Often, physicians who are appointed by a local or state governmental body in larger jurisdictions; duties include overseeing medicolegal death investigations (eg, postmortem examinations), ensuring identification of the decedent, and certifying the cause and manner of death on the legal death certificate.

— ***Medical Forensic Examination (MFE):*** The assessment/treatment of injuries and evaluation for sexually transmitted infections and pregnancy.

— ***Medicolegal Death Investigator (MDI):*** May hold titles such as death investigator, coroner, ME, deputy coroner, or coroner investigator; generally responsible for examining bodies, assessing scenes, and assisting in autopsies; serve as liaisons between the multiple disciplines involved in death investigation, assist surviving family members, collect medical and/or social history information on the deceased, and aid in determining the cause and manner of death.

— *Melanin:* Substance in the body that creates skin pigmentation.

— *Memorandums of Agreement or Understanding (MOA/MOU):* Legal agreements between 2 or more parties.

— *Mens Rea:* The guilty mind (ie, the mental intention to commit a crime).

— *Mental Illness:* A substantial disorder of thought, mood, perception, orientation, or memory that grossly impairs judgment, behavior, and capacity to recognize reality or ability to meet the ordinary demands of life.

— *Military Treatment Facility (MTF):* A hospital or clinic that is owned and operated by the armed forces.

— *Minority Health:* The various health characteristics of racial and/or ethnic minorities who may be socially disadvantaged due to potential discriminatory acts within the health care system.

— *Multidisciplinary Team (MDT):* MDTs typically include representatives from child protection agencies, prosecuting attorneys, forensic physicians, advanced forensic nurses with pediatric specialization, registered nurses, forensic interviewers, and child advocates.

— *National Response Framework (NRF):* Guides the national response to all types of emergencies.

— *Natural Disaster:* Catastrophic events caused by severe weather, global changes, or other nonhuman causes.

— *Near-Contact Wounds:* Produced when there is a gap between the gun muzzle and the skin, usually within a 1 or 2 centimeter range.

— *Nonconsensual Sexual Contact:* Penetration, attempted penetration, sexual touching, or inability to consent.

— *Nonintimate Stalking:* Absolutely no prior relationship between a stalker and their victim, but the stalker fixates on the victim after a brief encounter.

— *Nonmaleficence:* Physicians' obligation to not harm a patient.

— *Objection:* A procedure whereby a party asserts that a particular witness, line of questioning, or piece of evidence is improper.

— *Oral Swabs:* Swabs of the mouth that are effective for collecting DNA; obtained in cases of suspected orogenital contact by a perpetrator.

— *Outlaw Motorcycle Gangs (OMG):* Highly organized criminal groups that smuggle drugs and firearms and commit other violent crimes; primarily use motorcycles to run their illicit operations.

— *Patterned Injury:* An injury with a distinct pattern that may reproduce the characteristic of the object that caused the injury. The pattern may be caused by the impact of a weapon or other object on the body or by contact of the body with a pattered surface.

— *Penetrating GSW:* When a bullet enters the body but does not exit.

— *Perforating GSW:* When a bullet enters and then exits the body.

— *Perioral Swabs:* Collected from around the mouth without touching the lips.

— *Personal Relationship Workplace Violence:* When a partner/friend/family member of an employee enters the workplace and harms the victim.

— *Person-Centered Care:* Trauma-informed, holistic, just, respectful, compassionate, coordinated, evidence-based, and developmentally appropriate patient care.

— *Person-First Language (PFL):* A core competency for forensic nurses, PFL focuses on the person not the disability. Patients with ability challenges know their disability does not control or define them.

— *Petechiae:* Small, pinhead-sized spots caused by increased venous pressure in the capillary bed. The development of petechial hemorrhages in strangulation requires venous obstruction without obstruction of arterial flow. They can also result from nontraumatic causes, including forceful vomiting, coughing, childbirth, infection, and bleeding disorders.

— *Physical Disability:* A condition that affects a person's mobility, physical capacity, stamina, or dexterity which may include structural or functional impairments.

— *Physical Evidence Recovery Kit (PERK):* A special medical examination to collect evidence that may be helpful in a criminal prosecution or investigation of a sexual assault.

— *Physical Violence:* Ranges from abusive behaviors such as occasional slaps to regular, life-threatening beatings.

— *Polypharmacy:* The use of multiple drugs for treatment of 1 condition.

— *Positional Asphyxia:* Also known as "postural asphyxia;" a form of asphyxia occurring when the position of a person's body or external pressure prevents the person from breathing adequately.

— *Posttraumatic Stress Disorder (PTSD):* A condition caused by extensive trauma, initially known as "soldier's heart," that may include symptoms such as flashbacks and severe anxiety.

— *Prison Gangs:* Criminal organizations that have formed within the penitentiary system.

— *Prison:* A facility for criminals with felony sentencing greater than a year.

— *Processing Trauma:* A developmental process that varies greatly depending on the person's age, support systems, and the severity of the trauma.

— *Proliferative Phase:* Characterized by rebuilding the integument through supplying collagen and extracellular matrix.

— *Provider Fatigue:* A condition developed due to consistent high stress and working with patients/clients who experience trauma.

— *Psychological Violence:* Includes isolating tactics as well as academic, emotional, financial, technological, and verbal abuse.

— *Psychopathology:* The study of mental or behavioral disorders.

— *Range of Fire:* The factor that considers the distance of the barrel of the firearm to the patient. This range is classified as contact, near contact, intermediate, or distant.

— *Resiliency:* An effective way of addressing stress, creating and strengthening the ability to withstand, adapt to, and recover from stressful situations by using effective coping strategies to maintain a good state of mental health.

— *Restricted Reporting:* Allows the victim to receive medical, behavioral and advocacy support while not reporting to law enforcement or to a military unit or command.

— *Retraumatization:* Reliving stress reactions experienced as the result of a traumatic event when faced with a new, similar incident.

— *Risk-Taking Behavior:* A pattern of unnecessarily engaging in activities that are dangerous or highly subject to chance.

— *Rumination:* The process of continually thinking about the same sad or dark thoughts.

— *Scratch Mark Abrasion:* Long, superficial abrasions that may be as wide or narrow as the fingernail itself. Scratch marks may be caused by the assailant or may be a defensive wound caused by the victim trying to remove the hand(s) or object applying pressure to their neck.

— *Screening:* Medical tests used to check for health conditions before symptoms may be present.

— *Sensory Disabilities:* Affect 1 or more senses and occur across the lifespan; may also affect how a person gathers information because a reduction or loss of senses may result in communication difficulties.

— *Sex Trafficking:* The recruitment, harboring, transportation, provision, obtaining, patronizing, or soliciting of a person for the purposes of a commercial sex act, in which a commercial sex act is induced by force, fraud, or coercion, or in which the person induced to perform such act is not yet 18 years of age.

— *Sexual Assault Nurse Examiner (SANE):* Conducts the MFE while providing patient-centered care; addresses the medical, emotional, and forensic needs of the patient.

— *Sexual Assault Prevent and Response Office (SAPRO):* Responsible for oversight of the DOD's sexual assault policy; works to develop and implement innovative prevention and response programs.

— *Sexual Assault:* Any sexual contact or act performed by one person on another without consent, involving force, threat of force, refusal of consent, or the inability to provide consent.

— *Sexual Harassment:* Unwelcome verbal, visual, nonverbal, or physical conduct that is of a sexual nature or based on someone's sex.

— *Sexual Orientation:* An enduring emotional, romantic, sexual, or affectional attraction to another person; can be a fluid concept.

— *Sexual Violence:* Violence of sexual nature (eg, sexual harassment and assault).

— *Sexually and Gender Diverse:* Describes all members of the LGBTQIA+ community, including those who identify as nonbinary or whose identities, attractions, or behaviors do not align with traditional gender norms or current acronyms.

— *Simple Obsessional Stalkers:* The most common type of stalker; usually men focusing on an ex-wife, ex-lover, or former boss who feel like they were mistreated by the victim.

— *Smothering:* A form of asphyxia caused by closing the external respiratory orifices. This is caused either by the hand or by other means, such as blocking the cavities of the nose and mouth by introducing a foreign substance.

— *Social Determinants of Health (SDOH):* A person's overall health is determined based on where they are born, grow up, live, and work. SDOH also include access to education, health care providers, community resources, and economic stability.

— *Social-Ecological Model:* A violence prevention framework that provides a theoretical understanding of the effects of violence within and across systems.

— *Stalking and Harassment Assessment and Risk Profile (SHARP):* A computer-based program that contains 48 questions and generates 2 reports based on the patient's responses. The first report provides a stalking narrative and risk profile, while the second provides information about stalking risks and safety suggestions.

— *Stalking:* An interpersonal crime that is underscored by a persistent and repeated pattern of pursuit and harassment.

— *Stop the Bleed:* A program that provides courses on wound treatment.

— *Strangulation:* The external application of pressure to the neck resulting in alteration of consciousness.

— *Street Gangs:* Local or national gangs that can vary in membership size, ethnicities, and structure.

— *Stress:* A state of mental or emotional strain.

— *Subconjunctival Hemorrhage:* Capillary rupture and bleeding into the white portion of the eye (ie, sclera).

— *Subpoena:* A writ that sets the date, time, and location of the hearing requiring testimony.

— *Suffocation:* Obstruction or restriction of breathing by external mechanical forces; does not require blunt force.

— *Suspect Evidentiary Examinations:* Examinations routinely performed on the alleged perpetrators in a variety of cases, such as with sexual assault, child abuse, robberies, burglaries, homicides, and other interpersonal crimes, to gather and preserve evidence.

— *Special Weapons and Tactics (SWAT) Teams:* Police tactical units uniquely equipped to respond to high-risk scenarios.

— *Tactical Combat Casualty Care (TCCC):* United States military guidelines for trauma life support in combat medicine.

— *Tactical Emergency Casualty Care (TECC):* Training for emergency medical workers on how to safely respond to and care for patients in civilian tactical environments (eg, active shooter situations).

— *Tattooing:* Also known as "stippling;" embedded unburnt gunpowder grains after discharge.

— *Technology:* Machinery and equipment developed from applications of scientific knowledge.

— *Telehealth:* The use of information and communication technologies to improve patient outcomes through increased access to care and medical information. Forensic telehealth specifically aims to provide expert consultation, rapid evaluation, evidence collection, and timely response to community needs in underserved areas.

— *Testimony:* A statement made by a witness under oath, usually related to a legal proceeding.

— ***Trace Evidence:*** Materials left during commission of a crime (eg, hair, fiber, debris, dried fluids, secretions, or other traces of chemical or inert elements).

— ***Trauma:*** An event, series of events, or set of circumstances experienced by an individual as physically or emotionally harmful or life-threatening; has lasting adverse effects on the individual's functioning and mental, physical, social, emotional, or spiritual wellbeing.

— ***Trauma-Informed Care:*** A skill based on the 4 Rs: realization, recognition, response, and avoidance of retraumatization.

— ***Traumatic Brain Injury (TBI):*** An alteration in the normal function of the brain caused by external forces.

— ***Traumatic Experiences:*** An adverse event that leads to negative outcomes, often during childhood (eg, unstable housing; abandonment or neglect; domestic, sexual, physical, or emotional abuse; witnessing violence or national disasters).

— ***Trial:*** An examination, usually with testimony offered before a tribunal according to established procedures.

— ***Unrestricted Reporting:*** Allows the victim to receive medical, behavioral, and advocacy support and includes notifications to law enforcement or to a military unit or command.

— ***Verdict:*** An opinion rendered by a judge or jury on a question of fact.

— ***Victimization:*** The process of becoming a victim.

— ***Victimology:*** The study of the relationship between the victim, offender, and their intersection with the justice system.

— ***Voir Dire:*** The preliminary examination of a witness or juror by a judge.

Section II

OVERVIEW

Chapter 1

History of the Role of Forensic Nursing in the United States

Jessica M. Volz, DNP, CRNP, FNE A/P, FNP-BC, AFN-C, NE-BC, SANE-A, SANE-P, DM-AFN
Diana K. Faugno, MSN, RN, CPN, AFN-C, SANE-A, SANE-P, FAAFS, DF-IAFN, DF-AFN
Stacey A. Mitchell, DNP, MBA, MEd, RN, AFN-C, SANE-A, SANE-P, DF-AFN, FAAN
Sherry Arndt, BSN, RN
Patricia M. Speck, DNSc, CRNP, FNP-BC, AFN-C, DF-IAFN, FAAFS, DF-AFN, FAAN

Key Points

1. *The history of nursing began with a focus on maternal child survival up to 4 millennia ago in Persia, with additional records of deaconesses and nurse midwives in Europe in the 1300s.*

2. *Forensic nursing is heavily rooted in Sister Catherine McAuley's philosophy and model of careful nursing.*

3. *In her 1991 thesis, Virginia Lynch described a concept in nursing based on her experience and created the theoretical framework of forensic nursing in North America today.*

4. *Forensic nursing is a dynamic field at all educational levels, with opportunities to develop expertise in many sub-specialties founded on 3 pillars — legal, forensic science, and nursing.*

Introduction

The word "nurse" is derived from the Latin word "nutricius," meaning the nurture and sustenance of infants.[1] As such, nurses' interest in the survival of children is a common entry into the role. Nurses are frequently referred to as the *walking wounded*,[2] known for being honest, ethical, and caring for all types of patients, as well as learning to care for patients that are victims of violence. Forensic nursing is the intersection of nursing with the legal systems which utilizes borrowed elements of forensic science to assist patients who interact with the legal system.[3-7]

The first discovered documentation of medicine and forensic findings was in China and Mesopotamia, up to 6 thousand years ago.[8] Likewise, during the 13th and 14th centuries, Europeans recorded midwives and deaconesses in court records opining confirmation of virginity, sexual assault examinations, pregnancy examinations, and psychiatric care. Court records indicate that one nurse midwife, Emmeline La Duchesse, appeared in testimony records about virginity from the 1300s.[9,10]

By the 18th century, deaconesses documented victims of violence and midwives testified about rape routinely in court. They continued to verify virginity status of women planning to marry into royalty.[8,11,12] Many of these deaconesses were from the Catholic or Anglican European communities. The influence of Sister Catherine McAuley and her Sisters of Mercy spread the concept of *careful nursing*, a nursing model that focuses on the relational aspects of the nurse and their patients with the aim of providing excellent care. The mother of modern nursing, Florence Nightingale, trained specifically with the Sisters of Mercy. Sister Clare Moore, strongly influenced Nightingale's practice according to the memoirs she wrote while treating wounded British soldiers and other victims of violence in the Crimean War.[13] Meanwhile, the medical establishment of Great Britain created the first forensic psychiatry unit after a man accused of the attempted murder of King George III was found not guilty by reason of insanity and confined in a hospital instead of a jail.[7] In the late 1800s, hospitals housing mental health patients were akin to prisons and poorhouses.[14] In the early 1900s, nurses trained in careful nursing joined alongside the predominately male members of the asylum workers union to help transform the custodial asylum system.[15] Psychiatric mental health and corrections nursing experienced a unique path, different from hospital nursing care, making it more akin to forensic nursing today.

Throughout history, the role of forensic nursing evolved into a theoretical framework[5] based on Virginia Lynch's original supposition as related to forensic nursing theory,[16] concepts,[7] and various facets of practices.[17] Today, forensic nursing aligns with nursing core competencies (ie, domains), descriptions of practice, context for practice, and performance measures for content unique to the forensic nurse. The forensic nurse today has specific knowledge that is person-centered and trauma-informed, and is also based in quality, safety, professionalism, technology, and lifelong learning.[17] As such, in 1995, forensic nursing met the American Nurses Association's (ANA) criteria for specialty designation[18] and standards of practice were developed beginning in 1996.[19] The *Forensic Nursing Certification Board (FNCB) Core Competencies for Generalist and Advanced Forensic Nurses* have expanded, clarified, and aligned forensic nursing practices with general nursing core competencies.[17]

FORENSIC NURSING HISTORY IN THE UNITED STATES

In the United States, the first formal recognition of forensic nursing occurred when the American Academy of Forensic Sciences designated forensic nursing a role in 1989, largely because of the petitions for recognition from Lynch.[5] The field of forensic nursing's growth is largely due to media (eg, the TV show *CSI*), nursing interest, federal government funding, and market demands. Increasingly more educational opportunities have become available for nurses to expand their skill sets and roles in the forensic nursing area. The expansion of forensic nursing reflects the parallel growth with the nursing field,[20] and consequently, forensic nursing practice now includes care of patients in all settings across the lifespan according to educational achievement and license.[17]

The evolution of nursing and the role development in the 1960s promoted advanced roles in nursing and provided a path for nurses to work outside medical and hospital systems. The earliest programs responded to domestic violence and sexual assault, and they used advanced practice nurses and registered nurses for medical forensic care. By the 1970s, mental health nursing became an essential and necessary component in all nursing programs of study. In 1979, the surgeon general identified violent injury in youth as preventable with public health efforts.[21] Then, in 1991, the ANA published a position paper about violence against women.[22] In 1992, 74 nurses focused on the care of domestic violence and sexual assault patients met in Minneapolis, MN to form another organization recognizing forensic nurses – the International Association of Forensic Nurses. International forensic nurses formed country-specific organizations over the years, representing approximately a dozen countries. In 2018, the Academy of Forensic Nursing formed to give forensic nurses with comprehensive practices a platform for scholarly dissemination, including focuses such as domestic violence, sexual assault, human trafficking, death investigation, mental health, and corrections, among others.

FORENSIC NURSING TODAY

Forensic nurses care for and treat patients with intentional and unintentional injuries. Generalist forensic nurses represent the bedside nurse with specialized knowledge in forensic nursing; they are qualified to identify, document, treat under protocols, and refer patients in their care to advanced providers. Advanced forensic nurses are skilled as generalists, and with advanced education, they can collaborate with agencies to interpret clinical presentations and pathologies. They largely function as advanced providers of comprehensive care for patients with the licensed authority for long-term care. Today, many universities and colleges offer programs of study at the masters and doctorate levels. These programs prepare registered nurses to provide advanced specialized forensic nursing care. As a result, many hospitals and community-based forensic nursing programs offer a wide range of services today, including for patients who have experienced domestic violence, sexual assault, child or elder abuse, human trafficking, physical assault, and other forms of violence.

There are several professional organizations that serve forensic nurses:

— The Academy of Forensic Nursing

— The American Academy of Forensic Science

— The Academy on Violence and Abuse

— Futures without Violence

— International Association of Forensic Nursing

— Nursing Network on Violence Against Women International

Additionally, the FNCB now works "to provide professional certifications in Forensic Nursing Science that promote quality care to patients intersecting with the legal system."[23] The FNCB created the first comprehensive certifications for generalist and advanced forensic nurses in the nation. The organization's comprehensive examinations promise to guide the development of forensic nursing education and the competencies for sub-specialty micro-certifications in the future.

REFERENCES

1. Harper D. Etymology of nurse. Online Etymology Dictionary. https://www.etymonline.com/word/nurse

2. Conti-O'Hare M. *The Nurse as Wounded Healer: From Trauma to Transcendence.* Jones and Bartlett Publishers; 2002.

3. Speck PM, Peters S. Forensic nursing: Where law and nursing intersect. *Adv Nurse Pract.* 1999;11(10).

4. Speck PM, Aiken MM. Standards of practice for sexual assault nurse evaluators. Presented at: Sexual Assault Nurse Council Meeting (1st meeting of International Association of Forensic Nurses; August 13, 1992; Minneapolis, MN.

5. Lynch V, Duval JB. *Forensic nursing science.* 2nd ed. Mosby/Elsevier; 2011.

6. Lynch VA. *Clinical forensic nursing: A descriptive study in role development.* Thesis. University of Texas Arlington; 1991.

7. Kettles A, Woods P. A concept analysis of 'forensic' nursing. *Br J Forensic Pract.* 2006;8(3):16-27. doi:0.1108/14636646200600016

8. Payne-James J. History and development of forensic medicine and pathology. In: Payne-James J, Busuttil A, Smock W. *Forensic Medicine: Clinical and Pathological Aspects.* Greenwich Medical Media; 2003:3-12.

9. Cumston CG. Note on the history of forensic medicine of the Middle Ages. *J Crim Law Criminol.* 1913;3(6):855.

10. Marcus S, Higgins LA, Silver BR. Rape and representation. *Political Sci.* 1991.

11. Crane PA, Moreno M. Human Trafficking: What is the role of the health care provider? *J Appl Res Child.* 2011;2(1):4.

12. Shahar S. *The Fourth Estate: A History of Women in the Middle Ages.* Routledge Taylor & Francis Group; 1983:390.

13. Meehan TC. The Careful Nursing philosophy and professional practice model. *J Clin Nurs.* 2012;21(19-20):2905-16. doi:10.1111/j.1365-2702.2012.04214.x

14. Freeman H. [250 years of English psychiatry]. *Fortschr Neurol. Psychiatr.* 1996;64(8):320-6. doi:10.1055/s-2007-996401

15. Chatterton C. Women in mental health nursing: angels or custodians? *Int Hist Nurs J.* 2000;5(2)11-9.

16. Valentine JL, Sekula LK, Lynch V. Evolution of forensic nursing theory--introduction of the constructed theory of forensic nursing care: a middle-range theory. *J Forensic Nurs.* 2020;16(4):188-198. doi:10.1097/JFN.0000000000000287

17. Speck PM, Mitchell SA. *Forensic Nursing Core Competencies for Generalist and Advanced Forensic Nursing Practice.* The Forensic Nursing Certification Board; 2021.

18. American Nurses Association. Recognition of a nursing specialty, approval of a specialty nursing scope of practice statement, acknowledgment of specialty nursing standards of practice, and affirmation focused practice competencies. Congress on Nursing Practice and Economics. September 2005. Updated August 2017. https://www.nursingworld.org/~4989de/globalassets/practiceandpolicy/scope-of-practice/3sc-booklet-final-2017-08-17.pdf

19. *Forensic Nursing: Scope and Standards of Practice.* 2nd ed. American Nurses Association; 2017.

20. American Association of Colleges of Nursing. The Essentials: Core Competencies for Professional Nursing Education. 2021. https://www.aacnnursing.org/AACN-Essentials

21. US Department of Health, Education, and Welfare. Healthy People: *The Surgeon General's Report on Health Promotion and Disease Prevention.* Public Health Service; 1979:177. https://profiles.nlm.nih.gov/101584932X92

22. American Nurses Association. Violence Against Women: Statement of ANA Position. September 6, 1991. Updated March 24, 2000. Accessed December 20, 2021. https://www.nursingworld.org/practice-policy/nursing-excellence/official-position-statements/id/violence-against-women/.

23. Mission-Values-DEI. Forensic Nursing Certification Board. 2021. https://goforensicncb.org/mission_

Chapter 2

FOUNDATIONS OF FORENSIC NURSING

Patricia M. Speck, DNSc, CRNP, FNP-BC, AFN-C, DF-IAFN, FAAFS, DF-AFN, FAAN
Stacey A. Mitchell, DNP, MBA, MEd, RN, AFN-C, SANE-A, SANE-P, DF-AFN, FAAN

KEY POINTS

1. *The forensic nursing specialty reflects early nursing concepts of careful nursing, as represented by the relationships between the nurse, patient, environment, and health.*

2. *There are 2 levels of forensic nursing practice – generalist forensic nursing and advanced forensic nursing – guided by educational pedagogy and science.*

3. *Forensic nursing is informed by the 3 pillars of knowledge: legal, forensic science, and forensic nursing.*

4. *Forensic nursing pedagogy has guidance from forensic nursing core competencies, descriptions of practice, context for practice, core competencies for the practitioner, and content specific for foundational education.*

INTRODUCTION

Forensic nurses existed but were called "deaconesses" in the ancient world, they were primarily assistants to the physician, providing "healing and caring" with populations, such as soldiers, prisoners, families, slaves, and servants.[1] During the Renaissance, nurse midwives were also testimonial witnesses in French courts.[2] In the 18th century, nursing continued the care concept of *careful nursing* with soldiers, impoverished communities, and prisons.[3,4]

Nurses throughout the latter part of the 2nd millennium (17th to 20th century) nursed vulnerable populations. In 1991, Virginia Lynch introduced the concept of forensic nursing as a distinct role in the United States.[5] Conceptually, the role included 3 pillars of knowledge to inform forensic nursing practices with vulnerable populations. This was confirmed by the Forensic Nursing Certification Board Delphi study (Speck & Mitchell, 2022 unpublished at the time of this writing), which spanned 20 years. The Delphi study reflected the evolutionary conceptualization of the details of the practice and the theoretical framework for the role. The 126 educators participating in the study and subsequent 6 meetings established the elements from the experts necessary to define the practice and role of the forensic nurse, meeting the licensing regulations of registered nursing practices at the generalist and advanced nursing levels in state Boards of Nursing. The AACN *Essentials*[6] provided guidance for describing the practice, context for practice, core competencies, and content necessary for all forensic nursing practitioners. This includes those prepared and licensed as a registered nurse through a diploma, associate's degree, or bachelor's degree (ie, generalist forensic nurses), as well as those who are MSNs or DNPs with experience in physiology, pharmacology, and health assessment with differential diagnosis (ie, advanced forensic nurses). The 2 levels of practice reflect the licensure and scope of nursing practice in the United States but may not reflect preparation or licensure outside of it.

With a strong nursing foundation, the generalist or advanced registered nurse attends continuing education to build a narrow expertise in the care of a sub-specialty population in forensic nursing. The sub-specialties of forensic nurses include sexual assault, domestic violence, death investigation, corrections, legal consulting, child or elder abuse, and others. These roles often reflect existing registered nursing educational attainment and skills in working with specialty populations (eg, observation, objective documentation). They may refer concerns to the advanced provider, such as an advanced forensic nurse. The continuing education student learns about legal systems, evidence collection, and trauma-informed care principles[7] to attempt to mitigate the health outcomes in the traumatized individual.

The forensic nurse typically enters the forensic nursing role in the emergency department with a sub-specialty in sexual violence in adults and adolescents.[8] The generalist and increasing numbers of advanced forensic nurses in sexual assault care has evidence for increasing the justice outcomes with excellent adherence to evidence collection standards.[9] The impact on long-term health trajectory lacks evidence for the one-time patient encounter with a forensic nurse regardless of educational attainment.

FOUNDATIONAL FORENSIC NURSING PRACTICES

With preparation in leadership and systems thinking, the advanced forensic nurse prepares to practice under advanced nursing practice laws and state regulation, and some states allow independent practice. The advanced forensic nurse, through the intent of the *Essentials* "us[es] the unique knowledge and insight of the profession to inform any practice role and to impact the challenges in health care."[6] The advanced forensic nurse's education covers 10 domains as outlined in **Table 2-1**.[6] As forensic nursing clinical experience builds over time, the clinical expertise becomes useful to interprofessional coordinated care systems. Systems rely on the advanced forensic nurse to provide insight about forensic nursing populations and the evidence supporting their practices in programs. Whether general or advanced forensic nursing, the medical diagnosis and analysis about the forensic nursing practice parameters is a component of leadership in both generalist and advanced forensic nursing programs. All graduate-prepared forensic nurses demonstrate competency in the interpretation of the medical and health record, whether in short-term or long-term medical care delivered by the generalist or advanced forensic nurse, and make recommendations on diverse topics like nurse advocacy, medical treatment, and interprofessional care when working in legal systems.

Table 2-1. Forensic Nursing Core Competencies for Generalist and Advanced Forensic Nurses [9,10]

DOMAIN	BRIEF DESCRIPTION OF COMPETENCY SUMMARIES
Knowledge of Forensic Nursing Practice	— Integrate, translate, and apply established and evolving forensic nursing knowledge and knowledge from other disciplines — Enhanced knowledge leads to advanced practice and higher quality of care
Person-Centered, Trauma-Informed Care	— Focused care on the individual in complex contexts — Trauma-informed, holistic, just, respectful, compassionate, coordinated, evidence-based, and developmentally appropriate care
Forensic Populations	— Collaboration across disciplines to improve equitable population health outcomes for vulnerable populations
Forensic Nursing Scholarship	— Generation, synthesis, translation, application, and dissemination of forensic nursing knowledge to improve and transform health care

(continued)

Table 2-1. Forensic Nursing Core Competencies for Generalist and Advanced Forensic Nurses [9,10] *(continued)*	
DOMAIN	BRIEF DESCRIPTION OF COMPETENCY SUMMARIES
Quality and Safety in Forensic Settings	— Participate in the employment of established and emerging principles of safety and improvement of science to further quality forensic nursing care. — Quality and safety enhance care and minimize harm to patients and providers through system effectiveness and individual performance.
Interprofessional Relationships	— Participate in intentional collaboration across professions with multidisciplinary and interprofessional team members, patients, families, and communities.
Systems-Based Practice	— Lead within the complex interprofessional systems of health care — Coordination of care delivery, resources, and evaluation to provide safe, quality, equitable care to diverse populations
Informatics and Technology	— Utilization of information and communication technologies where informatics processes are used
Professionalism	— Participation in the formation and cultivation of sustainable professional and advanced forensic nursing identities — Accountability, perspective, collaborative disposition, and comportment that reflects forensic nursing's characteristics and values
Life-long Learning and Leadership	— Participation in activities and self-reflection to foster personal health, overcome barriers, build resilience and well-being — Continued lifelong learning to enhance forensic nursing expertise and lead in professional and advanced forensic nursing roles

© FNCB, 2022. Used with permission.

Launched in 2018, the Forensic Nursing Certification Board provides educational institutions with curriculum and content for forensic nursing programs.[9] The core competencies in forensic nursing build on the AACN *Essentials* core competencies and include trauma-informed care, knowledge that threads the brainstem response to trauma and stress to short- and long-term health sequelae, and whether disease formation or mental health adjustments to abnormal life events. Forensic nurses carry on the idea of *careful nursing* in the context of the intersection of forensic nursing and legal systems, utilizing borrowed elements of forensic science to guide concepts and practice. Forensic nurses are expected to know basic legal principles and understand their role in the legal system as health care professionals responsible for the overarching management of evidence collected following a crime. The management of evidence[11] includes but is not limited to: objective descriptions and documentation in electronic medical records and photography, evidence packaging, storage, and transfer; maintaining the integrity of the evidence storage over time; and preserving the chain of custody in health care systems.

SUMMARY

The foundations contributing to forensic nursing identify Level 1 and Level 2 practices, known as generalist and advanced forensic nurses. Interest in the representation of vulnerable populations who intersect with legal systems draws nurses from all disciplines to care for forensic nursing patients. The foundations supporting generalist forensic nurse practices guide development of new roles within unique populations, whether responding in a hospital or community-based system. The foundational knowledge that includes interprofessional team's approaches, coupled with the leadership skills of the advanced forensic nurse, guide the changing dynamics in the health care industry as the standardization of forensic nursing practice and education improves and aligns with forensic nursing foundational documents globally.

REFERENCES

1. Theofanidis D, Sapountzi-Krepia D. Nursing and Caring: An historical overview from ancient Greek tradition to modern times. *Int'l J Caring Sci*. 2015;8(3):791-801.

2. Cumston CG. Note on the history of forensic medicine of the Middle Ages. *J Crim Law Criminol*. 1913;3(6):855.

3. Meehan TC. The Careful Nursing philosophy and professional practice model. *J Clin Nurs*. 2012;21(19-20):2905-16. doi:10.1111/j.1365-2702.2012.04214.x

4. Strickler J. Florence Nightingale: Lighting the way for the future of nursing. *Lippincott Williams & Wilkins*; 2017:47(12)43-45. doi:10.1097/01.NURSE.0000526887.95058.3b

5. Lynch VA. *Clinical forensic nursing: A descriptive study in role development*. Thesis. University of Texas Arlington; 1991.

6. American Association of Colleges of Nursing. The Essentials: Core Competencies for Professional Nursing Education. AACN. 2021. Accessed November 11, 2021. https://www.aacnnursing.org/Portals/42/AcademicNursing/pdf/Essentials-2021.pdf

7. Simmons B, Grandfield K. Focus on forensic nursing education. *J Emerg Nurs*. 2013;39(6):633-634. doi:10.1016/j.jen.2013.06.010

8. Berishaj K, Boyland CM, Reinink K, Lynch V. Forensic Nurse Hospitalist: The comprehensive role of the forensic nurse in a hospital setting. *J Emerg Nurs*. 2020;46(3):286-293. doi:10.1016/j.jen.2020.03.002

9. The Forensic Nursing Certification Board. Forensic Nursing Core Competencies for Generalist and Advanced Forensic Nursing Practice. FNCB. 2021. Accessed December 11, 2021. www.forensicnursingcertificationboard.org

10. *Nursing: Scope and Standards of Practice*. 4th ed. American Nurses Association; 2021.

11. National Forensic Science and Technology Center. Crime scene investigation: A guide for law enforcement. 2013:180. Updated August 21, 2018. Accessed December 11, 2021. https://www.nist.gov/sites/default/files/documents/forensics/Crime-Scene-Investigation.pdf

Chapter 3

The Impact of Trauma on Health

Molly V. Cooper, MSN, RN
Callie Mersbergen, BSN, RN
Patricia M. Speck, DNSc, CRNP, FNP-BC, AFN-C, DF-IAFN, FAAFS, DF-AFN, FAAN

KEY POINTS

1. *Trauma activates the stress hormones. When the trauma ends, the body returns to homeostasis, but prolonged trauma can disrupt that process.*

2. *Traumatic events can lead to severe stress in children, affecting their memory, hormone and organ responses to stress, and their ability to form and maintain relationships.*

3. *A person's environment (eg, where they are born, live, etc.) is a determinant of health, influencing overall health and longevity.*

INTRODUCTION

The words "trauma" and "stress" are interchangeable in relation to health and wellness. The impact of trauma on health is present throughout the lifespan. The impact of traumatic events was first noted during the Civil War when many veterans were diagnosed with "soldier's heart." The term is now known as post traumatic stress disorder (PTSD) and includes an increased likelihood of cardiovascular disease.[1] Stress remains poorly understood as scientific explanations for stress outcomes are less than 30 years old. The association of stress with disease development provides a platform to understand the disease burden on society. Epidemiologists quantify victims from police reports, crime reports, and other government collection agencies, including the United States Census. This provides household and income data, which are 2 social determinants of health. Today, epidemiologists observe stress-related diseases associated with a lifetime of abuse as seen in **Figure 3-1.**[2]

THE STRESS RESPONSE

Almost 100 years ago, Selye[3] described the stress response by stating "the body never forgets." Selye's ***General Adaptation Syndrome*** (GAS) explains how the response to stress occurs and how chronic stress leads to physiological change and significant health problems (**Figure 3-1**). Trauma activates the stress hormones, and the body enters into ***fight or flight*** mode. When the trauma stops, the body returns to homeostasis; however, under repetition or severe traumatic stress, the chronic activation prevents a return to homeostasis. The chronic elevation of

Figure 3-1. An interactive map depicting how childhood trauma affects every system in our bodies.[2]

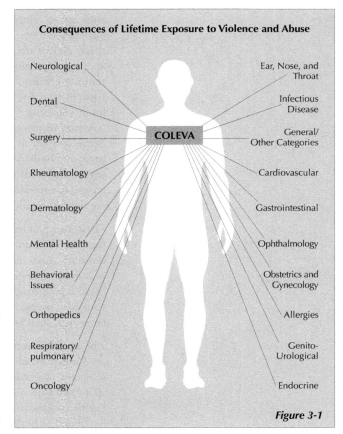

Consequences of Lifetime Exposure to Violence and Abuse

Neurological
Dental
Surgery
Rheumatology
Dermatology
Mental Health
Behavioral Issues
Orthopedics
Respiratory/pulmonary
Oncology

COLEVA

Ear, Nose, and Throat
Infectious Disease
General/Other Categories
Cardiovascular
Gastrointestinal
Ophthalmology
Obstetrics and Gynecology
Allergies
Genito-Urological
Endocrine

Figure 3-1

stress hormones results in neurologic and immune system injury. Inflammation from the trauma results in chronic health complications and increased risk-taking behaviors.[3] The association of stress and subsequent disease outcomes provides a foundation for understanding the disease burden on society, where health disparities demonstrate the stress burden in the disease profile of underserved populations.

Selye's GAS theory identified 3 stages of stress response: alarm reaction, resistance, and exhaustion. During experimentation, Selye noted a repeatable triad of stress response consisting of hypertrophy of the adrenal gland, atrophy of the lymph nodes, and peptic ulcers.[4] These common reactions are present whether stress is positive or negative and the body attempts to achieve a stable internal state of homeostasis.[5] Selye discovered that the physiologic responses of stressful situations activated the hypothalamic-pituitary-adrenal axis and named the glucocorticoid and mineralocorticoid hormones. Selye's work helped explain how increasing exposure to stress leads to the inability to maintain homeostasis.[6]

STRESS AND HEALTH

All human beings have body systems with checks and balances. When a person experiences no stress or positive stress (ie, eustress), there is *homeostasis* of body systems. When there is stress, the reptilian components of the vagal nerve sound an alarm and hormonal cascades occur. The body systems respond with the sole focus of preserving the heart, lungs, and brain. All other systems shut down, which is why patients with stress have cold hands and feet. The hormones influence the reactions of organs and increase the heart rate, dilate pupils, and improve awareness. Unfortunately, the hormones also stop all activity in organs related to digestion and elimination, which includes the gastrointestinal system, the urinary system, and other secretory organs. The brain also responds with heightened sensory awareness, imprinting smells and taste, visual and auditory events, and physical sensations. Short-term memory is blunted, and sensory memory is activated. Children without language development can describe what they heard, smelled, tasted, saw, and felt, but they do not have the ability to calculate temporal settings such as time and space. Adults attempt to put language to stress, often without success as language is an associative process; if the experience is new, there is no language to describe the traumatic stress. This type of stress is called *allostasis*. When the stress is repeated without time for recovery, the body experiences exhaustion, and the result is an allostatic loading.[7] The impact of the exhaustion phase is chronic vagal stimulus with coronary outcomes of vasoconstriction in all non-essential organs. Vasoconstriction denies oxygen to the cells, and the cells die, hence the shrinkage of organs in the brain and body. This cell death can lead to disease, including diabetes, hypertension, stroke, and cardiovascular and lung diseases. Some of the diseases are made worse by adaptive behaviors (eg, alcoholism, drug use, or smoking). All adaptations to trauma are normal reactions to abnormal events.

Environmental influences can positively or negatively affect the physiologic development of children. Stressful experiences cause hormone release, and cortisol, a stress hormone, has a negative impact when traumatic or repeated stress occurs. The cascade of hormones causes a dysregulation of the neurological and immune systems, affecting executive functioning, decision-making skills, and behavior. Chronic health problems may occur, including obesity and heart or lung disease, along with risk-taking behaviors, such as substance use, ultimately shortening life expectancy.[3]

The stressful events experienced in childhood that negatively impact a child's health are known as adverse childhood experiences (ACEs),[8] as shown in **Figure 3-2**. A screening tool scores ACEs and awards a single point to each experience of toxic stress in a child's life. In the identified areas, an increasing ACE score is associated with health complications later in life. An ACE score of 4 or greater indicates a serious likelihood of health complications,[8] as seen in **Figure 3-3**.

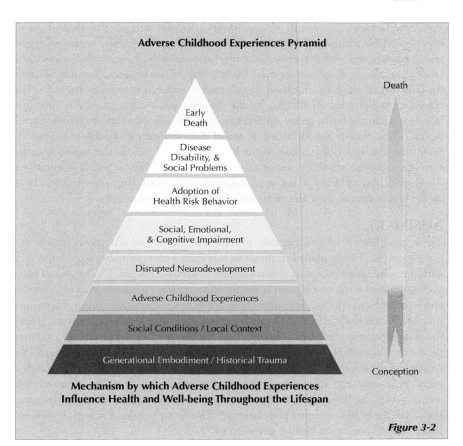

Figure 3-2. *Adverse childhood experiences pyramid (Image courtesy of the Centers for Disease Control and Prevention).*

Figure 3-3. *Lasting impact of adverse childhood experiences (Image adapted from the Centers for Disease Control and Prevention).*

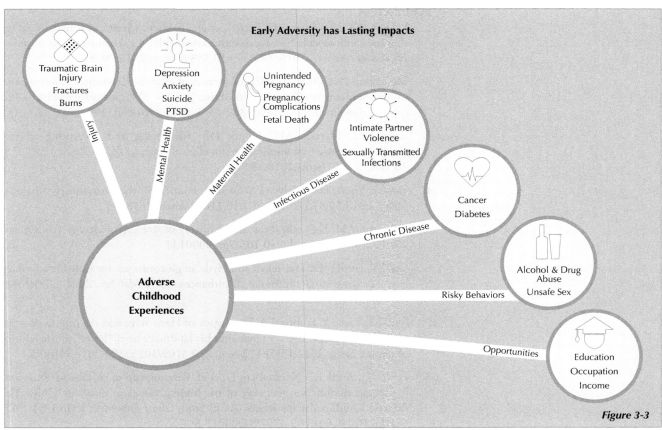

Protective factors in the family or community structure mitigate the stressful events experienced by a child. Children who have positive relationships with their peers and caregivers and who live in communities with stable housing, access to food, and readily available medical care are more likely to experience resilience in times of stress. An individual's access to education, health care providers, community resources, and economic stability are all affected by the geographical location in which they live. Where a person is born, grows up, lives, and works can thus influence their overall health. These factors are identified as ***social determinants of health***.[9] Oftentimes, these obstacles stem from characteristics historically linked to discrimination or exclusion (eg, race, age, ethnicity, socioeconomic status, disability, or sexual orientation). An individual with better access to resources to aid in mitigating adverse events is set up for higher success than an individual who lacks those resources.

SUMMARY

The human body responds naturally to traumatic events and oftentimes returns to a pre-stress state. Homeostasis is difficult to maintain with repeated or toxic stress and, with the subsequent increased allostasis, leads to chronic disease. The impact of stress and traumatic events on children is severe, affecting their memory, learning abilities, and relationships. A lack of resources can result in health disparities among communities, which negatively affects the health of certain populations who experience greater social or economic obstacles to health care. The medical model promotes providing illness care in emergent or urgent care centers rather than prevention measures for health and health care. Today, social determinants of health are often discussed in social, economic, and educational contexts, but public health attention must be directed toward the improvement of physical infrastructure and access to health care to guarantee the health of future populations.[10] The future promises attention to stress-reducing foci, leading to healthy populations.

REFERENCES

1. Pollard HB, Shivakumar C, Starr J, et al. "Soldier's Heart": A genetic basis for elevated cardiovascular disease risk associated with post-traumatic stress disorder. *Front Mol Neurosci*. 2016;9:87. doi:10.3389/fnmol.2016.00087

2. McCollum D. COLEVA — Consequences of Lifetime Exposure to Violence and Abuse. Academy on Violence and Abuse. January 2009. https://www.avahealth.org/file_download/inline/f89d58b2-1371-40a4-99c9-c4d2309eedf0

3. Jones CM, Merrick MT, Houry DE. Identifying and preventing adverse childhood experiences: implications for clinical practice. *JAMA*. 2020;323(1):25-26. doi:10.1001/jama.2019.18499

4. Tan SY, Yip A. Hans Selye (1907-1982): Founder of the stress theory. *Singapore Med J*. 2018;59(4):170-171. doi:10.11622/smedj.2018043

5. Robinson AM. Let's talk about stress: history of stress research. *Rev Gen Psychol*. 2018;22(3):334-342. doi:10.1037/gpr0000137

6. Seal SV, Turner JD. The 'Jekyll and Hyde' of gluconeogenesis: early life adversity, later life stress, and metabolic disturbances. *Int J Mol Sci*. 2021;22(7):3344. doi:10.3390/ijms22073344

7. Szabo S, Tache Y, Somogyi A. The legacy of Hans Selye and the origins of stress research: a retrospective 75 years after his landmark brief "letter" to the editor# of nature. *Stress*. 2012;15(5):472-8. doi:10.3109/10253890.2012.710919

8. Felitti VJ, Anda RF, Nordenberg D, et al. Relationship of childhood abuse and household dysfunction to many of the leading causes of death in adults. The Adverse Childhood Experiences (ACE) Study. *Am J Prev Med*. 1998;14(4):245-58. doi:10.1016/s0749-3797(98)00017-8

9. Healthy People 2030. Office of Disease Prevention and Health Promotion, Office of the Assistant Secretary for Health, Office of the Secretary, US Department of Health and Human Services. August 2020. https://health.gov/healthypeople

10 Agency for Healthcare Research and Quality. About SDOH in Healthcare. January 2020. Updated February 2020. Agency for Healthcare Research and Quality. https://www.ahrq.gov/sdoh/about.html

Burnout and Compassion Fatigue

Varsha N., JD, Mayo Clinic Trained and Certified Wellness Coach, Certificate Harvard Program Refugee Trauma, Harvard Medical School of Continuing Education Founder & Consultant, ROAR Training & Consulting, LLC

Key Points

1. *Burnout and compassion fatigue are 2 types of stress that are prevalent in nursing and include emotional, mental, and/or physical exhaustion.*

2. *Burnout occurs as a result of persistent stress caused by the work environment and includes fatigue, energy depletion, and reduction of professional productivity.*

3. *Patient safety and quality of care are negatively affected by burnout and compassion fatigue.*

4. *Implementation of self-care practices, combined with creating an awareness and increased education on burnout throughout organizations, is key to preventing compassion fatigue.*

Introduction

In our ever-growing complex health care system, frontline workers, especially nurses, are impacted by ongoing stress due to, "heavy workloads, long shifts…perceived job security…and lack of social support."[1] Burnout and compassion fatigue are 2 types of stress that are prevalent in nursing and include emotional, mental, and/or physical exhaustion. Professionals in nursing may find it necessary to take the appropriate steps to understand the profound implications of the impact of stress to improve outcomes for both nurses and their patients.

Burnout and Compassion Fatigue

Research[2] indicates that burnout occurs as a result of persistent stress caused by the work environment, and it includes fatigue, energy depletion, and reduction of professional productivity. Key contributors to burnout are high workloads, low staffing—contributing to long shifts—and low control, which can result in severe consequences for staff and patients. Over half of physicians and a third of nurses have been experiencing symptoms of burnout as it reached rampant levels in the United States during the COVID-19 pandemic.[3] When a nurse or physician is burnt out, it can double the odds of low work performance as they are completely spent mentally, physically, and emotionally.[4-6]

Both burnout and compassion fatigue carry a high risk of negatively impacting the social and physical well-being of nurses as well as critical outcomes of patient care. Efforts should be made by organizations to educate and destigmatize compassion fatigue as any medical professional can develop it. Furthermore, burnout and compassion fatigue impact nurses[7] across medical specialties, as demonstrated in a study of 100 oncology nurses reporting that there is a moderate risk for burnout and extremely high risk for compassion fatigue.In contrast to burnout, there is limited research on compassion fatigue, and it is an "understudied phenomenon that occurs in practicing nurses and [is] most likely to affect nurse educators in practice."[8] A key component of compassion fatigue is the stress resulting from professionals continuously working with patients/clients who experience trauma.[9] Medical professionals are especially vulnerable to compassion fatigue because of the close, ongoing contact with individuals who experience trauma and the empathy they must repeatedly demonstrate.

CONSEQUENCES OF COMPASSION FATIGUE AND BURNOUT

The quality of patient care depends greatly on the knowledge, skills, and well-being of nurses and can be negatively affected by burnout. In a systematic review, researchers concluded that in the majority of studies there was evidence that the well-being of nurses and their burnout are directly related to the patient's safety. Poor well-being (ie, depression, anxiety, poor quality of life, stress) and high levels of burnout were associated with reports of errors during patient care. When nurses experience these high levels of burnout, there are then higher rates of patient mortality, failures to rescue patients, and more prolonged hospital stays.[10,11]

An Iranian study[12] of 1200 health care workers noted an inverse relationship between burnout and safety culture, and that there was a direct negative effect on patient safety culture from burnout. So, burnout increases and the patient safety culture decreases. A study[13] on nurses at a university hospital in Korea found that 1 out of 5 nurses had experienced medical errors within the last 6 months, and they discovered that these participants also had moderate to high levels of burnout and emotional labor. The key characteristics to mitigate burnout and increasing the safety and quality of patient care are inclusion in decision-making, promotion of autonomy, and support by their teams, managers and leadership.[14-16]

EFFECTIVE STRATEGIES TO INCREASE EFFICACY OF SELF-CARE

Nurses work intimately with patients and are greatly impacted by the trauma experienced by their patients. They may not immediately understand the emotional, physical, and mental toll of caring for these patients. Self-care can be protective against the negative impacts of stress and it can be the strongest piece of armor to protect against compassion fatigue and burnout.[8] A study on student nurses experiencing compassion fatigue notes, "One way to explore difficult practices might be through reflective poetry which enables students and educators to share experiences in a meaningful way."[9] **Figure 4-1** displays a poem that demonstrates the emotional effect that a patient had on a nurse and highlights the impact of compassion fatigue, "a feeling of sadness was revealed…which conveyed psychological distress and unhappiness."[9]

Furthermore, a study[17] on mindfulness-based stress reduction (MBSR) in nurses found that using MBSR techniques like meditation, yoga, and journaling reduced burnout by 88.9%. As evidenced by these findings, these modalities of self-care have been helpful to professionals combatting stress. The implementation of self-care through these useful techniques, combined with creating awareness and increasing knowledge among organizations, is also key to the prevention of compassion fatigue.[18] Jack's study[9] on compassion fatigue, which highlights poems written by nursing students, concluded that "Positive practices such as shared reflection, use of creative teaching methods and exploration of feelings build resiliency and ways to cope." Building resiliency can be an effective way of addressing stress creating and strengthening the ability to withstand, adapt to, and recover from stressful situations by using effective coping strategies to maintain a good state of mental health.[19] The development of resiliency stems from harnessing personal strengths and support of friends, faith communities, and family.[19]

CASE STUDIES

Case Study 4-1

This nurse met with her 6th sexual assault survivor in a span of 2 weeks. She was taking over shifts for other nurses and getting very little sleep. The patient/survivor exhibited bruises, a

Figure 4-1. "The Professional Widow" by Kirsten Jack, 2017.[8]

It broke my heart to watch you suffer

"Chin up chick, you must get tougher"

Came the cries of camaraderie

"Concentrate now, that's an artery!"

I sought advice and found the strength

To keep my feelings at arm's length

Respect your boundaries, just pretend

Be your protector, not your friend

And leave you in your hour of need

Understand please, Just concede

I must be strong and let you go

To stand alone and beat your foe

But I will think of you today

And pray your fears have gone away

Forever in my heart & verse

You shaped my future as a nurse

Figure 4-1

sudden onset of vomiting, and bouts of crying. Upon speaking to the survivor, the nurse immediately thought of her own niece, who was roughly the same age as the patient, especially given the resemblance. The nurse visualized her niece suffering and felt tears welling up uncontrollably, intense sadness, and feelings of hopelessness upon hearing the details of the survivor's trauma. The nurse then rushed to exit the hospital room.

Discussion

The nurse could be experiencing both compassion fatigue and burnout. Her work schedule and long hours were contributing factors to her stress. The emotional impact of the survivor's experience and having feelings of hopelessness indicated that she was experiencing compassion fatigue. Practicing self-care (eg, mindfulness techniques, adequate sleep, healthy coping mechanisms) and turning to her support system could lead to positive outcomes of stress reduction. Furthermore, management can explore making modifications to her work schedule, such as reducing her work hours, create a supportive work environment aimed at alleviating the stress experienced, and enlist the help of their Employee Assistance Program.

SUMMARY

Although creating resiliency may take time to develop, nurses who are able to do so have self-care tools that combat both compassion fatigue and burnout to address ongoing complex health care situations, demanding hours, and high amounts of stress. Increasing the efficacy of self-care is dependent on the nurse first having an awareness of the negative outcomes of burnout and compassion fatigue and taking steps to address both types of stress. As nursing professionals continue to navigate the tumultuous landscape of health care, giving recognition to the negative impact of both types of stress can increase the professional efficacy of nurses and create positive outcomes for patient care.

REFERENCES

1. Søvold LE, Naslund JA, Kousoulis AA, et al. Prioritizing the mental health and well-being of healthcare workers: an urgent global public health priority. *Front Public Health*. 2021;9:679397. doi:10.3389/fpubh.2021.679397

2. Burn-out an "occupational phenomenon": international classification of diseases. World Health Organization. May 28, 2019. https://www.who.int/news/item/28-05-2019-burn-out-an-occupational-phenomenon-international-classification-of-diseases

3. Berg S. Half of health workers report burnout amid COVID-19. AMA Physician Health. July 20, 2021. Accessed June 13, 2022. https://www.ama-assn.org/practice-management/physician-health/half-health-workers-report-burnout-amid-covid-19

4. Reith TP. Burnout in United States healthcare professionals: a narrative review. *Cureus*. 2018;10(12). doi:10.7759/cureus.3681

5. Dall'Ora C, Ball J, Reinius M, Griffiths P. Burnout in nursing: A theoretical review. *Hum Resour Health*. 2020;18(1):1-41. doi:10.1186/s12960-020-00469-9

6. Dyrbye LN, Shanafelt TD, Johnson PO, Johnson LA, Satele D, West CP. A cross-sectional study exploring the relationship between burnout, absenteeism, and job performance among American nurses. *BMC Nursing*. 2019;18(1):1-57. doi:10.1186/s12912-019-0382-7

7. Jarrad RA, Hammad S. Oncology nurses' compassion fatigue, burn out and compassion satisfaction. *Ann Gen Psychiatry*. 2020;19(1):22. doi:10.1186/s12991-020-00272-9

8. Mullins N, McQueen L. Does compassion fatigue affect nurse educators in practice? *Nursing and Health*. 2017;5(1):18-20. doi:10.13189/nh.2017.050103

9. Jack K. The meaning of compassion fatigue to student nurses: an interpretive phenomenological study. *J Compassionate Health Care*. 2017;4(2). doi:10.1186/ s40639-017-0031-5

10. Hall LH, Johnson J, Watt I, Tsipa A, O'Connor DB. Healthcare staff wellbeing, burnout, and patient safety: a systematic review. *Plos One*. 2016;11(7):e0159015. doi:10.1371/journal.pone.0159015

11. Schlak AE, Aiken LH, Chittams J, Poghosyan L, McHugh M. Leveraging the work environment to minimize the negative impact of nurse burnout on patient outcomes. *Int J Environ Res Public Health*. 2021;18(2):610. doi:10.3390/ ijerph18020610

12. Khoshakhlagh AH, Khatooni E, Akbarzadeh I, Yazdanirad S, Sheidaei A. Analysis of affecting factors on patient safety culture in public and private hospitals in Iran. *BMC Health Serv Res*. 2019;19(1):1009. doi: 10.1186/s12913-019-4863-x

13. Kwon C, Lee B, Kwon O, Kim M, Sim K, Choi Y. Emotional labor, burnout, medical error, and turnover intention among South Korean nursing staff in a university hospital setting. *Int J Environ Res Public Health*. 2021;18(19):10111. doi:10.3390/ijerph181910111

14. Guirardello, EdB. Impact of critical care environment on burnout, perceived quality of care and safety attitude of the nursing team. *Rev Lat-Am Enferm*. 217;25:e2884. doi:10.1590/1518-8345.1472.2884

15. Sillero A, Zabalegui A. Organizational factors and burnout of perioperative nurses. *Clin Pract Epidemiol Ment Health*. 2018;14:132-142.doi:10.2174/ 1745017901814010132

16. Dall'Ora C, Saville C. Burnout in nursing: what have we learnt and what is still unknown? *Nurs Times*. 2021;117:43-44.

17. Vincent HL. *The Impact of Mindfulness-Based Stress Reduction Techniques on Nurse Burnout in an ICU*. Doctoral project. University of St. Augustine for Health Sciences; 2021. doi:10.46409/sr.TRAU8890

18. Peters E. Compassion fatigue in nursing: a concept analysis. *Nursing Forum (Hillsdale)*. 2018;53(4):466-480. doi:10.1111/nuf.12274

19. US Department of Health and Human Services. Individual Resilience. Public Health Emergency. Updated September 8, 2020. Accessed May 2, 2022. https:// www.phe.gov/Preparedness/planning/abc/Pages/individual-resilience.aspx

TRAUMA-INFORMED CARE

Michelle M. Tepper, DNP, MSN, AGNP-C, SANE-A, SANE-P
Elizabeth B. Dowdell, PhD, RN, AFN-C, FAAN
Patricia M. Speck, DNSc, CRNP, FNP-BC, AFN-C, DF-IAFN, FAAFS, DF-AFN, FAAN

KEY POINTS

1. *Trauma is universal, widespread, harmful, and costly to individuals and society at large.*

2. *Trauma-informed care is a skill based on the 4 R's: Realization, Recognition, Response, and Resist Re-traumatization.*

3. *Key principles in trauma-informed care include safety; trustworthiness and transparency; peer support; collaboration and mutuality; empowerment, voice, and choice; and sensitivity to cultural, historical, and gender issues.*

4. *The forensic nurse using trauma-informed care principles must seek permission to inquire about life circumstances and difficult life events. They should be aware of and avoid personal implicit and explicit biases.*

5. *To reach adversarial growth following trauma, stages of healing and recovery are necessary. These include disbelief, rumination, grief, reconciliation, and resolution.*

INTRODUCTION

Trauma is universal.[1] The definition of **trauma** is "an event, series of events, or set of circumstances that is experienced by an individual as physically or emotionally harmful or life threatening and that has lasting adverse effects on the individual's functioning and mental, physical, social, emotional, or spiritual well-being."[2] Persons, families, and communities experience trauma without regard to age, gender, socioeconomic status, race, ethnicity, or sexual orientation.

The effects of trauma are personal. They are based on a person's capacity to overcome trauma and create a path to reach their goals.[3] Hope is a major component of overcoming trauma.[4] With experience and practice, persons who have experienced trauma are said to be resilient. Many traumas result in adversarial growth, a phenomenon of acceptance of the event. Trauma results in a stress response, driven by the vagal nerve and hormone release. The neurobiological influences from trauma and subsequent stress result in acute and chronic changes in body and brain regions, which lead to long-term and, for some, permanent changes.[5] The seriousness of the impact of the stress response depends on the age and stage of development at the time of the trauma.[6]

PRACTICING TRAUMA-INFORMED CARE

Often, the patients seen by forensic nurses have a history of trauma, many times from their childhood. Adverse childhood experiences (see Chapter 16) can result in decisions that worsen health (eg, addictions and mental health). For the forensic nurse, it is important to recognize the presence of trauma symptoms and acknowledge the role trauma may play in an individual's life. By asking "What happened to you?" rather than "What is wrong with you?" forensic nurses can provide patients with an open opportunity to share their experiences. The 4 R's serve as a guide to practicing trauma-informed care. These guidelines, further explained in **Table 5-1,** include Realization, Recognition, Response, and avoidance of Re-traumatization.[2]

Table 5-1. The 4 Assumptions of Trauma-Informed Care*

ACTIONS	DESCRIPTION
Realization	Realize the widespread impact of trauma and understand that everyone has some trauma (eg, mass casualty [crashes, shootings, pandemic, weather events], government action/inaction [war, policy], racism [individual or structural], family trauma [abuse, exploitation, sexual violence, generational].
Recognition	Recognize the different expressions of trauma (eg, mental health, self-harm, depression, addictions, anger, fear, social phobias, aggression, and others).
Response	Use trauma-informed care principles to seek patient support for the inquiry (eg, What happened to you?).
Resist Re-traumatization	Ask the patient's preferences for your discussion about trauma (eg, May I speak to you about what happened?).

© Tepper, Dowdell, and Speck, 2021. Used with permission.

There are 6 key principles of trauma-informed care that should be practiced in provider-patient relationships: safety; trustworthiness and transparency; peer support; collaboration and mutuality; empowerment, voice, and choice; and sensitivity to cultural, historical and gender issues. These are further explained in **Table 5-2**.[1,2]

Table 5-2. The 6 Principles of a Trauma-Informed Approach in Organizations

PRINCIPLE	ACTION
Safety	Making sure people feel physically and psychologically safe in the environment
Trustworthiness and transparency	Conducting decisions with transparency and the goal of building and maintaining trust with all persons
Peer support	Providing patients with knowledge, experience, and emotional/social support
Collaboration and mutuality	Intentionally partnering with all persons and treating everyone equally
Empowerment, voice, and choice	Providing paths to success, building strength with support during trauma, perceptions of harm, and building resilience through healing
Cultural, historical, and gender issues	Acknowledging personal/structural implicit and explicit bias

Often, stereotypes and implicit biases interfere with person-centered care of forensic nurses. Judgement is an implicit assignment of stereotypes to a person's appearance, undermining patient safety. Biases hurt relationships, shut off avenues of communication, and diminish feelings of safety in patients. **Table 5-3** identifies different types of biases and gives examples of judgmental behaviors.[7]

Table 5-3. Cognitive Biases that Affect Provider Decision-Making[7]		
BIASES	DEFINITION	EXAMPLE
Aggregate Bias	Provider believes patients are exceptional without cause in comparison with patients for which guidelines were developed	Ignores that trauma is a factor in health
Confirmation Bias	Provider interprets and focuses on information that confirms their preconceptions	Is myopic in view of persons, not considering their lens
Fundamental Attribution Error	Provider blames patients for their respective situations rather than assess the factual circumstances	Judging persons for their situation; assigning blame for their condition
Overconfidence Bias	Provider believes they are more knowledgeable and/or skilled than they actually are, leading to action based on intuition, incomplete data, or in the absence of data	Discounting and minimizing persons' complaints and interpretation of their disease
Search Satisfying	Provider stops looking for other problems/diagnoses once one is identified	Convinced it's their way or the highway

© Speck, 2022, modified from McPeters et al, 2020. Used with permission.

RECOVERING FROM TRAUMA

Adversarial growth is the positive recovery goal of a person based on a series of predictable responses to trauma. The definition of adversarial growth is akin to posttraumatic growth, as both include positive psychological changes after the stages of recovery occur; however, reactions to trauma vary among people and cultures. The person's life experiences, core social structure response (eg, family), and larger community response can all influence their reaction to a traumatic event.[4] Their symptoms are not a psychological problem, but rather, they represent the person's unique coping style. People who have experienced trauma may be expressive or quiet, and their coping styles are not necessarily reflective of their experiences, as the body remembers the trauma it has endured.[8] The person's response is representative of trauma hormones and their impact on the body's systems.[6]

Regardless of the trauma they have experienced, all people need to express their feelings in a safe environment with supportive and caring providers. Symptoms expressed by trauma victims may include exhaustion, confusion, sadness, anxiety, agitation, numbness, dissociation, confusion, physical arousal, and blunted affect.[1,2] These are normal reactions to abnormal events of trauma. For some, a delayed or triggered response to trauma may be depression, persistent fatigue, anxiety, sleep disorders, fear of recurrence, and avoidance. When there is perceived culpability, shame is often a sensation that predicts a need for more intensive therapy.[4] It is normal for victims of trauma to experience intermittent distress with periods of relative calm or rest.

The stages of healing include disbelief, rumination, grief, reconciliation, and resolution.[1,2] Providers often find it necessary to implement trauma-focused cognitive behavioral therapy (CBT). CBT along with exercise and good nutrition make up the trio of interventions that promote healing. The elements of therapy include educating clients in the following ways[1]:

— Frame re-experiencing the event(s), hyperarousal, sleep disturbances, and other physical symptoms as physiological reactions to extreme stress.

— Communicate that treatment and other wellness activities can improve both psychological and physiological symptoms (eg, therapy, meditation, exercise, yoga).

— Refer certain clients to a psychiatrist who can evaluate them; if warranted, prescribe psycho-tropic medication to address severe symptoms.

— Discuss traumatic stress symptoms and their physiological components.

— Explain the links between traumatic stress symptoms and substance use disorders, if appropriate.

— Normalize trauma symptoms. For example, explain to clients that their symptoms are not a sign of weakness, a character flaw, being damaged, or going crazy.

— Support your clients and provide a message of hope—that they are not alone, and recovery is possible and anticipated.

SUMMARY

Trauma is universal, widespread, harmful, and costly. Trauma-informed care is a skill based on the 4 R's: Realization, Recognition, Response, and avoidance of Re-traumatization. Key principles in trauma-informed care include safety; trustworthiness and transparency; peer support; collaboration and mutuality; empowerment, voice, and choice; and sensitivity to cultural, historical, and gender issues. The forensic nurse's role is to implement trauma-informed care, seek the patient's permission to inquire about life circumstances and difficult life events, and avoid implicit and explicit bias.[9] Following trauma, a period of healing and recovery is necessary.

REFERENCES

1. Substance Abuse and Mental Health Services Administration. Trauma-Informed Care in Behavioral Health Services. *Treatment Improvement Protocol (TIP) Series 57.* US Department of Health and Human Services; 2014:342.

2. Trauma and violence. Substance Abuse and Mental Health Services Administration (SAMHSA). Updated March 22, 2022. https://www.samhsa.gov/trauma-violence

3. Masten AS, Tellegen A. Resilience in developmental psychopathology: contributions of the Project Competence Longitudinal Study. *Dev Psychopathol.* 2012;24(2):345-61. doi:10.1017/s095457941200003x

4. Muñoz RT, Hanks H. A structural model of adverse childhood experiences as antecedents of rumination leading to lower hope. *J Interpers Violence.* 2021;36(19-20):9790-9807. doi:10.1177/0886260519868195

5. LoBue C, Munro C, Schaffert J, et al. Traumatic brain injury and risk of long-term brain changes, accumulation of pathological markers, and developing dementia: a review. *J Alzheimers Dis.* 2019;70(3):629-654. doi:10.3233/jad-190028

6. Anda RF, Felitti VJ, Bremner JD, et al. The enduring effects of abuse and related adverse experiences in childhood. A convergence of evidence from neurobiology and epidemiology. *Eur Arch Psychiatry Clin Neurosci.* 2006;256(3):174-186. doi:10.1007/s00406-005-0624-4

7. Fargen KM, Leslie-Mazwi TM, Chen M, Hirsch JA. Physician, know thyself: implicit and explicit decision-making for mechanical thrombectomy in stroke. *J Neurointerv Surg.* 2020;12(10):952-956. doi:10.1136/neurintsurg-2020-015973

8. Selye H. *The Stress of Life.* McGraw-Hill; 1956:554.

9. Calow N, Bachmeier B, Lewis-O'Connor A. *Trauma, Violence, and Resilience Informed Care.* Academy of Forensic Nursing; 2021:7.

Chapter 6

FUTURE OF FORENSIC NURSING

Patricia M. Speck, DNSc, CRNP, FNP-BC, AFN-C, DF-IAFN, FAAFS, DF-AFN, FAAN
Stacey A. Mitchell, DNP, MBA, MEd, RN, AFN-C, SANE-A, SANE-P, DF-AFN, FAAN

KEY POINTS

1. *Roles and responsibilities in forensic nurse practices expanded to cover trauma in populations globally.*

2. *The maturity of the specialty of forensic nursing is dynamic and follows the nursing specialty nationally, influenced by the American Association of Colleges of Nursing (AACN) Essentials.*

3. *Legislation enhanced funding for programs nationally with expectations of continued funding for the general forensic nursing practice.*

4. *The impact of the COVID-19 pandemic reversed years of nursing practice restrictions and caused the growth of forensic telemedicine to address the needs of rural and remote populations of forensic nurses and their patients.*

5. *The Forensic Nursing Certification Board (FNCB) offers comprehensive certifications for generalist and advanced forensic nurses and is working with countries outside the United States to implement educational programs.*

INTRODUCTION

The first forensic nursing meeting in the United States was held in Minneapolis at the University of Minnesota and primarily consisted of forensic nurses in sexual assault care. The early growth was directly related to each scientific and health care organization's capacity to set standards[1] and to provide a location for common interests for the specialty of forensic nursing to develop. The roles of the forensic nurse[2] have since expanded and varied. They are dependent on the population, the patient's age and stage of development, and the type of intersection with the legal system. For instance, gunshot wound or domestic violence victims typically present to emergency departments and may be met by a forensic nurse or team of forensic health care professionals. The original conceptualization of *nurse clinician* was narrow among attendees at the first meeting. Nonetheless, the term *forensic nurse* was later adopted, as was the first definition that stated, "Forensic nursing is defined as the application of the nursing process to public or legal proceedings, and the application of forensic health care in the scientific investigation of trauma and/or death related to abuse, violence, criminal activity, liability, and accidents."[2]

Regardless, forensic nurses in sexual assault care dominated organizational activities through special interest groups (SIGs), oftentimes with interprofessional members. Active and diverse were other SIGs representing psyche-mental health (MH) forensic nursing, corrections, research, consultation, death investigation, and education. Divisions among forensic nurses and nurses that aligned with family violence advocates remained for decades. Funding domestic violence responses, shelters, and resources promoted these divisions in all states. The National Task Force to End Sexual and Domestic Violence recognized a need for similar funding for victims of sexual assault. The task force worked to combine funding for sexual and domestic violence, thereby growing the number of sexual assault nurse examiners (SANEs).[2] Other subspecialties continued to grow without the advantage of the federal government funding mechanisms. For those subspecialties, many found educational institutions supplied the opportunity to focus on their interests and practices. These early educators created forensic nurse graduate and doctoral programs that produced the first comprehensive generalist and advanced forensic nursing certifications. The focus on forensic nursing roles, graduate education for forensic nurses, and sexual assault care created schisms among early forensic nurses, and additional organizations were formed to address the needs of the growing diversity in communities of practice.

ROLES AND RESPONSIBILITIES

The state boards for nurses govern the roles and responsibilities of practicing nurses to protect the citizens in their respective states and territories. Some states oversee the forensic nurse role through specialty rules governing the practice of registered nurses. For example, Maryland confers a 'forensic nurse examiner' certificate with rules to govern education, location, and practice,[3] and Texas requires all emergency department nurses to attend 2 hours of forensic education.[4] There are other nuances in different states, but most do not require additional oversight by their state boards of nursing. Many states use existing licensing for the advanced nursing role where practice is with forensic populations; for instance, a nurse with a dual certification as a Family Nurse Practitioner with Psyche-MH may see human trafficking survivors and navigate the legal system on their behalf. As forensic nursing roles expand in all nurse practices, the AACN *Essentials*[5] defined and described the core competencies for each educational level. The *Essentials* served as the model for the *Forensic Nursing Core Competencies for the Generalist and Advanced Forensic Nurse*.[6]

Many of the skills necessary for practicing as a forensic nurse include infection control, medication management and accountability, quality improvement, objective documentation, anticipatory guidance, and communication. Many of these skills cross into forensic nursing practices, and as such, they are useful in forensic settings with patients intersecting with legal systems.

IMPACT ON NURSING EDUCATION

The first master's degree program in forensic nursing was opened in the 1990s, and the first doctorate in forensic nursing opened in 2004. There are now approximately 20 to 25 graduate programs in forensic nursing, growing annually with federal funding. The abeyance of new portfolio certifications from the American Nurses Credentialing Center (eg, AFN-BC)[7] left a gap in the community of forensic nursing practitioners, and it was the impetus for the FNCB to resurrect and move toward an examination of the 3 pillars (ie, legal, forensic science, nursing) of forensic nursing.

The impact of the *Essentials* on forensic nursing pulled the elements discovered in past meetings of forensic nursing educators forward, and from 2020 to 2021, forensic nursing educators and practitioners met several times to finalize the forensic nursing core competencies. They followed the same Delphi method used previously to reach consensus for domains and performance measures useful in future undergraduate and graduate educational curriculum and content. All elements in the FNCB Core Competencies[6] and content provided a platform for the FNCB Generalist and Advanced Forensic Nursing Certifications.[6] Over the span of 20 years, the work of more than 126 educators and practitioners solidified a future for forensic nursing.

IMPACT ON NURSING PRACTICE

As nursing roles expanded through continuing education, skill development, and acceptance, several new roles in forensic nursing emerged—telemedicine, flight forensic nursing, SWAT nursing, hospitalist nursing,[8] and risk management, to name a few. The cap on forensic nursing roles is limitless and needs only imagination. The common foundation is in the definition of forensic nursing, the comprehensive curriculum originated through collaboration, research, and consensus.

ADVANCEMENTS IN FORENSIC NURSING PRACTICE

While federal legislation focused on SANEs in the past, the focus of future legislation is on the generalist and advanced forensic nursing roles and their education in accredited schools and colleges of nursing.[9] As the specialty moves forward, the expectations of the forensic nurse are to master the broad common content for all forensic nurses, seek the comprehensive forensic nursing certification for the educational achievements, and then focus on obtaining further education and micro-certifications in forensic nursing subspecialties.

The COVID-19 pandemic impacted general patient care significantly. As such, restrictions on practice authorized forensic nurses to work with advanced providers to support remote and rural locations where inexperienced or new forensic nurses in sexual assault care existed. Telemedicine activities expanded the reach of forensic nursing support services, enabling acute patients who had experienced sexual assault to receive care during the pandemic. Forensic nurses needed to discuss "telemedicine-specific considerations... as well as guidance regarding practice assessment, financial feasibility, technical considerations, and clinical guidance to translate in-person visit skills into an effective virtual visit."[10] In order for this type of outreach to continue, forensic nurses must have a role in future legislation through education and nurse advocacy. Doing so is necessary to guarantee care to the rural and remote populations in their communities.

THE FUTURE — COMPREHENSIVE CERTIFICATIONS IN FORENSIC NURSING

Certifications are the foundation for professional advancement and recognition of expertise in a body of knowledge that is unique to the forensic nursing community of practice. The future of the role of the forensic nurse lies in the adoption of certification outcomes from the Delphi studies that defined not only the core competencies of the field but also the content necessary to help forensic nurses care for vulnerable populations.

Future forensic nurses will be able to attend accredited programs of study in universities and colleges at the bachelors, graduate, and doctoral program levels. Schools and colleges of nursing outside the United States plan to adopt the FNCB curriculum and tailor the legal pillar to their countries' laws on crime and nursing practices. These efforts by the FNCB will guide the future of forensic nursing for decades.

CASE STUDIES

Case 6-1

A forensic nurse was seeking continued education. She understood that attending an accredited school or college would be necessary for licensure and certifications. She was seeking a forensic nursing doctorate, as she enjoyed a relevant elective during her BSN coursework. One school advertised that they taught forensic nursing, but the teachers were not master's degree-prepared forensic nurses. She called her mentor to discuss her best option.

Discussion

The forensic nurse's mentor helped her to find accredited universities and colleges of nursing that promoted the fact that their students are eligible to receive a comprehensive certification as an Advanced Forensic Nurse upon completion of the program. They discussed the benefits of online education and the need for clinical hours that reflect all aspects of the forensic nursing practice. The choice was easy, as there was a forensic nursing graduate program in the nurse's community that met all aspects of the educational criteria for the certification she sought.

SUMMARY

For centuries, nurses have cared for people affected by trauma; this legacy continues through the practice of forensic nursing. Leaders in the field of forensic nursing are called upon to not only continually grow their own knowledge, but also to work with universities to create updated curricula to meet the needs of the contemporary patient. To expand their practice, forensic nurses should continually seek out leaders to mentor them and engage in continued education opportunities to prepare for future practice.

REFERENCES

1. American Nurses Association, International Association of Forensic Nurses. *Forensic Nursing Scope and Standards of Practice*. American Nurses Association; 1997.

2. Lynch V. Forensic nursing science: global strategies in health and justice. *Egypt J Forensic Sci*. 2011;1(2):69-76. doi:10.1016/j.ejfs.2011.04.001

3. Maryland Board of Nursing. Forensic Nurse Examiner. Updated August, 20, 2021. Accessed December 15, 2021. http://mbon.maryland.gov/Pages/forensic-nurse-examiner.aspx

4. Texas Board of Nursing. Education - Continuing Competency Requirements. 2021. Accessed December 15, 2021. https://www.bon.texas.gov/education_continuing_education.asp

5. American Association of Colleges of Nursing. The Essentials: Core Competencies for Professional Nursing Education. 2021. Accessed May 5, 2021. https://www.aacnnursing.org/Portals/42/AcademicNursing/pdf/Essentials-2021.pdf

6. Speck PM, Mitchell SA; The Forensic Nursing Certification Board. *Forensic Nursing Core Competencies for Generalist and Advanced Forensic Nursing Practice*. Forensic Nursing Certification Board; 2021.

7. American Nurses Credentialing Center. Advanced Forensic Nursing Certification. 2021. Accessed December 15, 2021. https://www.nursingworld.org/our-certifications/advanced-forensic-nursing-renewal/

8. Berishaj K, Boyland CM, Reinink K, Lynch V. Forensic nurse hospitalist: the comprehensive role of the forensic nurse in a hospital setting. *J Emerg Nurs*. 2020;46(3):286-293. doi:10.1016/j.jen.2020.03.002

9. *Murkowski, Hickenlooper Introduce Legislation to Improve Access to Medical Forensics for Victims of Violence*. Office of Senator Lisa Murkowski (R-AK); 2021.

10. Khosla S. Implementation of synchronous telemedicine into clinical practice. *Sleep Med Clin*. 2020;15(3):347-358. doi:10.1016/j.jsmc.2020.05.002

Section

BORROWED SCIENCE

Chapter 7

CRIMINOLOGY AND VICTIMOLOGY

Steadman L. McPeters, DNP, CPNP-AC, CRNP, RNFA
Alexis R. Del Grosso, BSN, RNC-MNN
Tanja Gavrilovic, DNP, PMHNP
Laquadria S. Robinson, MSN, APRN, PMHNP-BC
Lynn Ellen Shay, DNP, CRNP, FNP-C, CPM
Lauren C. Skinner, BSN, RN, CCRN, TCRN
Patricia M. Speck, DNSc, CRNP, FNP-BC, AFN-C, DF-IAFN, FAAFS, DF-AFN, FAAN

KEY POINTS

1. *Criminology is the study of crime and criminal behavior.*

2. *Victimology is a subscience criminology that studies the relationship between the victim and criminal in the culture of criminal justice.*

3. *Forensic nurses use criminology and victimology science to guide their practice and help navigate the patient's intersection with the legal system.*

4. *Forensic nurses develop and apply ethical personal philosophies to the trauma-informed, person-centered care of all patients intersecting with legal systems.*

INTRODUCTION

Both criminology and victimology focus on the unique relationship and intersection between the offender and the victim. Through the lens of forensic nursing, the borrowed science of criminology is essential in developing a plan of care for those whose cases intersect with legal systems. Forensic nurses are able to use their skills to interpret possible causes of legal offenses and the factors that encourage these crimes in global populations. Criminals often "...temporarily force their victims to play roles (almost as if following a script) [while a crime is in progress] that mimic the dynamics between predator and prey, winner and loser, victor and vanquished, and even master and slave."[1] In a systematic review of early-life risk factors, research showed that offenders often grow up in environments that promote crime for survival while victims often have traits that encourage vulnerability and environmental defenselessness.[2] Combined, these characteristics create an environment for crime to proliferate while simultaneously providing forensic nurses with a unique ability to provide care to this population.

CRIMINOLOGY

Criminology seeks to answer the questions of why people become criminals, what the social roots of crime are, and how crime affects victims and society as a whole. ***Criminology*** is the study of crime including causes, perpetrators' motivations, the effects on society, and prevention. Criminology studies deviant human behavior from a sociological perspective while considering the interplay of biology, psychology, anthropology, and philosophy. The study of criminology arose from the sociological intersection of criminals and victims and reflects the values of society in which it takes place. Numerous social, psychological, anthropological, and economic causes of violent crime exist.

Multiple philosophical theories of crime and delinquency guide the scientific study of criminology **(Table 7-1)**.[3,4]

Table 7-1. Theories Useful to Criminologists in Their Attempt to Explain Crime Causation[3,4]	
THEORY	DESCRIPTION OF THEORY
Rational Choice Theory	— Criminal behavior is an intentional choice — Criminals are not compelled or forced to commit crime — Criminal behavior is seen as more rewarding and less costly than non-criminal behavior
Sociological Positivism	— Behavior is the result of learning in the context of social structures, interactions, and situations
Biological Positivism	— Behavior is determined by biological factors beyond individual control
Psychological Positivism	— Psychodynamic theory: Early childhood experiences influence behavior later in life — Behavioral theory: Human behavior is developed through learning experiences — Cognitive theory: An individual's perception and how it is manifested influences behavior

VICTIMOLOGY

The term "victim" has ancient origins, dating back to the Hammurabi Code.[5] "Victimization is an asymmetrical interpersonal relationship that is abusive, painful, destructive, parasitical, and unfair."[1] *Victimology* is the study of the relationship between the victim and offender, as well as their intersection with the justice system.[4] As seen in **Table 7-2**, there are several theories in victimology that are used to explain how an individual may become a victim. While these theories explore how a victim's lifestyle or behavior could impact their risk of victimization, the blame for the crime still falls wholly on the perpetrator.

Table 7-2. Theories Useful to Researchers Studying Victimology[4]	
THEORY	DESCRIPTION OF THEORY
Mendelsohn's Theory of Victimization	— Victims had an unconscious attitude that led to their victimization — Identified several different types of victims: innocent victim, minor guilty victim due to ignorance, voluntary victim, victim who is more guilty than the offender, perpetrator who becomes a victim, and individual who falsifies victimization
von Hentig's Theory of Victimization (also known as Routine Activities)	— Victims are potentially negligent, provocative, and precipitate their own victimization (eg, individuals who have the same routine daily put themselves in the position to become a victim, creating vulnerability)

(continued)

Table 7-2. Theories Useful to Researchers Studying Victimology[4] *(continued)*

THEORY	DESCRIPTION OF THEORY
Lifestyle Exposure Theory of Victimization (also known as Deviant Place/Ecology)	— Certain lifestyles and risky choices may increase the chances of an individual becoming a victim (eg, walking alone at night)
Victim Precipitation Theory	— Analyzes the victim's involvement with the offender that led to the actual crime. — The victim is therefore an active participant in the crime; they act first, provoking the crime (eg, an armed robber is killed by their initial victim during the offense)

CRIMINOLOGY AND VICTIMOLOGY FORENSIC NURSING

The term *trauma-informed care* refers to how health care providers should respond to patients that have endured traumatic events or experiences that create feelings of helplessness, stress, overwhelming fear, or horror.[6] This type of care focuses on promoting safety and healing.[7] Forensic nursing was developed to provide patient-centered, evidence-based, trauma-informed, and equitable care to individuals affected by violence and trauma.[8] Forensic nurses borrow various theories from both criminology and victimology to navigate the patient's intersection with the legal system. Fully focusing on the patient's needs and having a nonjudgmental attitude are essential practices for providers applying person-centered care in a trauma-informed environment.

INTERPERSONAL RELATIONS

Nursing theorist Hildegard Peplau's *Interpersonal Relations Theory* emphasizes a therapeutic interpersonal process in which the nurse-patient relationship has a communicative character. This allows patients to use their experiences, feelings, thoughts, and complaints to freely express themselves.[9] Patients' expressions subsequently inform forensic nurses on how best to utilize their professional nursing expertise in establishing a therapeutic relationship. These interpersonal relationships impact the ability of forensic nurses to effectively address patients' care needs, which require complete information regarding their situations. Once established, this relationship promotes mutual respect and provides a patient with a sense of comfort and safety, allowing them to share, disclose, and discuss their situation more openly with the forensic nurse.[9]

As their healing begins, motivational interviewing methods may assist in helping patients gain confidence in their decisions by "strengthen[ing] personal motivation for and commitment to a specific goal by eliciting and exploring the person's own reasons for change."[10] When combined with criminology and victimology sciences, the *Interpersonal Relations Theory* helps promote trauma-informed principles in the establishment of essential trust required between forensic nurses and patients.[7]

NURSING CODE OF ETHICS

Forensic nurses follow the American Nurses Association's *Code of Ethics for Nurses with Interpretive Statements* (the Code)[11] to develop and apply ethical personal philosophies to the patient-centered and trauma-informed care of individuals intersecting with legal systems. The Code is a dynamic document that serves 3 purposes. First, it provides concise statements regarding the ethical values, obligations, duties, and professional ideals of nurses. Secondly, it sets nonnegotiable ethical standards for the nursing profession as a whole. It expresses nursing's understanding of its own commitment to society. The Code consists of 2 parts: provisions and their accompanying interpretative statements.[11]

Provision 1.1 of the Code dictates respect for human dignity as the foundational principle that underlies all nursing practice and acts as a driving force in forensic nursing.[11] Forensic nurses must set aside personal bias and prejudice in order to establish trusting relationships with patients and provide services according to individual needs, as stated in Provision 1.2.[11] This ethical guideline directly correlates to Peplau's Interpersonal Relations Theory[12] by emphasizing that nurse-patient relationships are based upon trust. This allows patients to openly disclose their situations, thus enabling nurses to obtain the necessary information to provide need-based care. Likewise, Leininger's transcultural theory[13] insists that nurses not only respect the differing cultural aspects that arise during care, but inform themselves regarding cultures that differ from their own culture of origin. Without the understanding of the patient's culture, holism in nursing care cannot be optimally be given. This is particularly true for forensic nurses who will encounter patients with very varied backgrounds.

CASE STUDIES

Case 7-1[14]

Theodore Kaczynski, also known as the infamous Unabomber, was a domestic terrorist that committed isolated, anonymous bombings from 1978 to 1995. His victims were random, and evidence was minimal, allowing him to elude police for over a decade. His targets included airlines, universities, retail establishments, personal residences, and public service offices. In total, his crimes killed 3 people and injured almost 24. Kaczynski was caught only when the FBI released an essay that he wrote to the public.

Discussion

The forensic nurse who may work with the individual victim, family, or community would use criminology and victimology theories to address concerns expressed by survivors. In this case, Passive Victim Precipitation Theory would be the "explanation" for Kaczynski's actions, as he believed these victims were ruining the "natural world." Understanding these theories of victimology can help a forensic nurse provide treatment as they are able to explain more of the "why" as well as provide medical care. Providing this information helps individuals overcome their traumas by accepting things they cannot change, such as them having no real fault in their injuries, and learning to move forward.

Case 7-2[15]

On September 15, 1963, at 16th Street Baptist Church in Birmingham, Alabama, a bomb exploded under the church's steps, killing 4 African American girls: Addie Mae Collins, Denise McNair, Carole Robertson, and Cynthia Wesley. Sixteenth Street Baptist Church was a predominantly African American church located in the most segregated cities in the United States and served as the headquarters for civil rights meetings and rallies. The criminals were members of the Eastview Klavern #13 Ku Klux Klan and were known for being violent.

Discussion

Applying the theories of victimization, the child victims of the bombing were vulnerable because of their "deviant" identities, reflecting the Lifestyle Exposure Theory of Victimization. This victimology also relates to observations of the perpetrators who held racist ideologies; they felt justified in their crime because they thought their victims to be lesser than them. Rational Choice Theory promotes the notion that criminals make choices based on their own self-interest, therefore justifying the outcome of their behavior. Through understanding these theories, a forensic nurse would be able to provide trauma-informed care for those who were critically injured as well as providing support for the families of the young girls. Especially in cases of racially driven attacks, forensic nurses must be able to understand "why" a patient was attacked. Criminology is also critical for caring for injured perpetrators, understanding the kind of person that you are caring for and what kind of beliefs they hold. Knowing this helps ensure that both patient and nurse are looked after.

SUMMARY

Criminology focuses on the study of criminals and the justice system, and criminologists use a number of theories to examine criminal behavior. Victimology is a sub-category in the science of criminology that studies the relationship between the victim and criminal, as well as the criminal justice system. Providers are guided by a number of theories that help them to better understand criminal behavior and victim experiences. Forensic nurses specifically use criminology and victimology sciences to navigate patients' intersections with the legal system by developing and applying ethical personal philosophies to the care of all patients.

REFERENCES

1. Rahman M. Violent men: trauma, humiliation and scenarios of harm. In: *Palgrave Studies in Risk, Crime and Society.* Palgrave Pivot; 2019:109-35.

2. Jolliffe D, Farrington DP, Piquero AR, Loeber R, Hill KG. Systematic review of early risk factors for life-course-persistent, adolescence-limited, and late-onset offenders in prospective longitudinal studies. *Aggress Violent Behav.* 2017;33:15-23.

3. Cullen FT, Agnew R, Wilcox P. *Criminological Theory: Past to Present.* 7th ed. Oxford University Press; 2021.

4. Burgess AW. *Victimology Theories and Applications.* 3rd ed. Jones and Bartlett Learning; 2019.

5. King LW. The Code of Hammurabi. 2008. Accessed January 27, 2022. http://avalon.law.yale.edu/ancient/hamframe.asp

6. HIV-prevention program fails rape survivors in Africa, group says. *AIDS Policy Law.* 2004;19(7):4.

7. Understanding the impact of trauma. In: *A Treatment Improvement Protocol (TIP): Trauma-Informed Care in Behavioral Health Services.* Vol 57. Substance Abuse and Mental Health Services Administration; 2014:59-90.

8. Valentine JL, Sekula LK, Lynch V. Evolution of forensic nursing theory--introduction of the constructed theory of forensic nursing care: a middle-range theory. *J Forensic Nurs.* 2020;16(4):188-198. doi:10.1097/JFN.0000000000000287

9. Gastmans C. Interpersonal relations in nursing: a philosophical-ethical analysis of the work of Hildegard E. Peplau. *J Adv Nurs.* 1998;28(6):1312-1319.

10. McKenzie KJ, Pierce D, Gunn JM. A systematic review of motivational interviewing in healthcare: the potential of motivational interviewing to address the lifestyle factors relevant to multimorbidity. *J Comorb.* 2015;5:162-174.

11. Steering Committee for the Revision of the Code of Ethics. *Code of Ethics for Nurses With Interpretive Statements.* American Nurses Association; 2015.

12. Sharma N, Gupta V. *Therapeutic Communication.* StatPearls; 2022.

13. Clarke PN, McFarland MR, Andrews MM, Leininger M. Caring: some reflections on the impact of the culture care theory by McFarland & Andrews and a conversation with Leininger. *Nurs Sci Q.* 2009;22(3):233-9. doi:10.1177/0894318409337020

14. The Unabomber. Federal Bureau of Investigation. Accessed May 5, 2022. https://www.fbi.gov/history/famous-cases/unabomber

15. Sixteenth Street Baptist Church. National Parks Service. Updated September 9, 2021. Accessed June 15, 2022. https://www.nps.gov/places/sixteenth-street-baptist-church.htm#:~:text=On%20Sunday%20morning%2C%20September%2015,galvanized%20the%20civil%20rights%20movement.

INTEGUMENT, HEALING, AND INJURIES

Catherine Carter-Snell, PhD, RN, SANE-A

Jessica M. Volz, DNP, CRNP, FNE A/P, FNP-BC, AFN-C, NE-BC, SANE-A, SANE-P, DM-AFN

Kathryn A. Swift, MSN, CRNP, FNE A/P, FNP-BC, CMSRN, SANE-A, SANE-P

Patricia M. Speck, DNSc, CRNP, FNP-BC, AFN-C, DF-IAFN, FAAFS, DF-AFN, FAAN

KEY POINTS

1. *The integumentary system is the largest organ system of the human body, and it contains 3 layers that protect against chemical, physical, and mechanical injury.*

2. *The healing speed of an injury reflects age, location, illness, and health, so the time of injury can only be estimated. Healing occurs in stages that overlap and are identifiable, aided by providing a moist, clean, and protected environment for the integument injury.*

3. *The BALD STEP guide allows the forensic nurse to methodically and thoroughly assess and document cutaneous injuries.*

4. *Consistent use of terminology is essential to accurate forensic nursing documentation.*

ANATOMY OF THE INTEGUMENTARY SYSTEM

In humans, skin (ie, integument) is the largest organ. Skin functions as protection against chemical, physical, and mechanical injury; helps regulate body temperature; provides sensation; aids in metabolic function; acts as a blood reservoir; and excretes some wastes.[1] It is known as the integumentary system and is composed of 3 layers: the epidermis, dermis, and hypodermis.

The epidermis is the outermost layer that contains several layers of different types of cells, namely keratin, which provides structure and protection, and melanocytes, which produce the chemical melanin that creates skin pigment. Each layer of the epidermis contains structures that are necessary for its functioning and health such as hair, hair follicles, nails, and glands.

The dermis is the only layer that is vascularized and has 2 layers itself. It is relatively dense and contains the largest number of structures, including the hair root, sensory nerve fibers, sweat glands, sebaceous (ie, oil) glands, and capillaries. These structures provide a place for hair growth to occur, the sensation of touch to originate, and the required physical space for the structures to maintain their health. The secretory glands of this layer include sweat glands, sebaceous glands, and ceruminous glands. These glands help regulate temperature, inhibit bacterial growth, control moisture, and aid in secretion of waste products.[1]

The hypodermis represents the innermost layers of skin before the fascia separation for underlying adipose tissue, muscle, and bone.

INJURY AND HEALING

The estimated time of injury to the skin varies and is dependent on an individual's age, location, illness, and health.[2-4] The stages of wound healing typically proceed in an organized and linear way.[2] There are 4 stages of healing following disruption of the integument: hemostasis, inflammation, proliferation, and maturation.[2] Although the stages of wound healing are oftentimes linear, wounds can progress backward or forward depending on internal and external patient conditions.[4]

Furthermore, the stages of healing are known by the characteristics of the stage, not the timing.[3] The first phase, *hemostasis*, is characterized by constriction of blood vessels and capillaries where coagulation occurs. Fibrin is a binding agent, and platelets are a clotting agent. This stage for minor wounds is rapid, lasting seconds. In severe rupture of larger vessels, procoagulants and prothrombin assist in the development of a clot to stop bleeding.

The second stage of wound healing is the *inflammatory phase*, which begins with swelling to control bleeding and prevent infection.[2,4] During this phase, damaged cells and pathogens are removed from the wound area. Most inflammation phase activities occur in the first 48 hours following a wound. White blood cells, growth factors, and enzymes create swelling, and the outward appearance is a hot, painful redness, only becoming problematic if persistent or creating an entire body system response (eg, cellulitis or sepsis).

The third stage, called the *proliferative phase*,[2,4] is characterized by rebuilding the integument through supplying collagen and extracellular matrix. In this phase, the wound contracts and grows new blood vessels and nerves. Granulation tissue is the result of myofibroblasts, and when sufficiently healed, epithelialization is continuous through the next phase, maturation. In this phase, the wound closes and is thick, where the building blocks of collagen and fibrinogen are aligned with Langer's lines (ie, tension lines).

Most injuries are in the final phase, *maturation*, for 1 month to 6 weeks.[2,4] Along the healing trajectory, venous disease, infection, metabolic diseases, or old age may interfere in the rapid wound healing necessary to create a linear model for wound healing.[3] Of note, keeping a wound moist, clean, and protected promotes rapid healing in all ages[1] and may be the single cause for rapid healing following rape injury in the vestibular tissue.[4]

BALD STEP: AN INJURY AND PHYSICAL FINDINGS GUIDE

Figure 8-1. Bruises vs. Ecchymosis (© C. Carter-Snell, 2014. Used with permission).

Physical findings after trauma vary with the types of contact. Factors such as resistance or being restrained are likely to increase risk of injury, while intoxication or decreased levels of consciousness are associated with lower risks of injury.[4] Additionally, there are numerous findings that mimic injury. The appropriate use of injury terms also indicates the mechanism of injury. Application of blunt force results in injuries such as bruises, bites, avulsions, abrasions, lacerations (ie, splitting the skin), and acute deformities of limbs such as sprains or strains.[2,4] Tenderness may be an early indicator of deeper tissue trauma that could appear a few days later. Bruises are often mistakenly called ecchymosis, and co-morbid disorders such as low platelets promote ecchymotic spread. While ecchymosis is explainable, it is not trauma and instead reflects gravitational drainage from a distant source of impact as noted in **Figure 8-1**.

Lacerations, unlike bruises, release blood from the confined space and have characteristics such as irregular edges or cross-bridging of hair or connective tissue inside of the wound. Penetrating forces applied to skin, such as knives, result in injuries described as incisional wounds or puncture type injury. The characteristic includes straight edges on both sides of the injury and little to no cross-bridges as the object cleanly slices the tissue.

Conducting research about injuries is challenging because there is inconsistent use of terminology, making it difficult to determine a pattern injury (ie, one injury reflecting an identifiable object) and patterns of injury (ie, multiple injuries over time) in research. Research helped identify the types of injuries that result from various forms of trauma. That knowledge led to the development and dissemination of BALD STEP[5] to replace TEARS in an attempt to more comprehensively and systematically document injuries. The BALD STEP guide acts as a checklist for forensic nurses while they look for specific characteristic findings. The checklist allows for a comprehensive testimony about looking for all characteristics of wounds. The BALD STEP abbreviations on the trauma gram indicate the type of injury or finding, along with the measurements and color or other injury characteristics, creating a comprehensive objective documentation that enhances communication and understanding among professionals (**Table 8-1**).[6]

Table 8-1. BALD STEP©*					
B	BL	Bleeding	**S**	SW	Swelling
	BI	Bite		ST	Stain *(+ FL if fluorescent)*
	BU	Burn	**T**	TE	Tenderness
	BR	Bruise		TR	Trace evidence *(specify)*
A	AB	Abrasion	**E**	ER	Erythema
	AV	Avulsion	**P**	PA	Patterned injury *(draw shape)*
L	LA	Laceration		PT	Petechiae
D	DE	Deformity *(acute)*		PE	Penetrating injury + descriptor: I=incised, S=stab, P=puncture, G=Gunshot *(known)*

* Include measurements, color/characteristics for each injury and draw shape if appropriate.

BALD STEP© Guide to Physical Findings in Trauma (used with permission). Carter-Snell, 2011. (bit.ly/BALDSTEP) May be reproduced. Also available in French.

CASE STUDIES

Case Study 8-1

This 2-year-old boy presented to the emergency department (ED) accompanied by Child Protective Services (CPS) for a welfare check. According to CPS, the child's parents were involved in a domestic dispute in which the police were required to intervene. While at the home, the police noted that the child had multiple concerning areas of discoloration to his back, left thigh, and bilateral upper arms. The forensic nurse used the BALD STEP guide to assess the child and focus on the areas of concern. After thorough examination and documentation of each area, including any injury's size, shape, and color, it was found that these areas are consistent with congenital dermal melanocytosis, previously called Mongolian Spots. There were no additional areas of concern found on the child's body.

Discussion

In many cases, children like this one present without history. Regardless, the forensic nurse used the BALD STEP tool to assess areas of concern. This provided the nurse with descriptive information, leading to a medical diagnosis.

Case Study 8-2

This 87-year-old homeless woman walked into the ED complaining of sexual assault. As a frequent user of the ED, the provider decided to call the forensic nurse for sexual assault care. The woman was then referred to an advanced provider. The findings were vestibular burns from use of creams for hygiene, complicating the presentation, and the diagnosis of severe contact dermatitis which is a type of vulvar disease from type 2 diabetes.

In this case, the generalist forensic nurse recognized that there was a disease process and referred the patient to the advanced provider for the definitive diagnosis. Before the referral, the generalist forensic nurse requested an order for a urine sample and obtained the self-collected sterile 4x4 cotton wipe for evaluation by the forensic laboratory. The laboratory results found no additional DNA in the sample, and the sexual assault complaint was unfounded by the coordinated community response team and multidisciplinary team.

Discussion

Persons who are often vulnerable to the environmental elements without access to resources have chronic diseases which are not easily managed. In this case, the forensic nurse recognized the need for follow-up and referred the patient to a primary care provider. However, homeless individuals rarely follow up, but rather they are likely to be seen at another ED for an acute problem.

SUMMARY

The integumentary system is the body's first line of protection from external environmental dangers, and thus it commonly reflects injury. Specialized knowledge for the forensic nurse about integument anatomy and its functions ensure accurate identification and objective documentation of injury on all tissue types. The healing process of the integumentary system is linear, and it generally takes approximately 6 weeks for healthy young people but longer for older persons and those with comorbidities.

The BALD STEP tool standardizes the assessment of cutaneous injury and promotes objective documentation that is systematic, avoiding omission of findings. Additionally, BALD STEP establishes standardized terminology that is consistent with the mechanism of injury and wound characteristics, improving communication between professionals and enhancing quantification of language for researchers interested in patterns of injury.

REFERENCES

1. How does skin work? Institute for Quality and Efficiency in Health Care. September 28, 2009. Updated April 11, 2019. https://www.ncbi.nlm.nih.gov/pubmedhealth/PMH0072439/

2. Broughton G 2nd, Janis JE, Attinger CE. The basic science of wound healing. *Plast Reconstr Surg.* 2006;117(7):12s-34s. doi:10.1097/01.prs.0000225430.42531.c2

3. Grey JE, Enoch S, Harding KG. Wound assessment. *BMJ.* 2006;332(7536):285-288. doi:10.1136/bmj.332.7536.285

4. Takeo M, Lee W, Ito M. Wound healing and skin regeneration. *Cold Spring Harb Perspect Med.* 2015;5(1):a023267. doi:10.1101/cshperspect.a023267

5. Carter-Snell C. Understanding women's risks of injury after sexual assault. Dissertation. University of Alberta; 2007. https://central.bac-lac.gc.ca/.item?id=NR32932&op=pdf&app=Library&oclc_number=502629533

6. Carter-Snell C, Lewis-O'Connor A. Forensic nursing in the healthcare setting In: Price B, McGuire K, eds. *Core Curriculum for Forensic Nursing.* International Association of Forensic Nurses; 2016:49-93.

GUNSHOT WOUNDS

Christine Foote-Lucero, MSN, RN, CEN, SANE-A, SANE-P, AFN-C

ACKNOWLEDGEMENT:
Dr. William Smock, a national educator for forensic nurses and law enforcement on gunshot wounds, consulted on this chapter.

KEY POINTS

1. *Documentation for a patient affected by a gunshot wound (GSW) should include detailed written descriptions of the injury and a series of photographs taken from various angles.*

2. *Physical characteristics of GSWs can vary due to a number of factors, including the range of fire and entrance/exit location of the bullet.*

3. *Evidence collection requires careful documentation and management, as there can be legal repercussions to mishandling evidence for a case.*

INTRODUCTION AND EPIDEMIOLOGY

Unintentional gun death occurs 4 times more often in the United States than in any other comparably developed countries. In 2019, there were 39 707 firearm-related deaths (ie, 109 people died from a firearm-related injury each day in the United States). Firearm-related injuries are in the top 5 leading causes of death for people ages 1 to 64 in the United States. Men account for 86% of all victims of firearm death and 88% of nonfatal firearm injuries. Rates of firearm violence also vary by age, race, and ethnicity. Firearm homicide rates are highest among teens and young adults (15 to 34 years of age), as well as among Black, American Indian/Alaskan Native, and Hispanic populations. Firearm use in suicide attempts is usually lethal. Firearm suicide rates are highest among adults 75 years of age and older and among American Indian/Alaskan Native and non-Hispanic white populations.[1]

GSWs are complex, penetrating injuries that are often encountered by health care professionals that work in the emergency department (ED) and other acute care and forensic settings. Forensic nurses who interact with patients experiencing a GSW also perform life-saving measures and function in an important role in the identification, collection, and preservation of forensic firearm evidence. Forensic nurses need an "understanding of the potential pitfalls of consent, gathering and preserving evidence, chain of custody, reporting, documentation, and photographing injuries… not just for the patients but also for the health care provider responsible for their care, the institution where the patients receive their care, and the safety of the community."[2] Legal systems use descriptions of GSWs and characteristic injury patterns to create narrative in adjudication.

FIREARM BASICS

All firearms use gunpowder, which propels 1 or more projectiles at a high rate of speed. There are 4 basic types of firearms: revolvers, pistols, shotguns, and rifles. Revolvers and pistols are typically referred to as handguns, while shotguns and rifles are typically referred to as long guns. Basic differences between these firearms include the rounds (ie, projectiles) carried, rate of fire, features of the barrel, and function. The barrel is a tube of variable length depending on the type of firearm. For example, rifles have a rifled (ie, grooved) barrel, while handguns have a smooth barrel.[3]

SCENE SAFETY AND IMMEDIATE CARE

Rapid patient assessment is essential for identifying life-threatening injuries. Nurses entering a scene where there is a GSW victim must ensure that it is safe to approach and that there are no active shooters present. Scenes must first be secured by the proper authorities, such as police, prior to medical evaluation and intervention. In the hospital setting, policies that ensure staff safety are of primary importance, such as having security personnel perform a weapons search upon patients and visitors entering the building and/or securing patient belongings while following evidence management guidelines for health care institutions.[4] The priority treatment for a GSW, aside from ensuring that the patient has an airway and is breathing, is to control their bleeding by applying direct pressure to any actively bleeding wound.[2,5] For a bleeding extremity, a tourniquet may also be used by a specially trained nurse. The ***Stop the Bleed*** program provides courses on wound treatment that can be useful in community settings.[5]

Patients affected by gun violence suffer challenges to both their emotional health and physical ability. Nurses should consult social services and/or mental health professionals during hospitalization and post-discharge follow-up to ensure comprehensive safety planning, mental and emotional support, community support and resources, and violence intervention services.

DOCUMENTATION AND REPORTING

Rapid objective documentation of injuries is important because many of the techniques performed during resuscitation and wound cleansing alter the appearance of wounds. Life-saving measures and procedures like surgery, excision, or suturing also change GSW appearances. Like all wounds, GSWs change as the injury heals over time; therefore, the most accurate and systematic description of wounds is likely from the initial evaluation upon patient arrival.

Forensic nurses are taught to objectively document injuries with specific descriptions such as the shape, body location, proportion/size, color, and patterns, and the presence of any foreign material should also be noted. A measuring device such as the American Board of Forensic Odontology (ABFO) ruler is a common reference in documentation and photography. Terms such as "penetrating" and "perforating" are often used to describe GSWs with a specific meaning. When a GSW is described as ***penetrating***, the bullet enters the body but does not exit, and when a GSW is described as ***perforating***, the bullet enters and exits the body. Differentiation between entrance and exit wounds is difficult, and information from patients or witnesses is often false or inaccurate. Unless the forensic nurse is specifically trained in identifying these details, the interpretation of GSWs (eg, entrance and exit, direction of fire, or type of firearm or ammunition) is typically a function of medical examiners and law enforcement.[6]

In addition to written documentation, body diagram maps and photographs are standard forms of documentation. Department and/or hospital policies guide procedures for image security and storage. "Bookend" photographs identifying the patient, case number, date, and time with labels indicating either ***Start Series*** (initial photo of the series) or ***Ending Series*** (final photo of the series) improve the completeness of the record. The rule of thirds, fourths, or fifths creates a series of photographs for each wound: an orientation photo that shows the gross anatomical location of the wound location, including the body part; gradual proximity photographs; and specific magnified photograph of the wound with a measuring tool (also referred to as a reference or standard). All photographs should be taken at a 90° angle to the wound, which is often difficult on curved surfaces.

Many local and state jurisdictions require EDs to notify local law enforcement of GSWs. Always follow mandatory reporting laws. Law enforcement investigations often ensure that no other victims need assistance. During an active police investigation for a mandatory report situation, HIPAA is waived and allows hospital personnel to communicate with hospital security or police about the patient(s) in question. The report in the patient's medical record should include the date, time, and person reported to (ie, the police officer's name and badge number).

When possible, the medical history is directly obtained from the patient. It is important to document this history using direct quotes from the patient and to record any information necessary for medical care, evaluation, and treatment. Questions that are not related to medical inquiry should be avoided as the medical history will be different from the interview obtained by law enforcement. The forensic nurse should ask the patient about their body position at time of shooting (ie, standing, sitting, or lying down); range of fire (ie, estimated distance from shooter); and interposing factors (ie, any objects between the shooter and patient). The information gathered contributes to the appearance of the wound. If the patient recalls, also document the time of injury and the number of gunshots heard. As part of a safety assessment, the forensic nurse should ask questions related to the safety of the patient, providers, and staff. If gang or trafficking activity, domestic violence, or other violent crimes have occurred, there is a risk that someone will re-attempt to end the patient's life while they are in the hospital. Regardless of the patient's victim/suspect status, forensic nurses have the obligation to ensure that all GSW patients receive thorough, appropriate, and unbiased interventions in a trauma-informed environment.

GUNSHOT WOUND INJURY

Many features of the GSW depend upon the range of fire. **Range of fire** is the factor that considers the distance of the barrel of the firearm to the patient and is classified as contact, near contact, intermediate, or distant. When the muzzle of the weapon is held firmly (hard contact) or loosely (loose contact) against the skin, a **contact wound** results. The wound edges sear with hot gases, and soot from the flame is either embedded (hard contact) or deposited (loose contact) in the circumference of the wound. Hard contact wounds have no space between the muzzle and the skin. **Near contact wounds** are produced when there is a gap between the gun muzzle and the skin, usually within a 1 or 2 centimeter range. Seared skin and soot may be noted on both types of wounds and is easily wiped off, and often a muzzle imprint is observed. The injuries appear stellate in contact wounds when bone is under the injury, and in these types of injury, the gases exiting the barrel cause the expansion of subcutaneous tissue, resulting in tearing or lacerating of skin. **Intermediate range wounds** cause powder "tattooing," or stippling, as a result of embedded gunpowder grains in the skin. The range is anything greater than near contact and up to 90 centimeters for handguns or 110 centimeters for newer high-velocity cartridges. Tattooing appears as red or brown punctate lesions around the wound entrance that cannot be wiped away because it is caused by abrasions, not a powder burn. **Distance wounds** occur when the distance to the weapon exceeds that of an intermediate wound and is far enough that there is no soot deposition or tattooing. Body position at the time of the shooting, the area of the body that was shot, muzzle attachments, type of gunpowder, barrel length, and caliber can all influence the characteristic appearance of a GSW.[7]

Entrance wounds vary widely in size but are usually round with an abrasion collar or abrasion ring. Abrasion characteristics include an area of abraded tissue around the entrance where the bullet scrapes the skin as it penetrates the dermis; however, abrasion collars are not typical for the soles of the feet or the palms of the hand. Exit wounds are generally larger and more irregular than entrance wounds; however, the size of wounds is necessary for documentation, but size is never the sole determinant of whether a wound is entrance or exit. Exit wounds appear round, oval, slit-like, stellate, or crescentic shaped.[3] Deformation and instability of the bullet as it moves through the tissue accounts for the general appearance of the exit wound.

GUNSHOT WOUND EVIDENCE COLLECTION

Evidence storage and transfer are guided by evidence management guidelines. Hospital procedures are the first step in ensuring admissibility of the evidence during adjudication. The forensic nurse who removes a patient's clothing uses paper bags, not plastic, and each item of clothing is stored in its own bag. When removing clothing, take careful notice not to cut through any bullet holes of the clothing with trauma shears. Once the evidence is labeled and sealed, the forensic nurse signs their name or initials and labels the time and date on the tape over the edges. Bullets are removed using gauze or hemostats covered with suture booties to avoid damage to the bullet's surface during handling. Evidence should be kept in its original state unless medical treatment is necessary. Careful documentation of any procedure altering the original condition of the evidence is important.

Evidence management begins with identification, and all involved parties must take steps to ensure preservation of the evidence. The ***chain of custody (COC)***, also termed "chain of possession," is a core principle in evidence management that requires logarithmic documentation of possession of evidence. Accounting for all evidence at all times is prudent because legal action may be taken if individuals tamper with evidence or evidence is misplaced. The COC protects evidence from tampering and contamination. This form also ensures that collection and/or acceptance of the evidence is properly documented, that evidence is never left unattended, and that evidence is stored in a secure location until transfer to legal authorities.

CASE STUDIES

Case Study 9-1

A 26-year-old female arrived at the ED reporting a GSW. She was awake, alert, and talking. Bleeding was controlled. She was brought back to a treatment area and assessed. The generalist forensic nurse consultant arrived to see the patient. A history was obtained and documented, and this was used to guide evidence collection. The patient's statements were documented in quotes. She indicated she was shot by a stranger while walking along the street at approximately 10 to 15 feet distance. A physical examination revealed she had 2 gunshot wounds: the first wound was to the base of her left index finger, and the second wound was to the dorsal aspect of her left hand. The first wound was round with inverted tissue. There was no soot, stippling, muzzle imprint, seared skin, or abrasion collar noted. The forensic nurse recognized that abrasion collars would not be an expected finding, and it was an entrance wound on the palm of the hand. The second wound was irregular, and an outward protrusion of tissue was noted. The forensic nurse recognized that the first wound was consistent with an entrance wound and would also be likely in the event the patient put her hand up to cover her face if threatened with a gun (defensive injury).

Discussion

The patient's wounds were photographed before and after cleaning. The forensic nurse's documentation of the wounds was then used by the advanced provider, who ordered imaging to evaluate for fractures and arrive at a differential medical diagnosis for billing. The advanced provider also consulted a hand surgeon, and they scheduled surgery for the patient.

The patient ultimately endorsed being shot at close range by her boyfriend during a heated argument and that she had put her hand up to protect herself as an instinctual reaction when he pulled a gun out. There was no bullet to collect as evidence since this was a perforating wound. The generalist forensic nurse provided lengthy patient education on interpersonal violence and the concern for lethality in the patient's current relationship with gun violence. The advanced provider ordered an updated tetanus immunization, and the forensic nurse helped the hospital social services develop safety planning including shelter arrangements. Because the patient had an active police investigation, the forensic nursing report was released to law enforcement according to jurisdictional mandates. Finally, the forensic nurse discussed wound healing and validated the patient's understanding about injury and the recommended referrals for community resources and counseling.

SUMMARY

GSWs are undoubtedly complex injuries. The application of the nursing process combined with the principles of forensic science are imperative during the care of patients affected by a GSW. This requires that nurses protect the forensic evidence that links health care to criminal justice. Interpretive errors regarding GSWs are common in the healthcare field, therefore objective and descriptive documentation is crucial. Nurses must realize that oversimplification and assumptions regarding GSWs may compromise patient care and legal proceedings. When possible, generalist forensic nurses should be incorporated into the care of all patients affected by violence.

REFERENCES

1. Violence Prevention: Fast Facts. Centers for Disease Control and Prevention. Updated May 4, 2021. Accessed April 20, 2021. https://www.cdc.gov/violence prevention/firearms/fastfact.html#:~:text=In%202019%2C%20there%20 were%2039%2C707,firearm%2Drelated%20injuries%20than%20die

2. Reed GD, Symonds A, Stier A, Peluso S, Watson SO. Prosecutor preference for forensic nurse testimony: outcome of expanding a forensic program. *J Emerg Nurs.* 2020;46(3):310-317. doi:10.1016/j.jen.2020.02.014.

3. Gitto L, Stoppacher R. Gunshot wounds. PathologyOutlines.com, Inc. 2021. Updated August 24, 2021. www.pathologyoutlines.com/topic/forensicsgunshot wounds.html

4. National Institute of Standards and Technology. Evidence management. 2014. Updated October 25, 2021. www.nist.gov/topics/forensic-science/inter disciplinary-topics/evidence-management

5. American College of Surgeons. Stop the Bleed. 2021. www.stopthebleed.org

6. American College of Surgeons Committee on Trauma. *Advanced Trauma Life Support (ATLS) Student Course Manual.* 10th ed. American College of Surgeons; 2018.

7. Stefanopoulos PK, Pinialidis DE, Hadjigeorgiou GF, Filippakis KN. Wound ballistics 101: the mechanisms of soft tissue wounding by bullets. *Eur J Trauma.* 2017;43(5):579-586. doi:10.1007/s00068-015-0581-1.

Chapter 10

THE PSYCHOLOGY OF TRAUMA

Theresa Fay-Hillier, DrPH, MSN, PMHCNS-BC
Maud D'Arcy, BSN, RN
Melanie Alexander, RN, MSN

KEY POINTS

1. *The age of a child at the time of a traumatic event (or events) influences their ability to process trauma.*

2. *Exposure to childhood trauma increases susceptibility to psychopathologies, including posttraumatic stress disorder (PTSD) and substance abuse.*

3. *Forensic nurses mitigate trauma and promote healing by practicing trauma-informed and person-centered care.*

INTRODUCTION

Trauma can be experienced throughout life, but it more commonly occurs during childhood. By age 16, more than two-thirds of children have experienced at least 1 traumatic adverse event.[1] In addition to known adverse childhood traumatic experiences (eg, unstable housing; abandonment; domestic, sexual, physical, and emotional violence; and neglect), witnessing violence or natural disasters is also a traumatic experience for children.[1] Children who experience one type of violence, such as physical abuse, are at greater risk for experiencing other forms of violence.[2] The Adverse Childhood Experiences (ACEs) study examined the connections between traumatic events during childhood and adverse health outcomes. The ACEs study found that as the number and intensity of traumatic events in childhood increased, adults died earlier than anticipated because they developed chronic physical and mental health diagnoses.[3] Health Outcomes of Positive Experiences is a framework identifying protective factors that can positively impact the outcomes of children who have encountered ACEs.[4] The subjective impact and the resources available to support the person mitigates the impact of the trauma. There is greater risk for negative emotional and psychological consequences when the individual identifies feelings of immobility and helplessness during the trauma or has triggering memories of trauma. Children often have cognitive distortions or personal interpretations about what happened during an adverse event. When adults intervene, their language tends to influence the child's description of what happened to them. Explaining that adverse events occur and providing adequate support allows children to process the event without blaming themselves. Eventually, often in adulthood, children are able to fully process the event and realize that they were powerless in changing the perpetrator's behavior or environment.

RECOVERY

Recovery requires processing, so after an adverse event, children may withdraw to protect themselves and feel safe by sleeping more or crying often. They may also project anger toward playmates and pets. Following trauma, preschool-aged children may experience fear and separation anxiety when away from family members, leading to crying more frequently. Elementary school children typically express an anxious fear and may show feelings of guilt or shame with suicidal ideation, which is expressed through risky behavior. Middle and high aged school children who experience ACEs are at risk for developing eating disorders, becoming suicidal, and engaging in lethal risky behaviors such as drug use and unsafe sexual behaviors.[1]

As shown above, processing trauma varies greatly depending on the person's age, support systems, and the severity of the trauma. Symptoms of anxiety generally appear when there is a lack of trauma resolution or if triggering occurs frequently, and recovery often occurs later in adulthood with maturity and experience in overcoming other traumas. Although some children are able to recover from traumatic experiences, other children develop maladaptive intrapsychic and behavioral sequelae as part of their post-trauma symptoms.[5] The patterns follow a continuum of trauma resolution learning with patterns of reenactment, repetition, and displacement. Developing a trauma-learning pattern occurs when the repetitive traumatic events are not discovered or disclosed and the person lacks the opportunity to process trauma in a supportive environment.

MENTAL HEALTH AND ADDICTIONS

Almost 1 in 5 children in the United States experience traumatic events involving harm or the threat of harm, wherein exposure to interpersonal violence, physical abuse, and/or sexual abuse heightens the risk of psychopathology.[6] The continuous neurocognitive brain patterns are incomplete in children, and adverse experiences create a negative impact on brain development following trauma exposure. Children often respond with protective mechanisms, such as recognition of potential threats and intensified emotional responses to threats.[6,7] These mechanisms are adaptive and sometimes helpful; however, they may remain a pivotal adaptation that connects childhood trauma to the internalization and externalization of psychopathology. These reactions are medicalized and include co-occurring PTSD, mood disorders, and substance abuse, among others.[6,8] *Complex trauma* refers to prolonged or multiple occurrences of interpersonal victimization, further complicating symptoms and diagnoses of trauma and stress-related disorders.[7]

Victimization contributes to adolescent substance abuse, particularly binge drinking.[8,9] For many teens, drug use is a coping strategy used to assuage negative emotions and fear sensations. Common motivations for substance abuse are to manage emotional dysregulation associated with traumatic stress by reducing negative affect, raising positive affect, or altering an emotion.[8] Trauma-exposed adolescents and adults also have an increased risk of psychiatric comorbidities. Substance abuse and depression are more frequently diagnosed with PTSD rather than PTSD alone.[8,9] These complex adaptations are treatable with early interventions. Therapies such as cognitive behavioral therapy are employed to mitigate risk factors and prevent the onset of psychopathology.[6] Trauma-focused cognitive behavioral therapy is used more often for persons with polyvictimization with coercive and toxic relationships.

MITIGATION OF TRAUMA

The provision of trauma-informed, person-centered care mitigates mental stress in the health care setting. Trauma-informed, person centered care, when universally applied, prevents retraumatization by focusing on these key principles: physical and emotional safety; trustworthiness and transparency; peer support; collaboration and mutuality; empowerment and choice; and sensitivity to cultural, historical, and gender issues.[10] Building a trusting foundation is essential for easing patients' emotional burden. Practicing trauma-informed care may involve screening for ACEs and providing mental health outpatient resources as well as the general care techniques used in every patient interaction. This includes the forensic nurse introducing themselves and seeking permission for all activities as they explain their role in the patient's care. Using open, non-threatening body language to promote feelings of control and safety and provide anticipatory guidance ensures a consistent message, minimizing surprises and setting appropriate expectations for care. Asking permission before touching patients reduces the chances of re-traumatization and dysregulation.[6] In trauma-informed care environments, privacy is protected to mitigate trauma by respecting the patient's wishes regarding who is present during their assessment.

CASE STUDIES

Case Study 10-1

This 10-year-old patient was admitted to an acute psychiatric treatment facility for stabilization after experiencing suicidal ideation, flashbacks, and aggressive behavior. She had a significant prior mental health history and was previously hospitalized in a long-term care facility for similar symptoms. In utero, she was exposed to drugs and alcohol. Her parents both had HIV and eventually succumbed to AIDS. Her mother died 2 months prior to her hospitalization. Before his death, the patient's father forced her mother to perform sex work, and the patient herself was a survivor of sexual assault by one of her father's friends. In addition to sexual abuse and drug and alcohol exposure, the patient witnessed extensive domestic violence and experienced housing instability throughout her life. She had tried multiple medications over the course of treatment, and at the time of admission, she was prescribed sertraline, clonidine, and desmopressin for impulse control, major depressive disorder, and PTSD symptoms. Her treatment team was focused on stabilization of acute symptoms, medication management, and coordination of care upon discharge. Child Protective Services (CPS) was actively involved in her case, and the patient was placed in the custody of her maternal grandmother. Her grandmother became active in her care and provided her with safe and stable housing.

Discussion

Using the work from the ACEs study, the forensic nurse instructed the psychiatric staff on the risk factors encountered by the patient and the importance of providing early interventions to modify the impact of the maltreatment encountered by the patient.[4,11] In addition to the patient being exposed in utero to drugs and alcohol, unstable childhood parenting, and the death of both parents, the violence witnessed and experienced increased her risks of developing psychiatric disorders. The forensic nurse educated staff on the importance of building protective factors (such as providing a stable home life) and supporting CPS in providing outside resources and addressing the patient's safety. Furthermore, the forensic nurse ensured that the staff consistently provided trauma-informed and patient-centered care to build trust and begin the process of empowering the patient in her recovery process.[10]

Case Study 10-2

This 30-year-old patient was a victim of sexual assault by a family friend from the age of 10 to 13 but never shared the assault with anyone. Being unaware that the family friend was a pedophile, the patient's single mother admired the friend and frequently encouraged her daughter to spend time with him. The man was wealthy and frequently offered to assist with paying bills and providing the family with expensive gifts. In high school, the patient began experimenting with drugs and became sexually promiscuous. By the age of 16, she had dropped out of school and was actively prostituting herself, using and selling drugs, and seeking children to traffic. By age 20, she was convicted of sexually assaulting a 10-year-old child.

Discussion

In this case, the forensic nurse provided and encouraged staff to provide trauma-informed, person-centered care to prevent retraumatization.[10] The forensic nurse educated the staff about the impact of complex traumatic experiences on the development of the trauma learning pattern, which ultimately evolved into a pattern of displacement.[5,7] Early interventions and treatment of PTSD would have provided an opportunity for the patient to recover prior to evolving into a serial pedophile. Although the patient is accountable for the criminal activity and abuse of children, the forensic nurse and the staff remembered the importance of providing appropriate support.

Additionally, the patient did not have the opportunity to process the sexual assault after the event. The patient's mother was not aware that the family friend was a pedophile. The forensic nurse explained to the staff that the patient (who is now an adult) had the opportunity to fully process the traumatic experiences.

SUMMARY

It is the forensic nurse's responsibility to clearly outline the parameters of mandated reporting. Trauma is universal, and using trauma-informed, patient-centered techniques in the care of all patients has the potential to create safe spaces that are transparent and supportive, thereby minimizing harm to facilitate patient healing.

REFERENCES

1. Understanding child trauma. April 29, 2020. Updated October 8, 2021. Accessed October 8, 2021. https://www.samhsa.gov/child-trauma/understanding-child-trauma

2. Gartland D, Conway LJ, Giallo R, et al. Intimate partner violence and child outcomes at age 10: a pregnancy cohort. *Arch Dis Child.* 2021;106(11):1066-1074. doi:10.1136/archdischild-2020-320321

3. Felitti VJ, Anda RF, Nordenberg D, et al. Relationship of childhood abuse and household dysfunction to many of the leading causes of death in adults: the Adverse Childhood Experiences (ACE) Study. *Am J Prev Medicine.* 1998;14(4):245-258. doi:10.1016/S0749-3797(98)00017-8

4. Sege R, Bethell C, Linkenbach, J, Jones JA, Klika B, Pecora PJ. Balancing adverse childhood experiences (ACEs) with HOPE: new insights into the role of positive experience on child and family development. Center for the Study of Social Policy. 2017. Accessed May 10, 2022. https://cssp.org/wp-content/uploads/2018/08/Balancing-ACEs-with-HOPE-FINAL.pdf

5. Burgess AW, Hartman CR, Clements PT. Biology of memory and childhood trauma. *J Psychosoc Nurs Ment Health Serv.* 1995;33(3):16-26. doi:10.3928/0279-3695-19950301-04

6. McLaughlin KA, Lambert HK. Child trauma exposure and psychopathology: mechanisms of risk and resilience. *Curr Opin Psychol.* 2017;14:29-34. doi:10.1016/j.copsyc.2016.10.004

7. Dye H. The impact and long-term effects of childhood trauma. *J Hum Behav Soc Environ.* 2018;28(3):381-392. doi:10.1080/10911359.2018.1435328

8. Cole J, Sprang G, Silman M. Interpersonal trauma exposure, trauma symptoms, and severity of substance use disorder among youth entering outpatient substance abuse treatment. *J Child Adolesc Trauma.* 2018;12(3):341-349. doi:10.1007/s40653-018-0239-3

9. Garami J, Valikhani A, Parkes D, et al. Examining perceived stress, childhood trauma and interpersonal trauma in individuals with drug addiction. *Psychol Rep.* 2019;122(2):433-450. doi:10.1177/0033294118764918

10. Fleishman J, Kamsky H, Sundborg S. Trauma-informed nursing practice. *OJIN: The Online Journal of Issues in Nursing.* 2019; 24(2): Manuscript 3. doi:10.3912/OJIN.Vol24No02Man03

Forensic Science and Evidence

Jessica M. Volz, DNP, CRNP, FNE A/P, FNP-BC, AFN-C, NE-BC, SANE-A, SANE-P, DM-AFN

Joyce P. Williams, DNP, MFSA, RN, FAAFS, DF-IAFN, FAAN

Jennifer L. Johnson, DNP, APRN, WHNP-BC, AFN-BC, SANE-A, SANE-P, AFN-C, DF-AFN

Stacey A. Mitchell, DNP, MBA, MEd, RN, AFN-C, SANE-A, SANE-P, DF-AFN, FAAN

Patricia M. Speck, DNSc, CRNP, FNP-BC, AFN-C, DF-IAFN, FAAFS, DF-AFN, FAAN

Key Points

1. *Legislation often funds forensic science agencies, establishes best practice standards, and creates consensus among professionals that accredit forensic science agencies, such as laboratories.*

2. *Management of evidence in health care settings reflects forensic science theories, principles, and research necessary to improve justice outcomes.*

3. *Forensic nurses have a responsibility to implement evidence-based forensic science and evidence management to promote justice for patients intersecting with health care and legal systems.*

Introduction

Evidence management is an important part of criminal justice system outcomes. *Forensic science* is the application of scientific principles and methods to matters of law and is comprised of a broad array of science, math, and engineering disciplines. Forensic nurses are not forensic scientists,[1] but they do work with forensic scientists. Recent legislation has worked to authorize additional funds to train more forensic examiners and provide additional technical resources to service providers.[2]

The Advancing Justice through DNA Technology Act of 2003 addressed the acquisition of DNA identification records and laboratory accreditation, while the National Institute of Justice's publication of *National Best Practices for Sexual Assault Kits: A Multidisciplinary Approach* created a standard for sexual assault examiners nationwide when collecting evidence.[3,4] Forensic science is broken down into many disciplines that all aim to interpret clues and gather evidence using a wide range of tools and methodologies that require specialized training and expertise.[5] Sub-disciplines in forensic science include forensic biology, forensic anthropology, forensic odontology, forensic pathology, medicolegal death investigation, forensic toxicology, controlled substances, fire and arson investigation, impression and pattern evidence, firearms and toolmarks, bloodstain pattern analysis, questioned documents, trace evidence, crime scene investigation, and digital evidence.

Basic Principles of Evidence

Identification

The first step in the identification of evidence is knowing that it may yield probative value through existing DNA, hair, fiber, residue, or other chemical elements to support or refute narratives of a crime. The evidence is objective, and the analysis requires that once identified, the element or item is preserved for analysis by the forensic scientist.

There are a number of types of evidence that the forensic nurse will encounter in their daily practices. A high index of suspicion is necessary to observe a person, their behavior, and reactions to medical procedures to understand the complexity of forensic nursing. Once the forensic nurse is called to a patient's bedside, everything is possible evidence and subject to careful handling and documentation. **Table 11-1** identifies types of evidence.

Table 11-1. Types of Evidence and Sampling Recommendations

TYPE OF EVIDENCE	EXAMPLES	SAMPLING
Trace Evidence	Trace items such as hair, fiber, debris, dried fluids, secretions, or other traces of chemical or inert elements	Uses tools and methods to identify, document location, and collect so the samples are preserved (eg, bindle folding)
Biological Evidence	Body fluids such as saliva, breast or vaginal fluids, ear wax, sweat	Uses tools and methods to capture samples for preservation (eg, cotton tipped applicator, where drying or freezing is preferred method for storage)
Technology Evidence	Electronic devices, photography, electronic records (eg, pornography)	Preservation of the technology; even if destroyed, oftentimes still in the "cloud"
Verbal Evidence	Anything said is verbal evidence. Documentation includes what patients say in quotes. Bias is a risk for the forensic nurse who is not objective.	HIPAA protects patient records, but not during an active criminal investigation. Other protections for records govern release.

PROCUREMENT

Taking any item into custody requires that the health care provider understands the preservation of samples weighed against the potential for blood-borne pathogens and hospital protocol. While not exclusive, adjustments may be necessary to take some evidence into custody. For instance, sharp items require safety in handling without disturbing the evidence on the sharp object. High value items, such as drugs or jewelry, require special handling and packaging to prevent theft.

PRESERVATION

Storage facilities in health care organizations often have a locked closet. To preserve evidence, the environment must be temperature-controlled and have an indexing system to help staff easily find objects in the closet. For instance, when someone checks evidence into the closet, the log identifies the person opening the door, the time the door opened, and the location of the item (ie, shelf number and numbered space). Every person who enters the closet must be documented. Temperature should also be recorded in the log. If the evidence is in a refrigerator, the same level of documentation is required, as demonstrated in **Table 11-2-a** and **b**.

Table 11-2-a. Biological Evidence: Short-Term Storage Conditions[6]

TYPE OF EVIDENCE	FROZEN	REFRIGERATED	TEMPERATURE CONTROLLED	ROOM TEMPERATURE
Liquid Blood	Never	Best	Less than 24 hours	
Urine	Best	Less than 24 hours		
Dry Biological Stained Item			Best	Acceptable

(continued)

Table 11-2-a. Biological Evidence: Short-Term Storage Conditions[4] *(continued)*

TYPE OF EVIDENCE	FROZEN	REFRIGERATED	TEMPERATURE CONTROLLED	ROOM TEMPERATURE
Dry Biological Stained Item			Best	Acceptable
Wet Bloody Items (if cannot be dried)	Best	Acceptable	Less than 24 hours	
Bones	Acceptable		Acceptable	Acceptable
Hair			Best	Acceptable
Swabs with Biological Material		Best (wet)	Best (dried)	
Vaginal Smears			Best	
Feces	Best			
Buccal Swabs			Best	Less than 24 hours

Table 11-2-b. Biological Evidence: Long-Term Storage Conditions[6]

TYPE OF EVIDENCE	FROZEN	REFRIGERATED	TEMPERATURE CONTROLLED	ROOM TEMPERATURE
Liquid Blood	Never	Best		
Urine	Best			
Dry Biological Stained Item			Best	
Bones			Best	
Hair			Best	Acceptable
Swabs with Biological Material			Best (dried)	
Vaginal Smears			Best	
Feces	Best			
Buccal Swabs			Best	
DNA Extracts	Best (liquid)	Acceptable (liquid)	Acceptable (dried)	

TRANSFER

Transfer of any kind of evidence requires a chain of custody (COC). The COC is a logarithmic documentation trail of possession and location of the item to be used in court. A break in the COC results in denial of evidence submission during trial. If there is a suspicion of intent in mishandling evidence, oftentimes a break in the COC results in a mistrial.

FORENSIC NURSING ORGANIZATIONS

There are a number of national and international organizations serving forensic nurses. One of these organizations is the *American Academy of Forensic Sciences* (AAFS). In 2022, the AAFS membership voted to accept the "Forensic Nursing Science Section" as its 12th discipline, a full 40 years since accepting forensic nursing as a specialty role. This section represents nurses who provide medical-forensic examinations, testimony, training, education, and/or research in forensic nursing.

The Academy of Forensic Nursing (AFN) was established in 2018 and now serves over a thousand forensic nurses, partnering with a number of organizations that support generalist and advanced forensic nursing practices. Its vision is "to respond to trauma with care," and its mission "is to link research to practice through dissemination of scholarship, education, and service to those affected by and responding to trauma."[7] The AFN's partnerships disseminate education globally and promise to improve care of patients intersecting with legal systems around the world.

The International Association of Forensic Nurses (IAFN) was established in 1993 and has over 6000 members, primarily sexual assault nurse examiners (SANEs). The IAFN mission is "To provide leadership in forensic nursing practice by developing, promoting, and disseminating information internationally about forensic nursing science."[8] The IAFN receives millions of dollars in funding from the federal government for SANEs and SANE practices. The IAFN offers SANE-A (focused on adult/adolescent populations) and SANE-P (focused on prepubescent/adolescent populations) certification examinations through the Commission for Forensic Nursing Certification twice each year.

The Forensic Nursing Certification Board (FNCB) was reestablished in 2018. The FNCB vision is serving all forensic nursing communities and organizations. The FNCB has a desire to "improve the quality of care, and thus safety and satisfaction, in patients who intersect with the legal system, through certification of forensic nurses."[9] The FNCB provides certification to the Generalist Forensic Nurse (GFN-C) and the Advanced Forensic Nurse (AFN-C). The FNCB Generalist and Advanced Forensic Nursing certifications have a comprehensive foundation, common to all forensic nurses regardless of sub-specialty, and are grounded in research and consensus-building among forensic nursing educators and practitioners globally.

In January 2014, the Organization of Scientific Area Committees for Forensic Science (OSAC) was established to define minimum requirements, best practices, standard protocols, and other guidance to help ensure that the results of forensic analysis are reliable and reproducible. Its objectives support the development of quality benchmarks in and enhance consistency across the forensic science community. In October 2021, the OSAC launched a new subcommittee on forensic nursing. This committee's charge is to draft standards to improve the quality of care for victims of violence.

CASE STUDIES

Case Study 11-1

A reproductive-aged person presented to the emergency department (ED) at a local hospital and reported to the nurse that they were assaulted just prior to arrival. They reported that they had not bathed, and they were wearing the same clothing before and after the assault. The patient was undressed for medical evaluation because they reported having severe back pain and a possibly fractured rib. The ED nurse recognized that the patient's body and clothing might contain valuable evidence.

Discussion

Identification of evidence is the first step of the evidence management process in the ED. Forensic nurses use the Evidence Management Guidelines from the Department of Justice and other publications to ensure policy and procedure is followed. Proper protocol for the identification, collection, packaging, documentation, storage, and transfer of evidence from the ED to the appropriate agency (eg, law enforcement or laboratory personnel) is crucial. In this case, these steps would include: photographing the clothing and checking for rips or tears; placing each article of clothing into evidence bags and clearly marking them; performing an examination of any physical injuries as well as a sexual assault examination; and swabbing for any DNA evidence.

Case Study 11-2

An older patient was in primary care for blood pressure management. The nurse noticed an injury and requested the patient's permission to ask about what happened. The patient disclosed that their child, who had been struggling with their mental health and drug dependence, was responsible for the injury. The forensic nurse recognized that the patient's verbal history of the crime as evidence.

Discussion

Forensic nurses recognize that patient's reporting of intentional injury has the potential to be used as *medical exception to hearsay* in court. Sometimes, the verbal evidence is the only evidence allowed in court. Therefore, documentation that captures the direct quotes of the patient helps transfer verbal evidence without opinion to the trier of fact (judge and jury). Therefore, the forensic nurse should be sure to carefully detail the history of crime using direct quotes as often was possible.

SUMMARY

Evidence management requires practitioners to follow best practices and ensure integrity, prevent loss, and reduce premature destruction of biological evidence from collection through post-conviction.[6] All forms of evidence, whether biological, forensic DNA, or trace, must be identified, properly preserved, documented, and managed in compliance with the COC procedure.[6] The growth of forensic nursing over the last 40 years met a need in the health care industry to improve the care of patients intersecting with legal systems while in their organizations and institutions.

REFERENCES

1. Speck PM, Ekroos R, Gill-Hopple K, Faugno D. *Resources for evidence management in health care settings.* Evidence Technology Magazine; 2019.

2. Murkowski, Hickenlooper Introduce Legislation to Improve Access to Medical Forensics for Victims of Violence. August 23, 2021. United States Senator for Alaska: Lisa Murkowski. https://www.murkowski.senate.gov/press/release/murkowski-hickenlooper-introduce-legislation-to-improve-access-to-medical-forensics-for-victims-of-violence

3. Advancing Justice Through DNA Technology Act of 2003, S 1700, 108th Cong (2003). https://www.congress.gov/bill/108th-congress/senate-bill/1700

4. SAFER Technical Working Group, *National Best Practices for Sexual Assault Kits: A Multidisciplinary Approach.* Department of Justice Office of Justice Programs; 2017.

5. Committee on Identifying the Needs of the Forensic Sciences Community, National Research Council. *Strengthening forensic science in the United States: A path forward.* The National Academies Press; 2009.

6. Technical Working Group on Biological Evidence Preservation. *The Biological Evidence Preservation Handbook: Best Practices for Evidence Handlers.* 2nd ed. US Department of Commerce and National Institute of Standards and Technology; 2014:73.

7. Academy of Forensic Nursing. 2020. www.goafn.org

8. About Us. International Association of Forensic Nurses. 2021. https://www.forensicnurses.org/page/Overview

9. Mission. Forensic Nursing Certification Board. 2021. https://goforensicncb.org/mission

NAVIGATING THE LEGAL SYSTEM

Laura Zimm, JD

KEY POINTS

1. *Forensic nurses must have an understanding of the structure of the court system, including the roles of all participants.*

2. *Understanding the various court hearings and witness expectations is an important component of the forensic nursing role.*

INTRODUCTION

In court, medical evidence is an important component of a case. This medical evidence receives greater scrutiny by the court parties (eg, judge, plaintiff, and defendant attorneys) than any other evidence. Understanding the court system and its participants helps the forensic nurse prepare any documents and potential testimony for legal cases. Familiarity with the various types of court hearings and the expectations of witnesses is an important aspect of the forensic nursing role.

THE STRUCTURE OF THE COURT SYSTEM

CIVIL COURT

The American legal system has 2 basic components: civil and criminal court. Forensic nurses are often involved in *civil cases*, which are lawsuits filed on behalf of 1 private party (eg, an individual) against another. Often, a party is injured in some way, such as a car accident or an injury at work, for which they receive medical treatment after an evaluation. As part of their practice, forensic nurses complete said medical evaluation and any appropriate intervention with the expectation that they will carefully document any injuries and subsequent care. Based on this, forensic nurses provide depositions (ie, statements under oath) in which court parties question them in an office setting with a court reporter present. Civil cases can proceed to jury, court, or trial if they are unresolved after the deposition and pretrial discussions.

CRIMINAL COURT

Forensic nurses are also called to testify in criminal court cases. *Criminal cases* require probable cause in order to criminally charge a party with a crime. While practicing, a forensic nurse may be involved in the treatment of patients who are victims of child abuse, domestic violence, or sexual assault; thus, it is imperative for forensic nurses to carefully document any findings. The objective assessment of superficial injury and documentation of the patient's provided injury history helps the presentation of facts in court. In addition, the identification, collection, and maintenance of evidentiary samples or items (eg, clothing, photographs, etc.), whether brought by the patient or collected from the patient, are of paramount importance. All of the submitted evidence that is collected by the forensic nurse is carefully reviewed for maintenance methods and chain of custody by the criminal court. *Chain of custody* is a term referring to the tracking of evidence from identification through maintenance and disposal.

Court Hearings and Witness Expectations

Whether it is civil or criminal court, the roles of the participants remain similar. The judge oversees the case, which includes the scheduling, admission of evidence, and conduction of the trial. An attorney presents the case. In criminal cases, this is a prosecuting attorney with the local prosecutor's office. There will also be an attorney defending the person who is charged with a crime. In criminal cases, this is a criminal defense attorney, often a public defender. In civil cases, these roles are filled by private attorneys hired by the respective parties – the plaintiff who claims harm and the defense who is charged with creating the harm. In the courtroom, there will always be a bailiff who is an officer of the court and security personnel. The bailiff is responsible for keeping everyone safe and helping to move the court calendar along. There is also often a court clerk in the courtroom who is responsible for documenting scheduling hearings and accepting any documents to be provided to the judge.

The Legal Framework

Whether a case is brought in civil or criminal court, there is a universal right to have a jury trial in the United States. Before the trial, there are numerous steps in the process. The forensic nurse's work receives scrutiny in an evaluation process every step of the way. The steps begin with a review to determine if there is enough evidence to go forward. The parties look at the basis of the allegations and the details of how they arose. All medical documentation is important and informs the decision to move forward. Medical evidence collection is best completed by a forensic nurse with training or education in forensic nursing. Evidence kits (eg, rape kits and drug-facilitated sexual assault kits) require scrupulous attention to detail. The objective documentation by forensic nurses of superficial injuries (eg, location, color, discharge, margin measurements) is closely reviewed by the legal parties. The same attention to medical testing (eg, scans, x-rays, ultrasounds) occurs. If there is enough medical forensic evidence properly collected and documented with a clear chain of custody to bring a case, then the case is scheduled on a court calendar. At that time, the accused responds to the allegations. In criminal cases, the accused may plead guilty or not guilty. If the accused pleads not guilty, the case will be set for a trial. In civil cases, the defendant must respond to the allegations of harm.

Both civil and criminal cases are set for numerous pre-trial hearings to sort out evidentiary issues. In criminal cases, this may involve asking the court to suppress evidence. The forensic nurse's training and experience will be challenged during voir dire (the preliminary examination by a judge). Other challenges may include confronting the use of any specialized equipment (eg, colposcope or photography) and the process of evidence collection (eg, whether the person collecting the evidence was qualified to do so). Testimony is often taken at these suppression hearings, or it is briefed in writing. The defending party may also dispute the admission of any expert testimony, including from a forensic nurse. Challenges to the forensic nurse often involve the witness's training and experience and include any protocol variances. Ultimately, the judge decides what evidence is admitted into the court or jury trial.

Trials

After a number of pre-trial meetings, the case is ready for trial. Court cases often take place a year or more after the filing of the case. There are 2 kinds of trials: court and jury. During a **court trial**, the attorneys present their cases to the judge, and the judge is the "fact finder" who makes decisions on the civil claim or the criminal charges. During a **jury trial**, the attorneys present their cases to a panel of jurors. In criminal cases, there are 12 jurors, while in civil cases, there are 6 jurors. The jury then assesses the facts and evidence presented and makes the final decision regarding the civil claim or the criminal charges.

WITNESSES

Witnesses testify in open court at both court and jury trials. The calling attorney or judge serves a subpoena to the witness. The subpoena sets the date, time, and location of the hearing requiring testimony, along with a contact person. The medical testimony is often technical and confusing for the jurors and legal parties alike, so the best witness is a professional who *teaches* the fact finder about their subject. Someone with a professional, non-defensive attitude carries weight with the fact finder. The forensic nurse should not advocate for either party but educate the court about what they did and/or what they know.

There are 2 basic types of witnesses: fact witnesses and expert witnesses. A **fact witness** is someone who was involved in the incident. Health care providers who care for victims of crime are fact witnesses. The fact witness describes what they saw and did during an examination and what they observed afterwards. Often, a forensic nurse, after the delivery of the incident facts, also serves as an expert witness. An **expert witness** is someone who is called upon to give their educated opinion on a topic. The attorney who calls the witness will tell them which type of witness they are. It is important for any witness to meet with the subpoenaing attorney to talk about the anticipated testimony. The attorney-witness discussion might include determining the witnesses' role and opinion (if expert), confirming what information and/or files they should bring with them, and discussing the expectations of cross-examination. The jury holds the forensic nurse in high regard, whether they serve as a factual or expert witness, because their knowledge is based on their education, role, and experience. The successful forensic nurse remains unbiased at all times and remains an impartial witness in court.

Furthermore, any inconsistencies in the patient's report will be questioned, so documenting quotations in the medical record helps the witness while testifying. In addition, any prior testimony or written work that is perceived as biased is subject to questioning. If the patient's account or statement is unclear and the forensic nurse did not clarify through inquiry, then the the forensic nurse may be asked to explain the lack of inquiry. Any possible alternative causes of the injury will likely be brought up in court as well; therefore, the forensic nurse should remain objective and readily acknowledge any of those alternatives. During the testimony, the methods used to collect data and any deviation in the collection of evidence will also be discussed. The forensic nurse's training, education, and experience should be clearly stated to help show the basis for their ability to collect evidence.

RULES OF COURT

The rules of court apply to all court proceedings and dictate what evidence is admitted. The witness should confirm what they are prohibited from testifying on during their pre-trial meeting with the attorney, and they should remain alert to the judge's instruction to not testify about said topics. In criminal court, there are court rules generally forbidding testimony about certain topics (eg, prior sexual assault allegations, prior criminal charges, and incarceration). The forensic nurse must understand that violating the court rules will result in a mistrial, starting over with a new jury, or reversal of a conviction upon appeal.

CASE STUDIES

Case Study 12-1

This forensic nurse was called to criminal court as a fact witness. In court, they made a statement indicating that they believed the victim and assumed that the victim was telling the truth, as was reflected in the forensic nurse's documentation. The defendant's attorney made an objection to this statement, which the judge sustained as an improper opinion. The jury was then told to disregard the forensic nurse's statement.

Discussion

The forensic nurse provided an opinion about a fact in the case, therefore providing an opportunity for appeal if the jury convicted the accused. Forensic nurses, when called as fact witnesses, should not give opinions while on the stand, only factual statements.

Case Study 12-2

This advanced forensic nurse was called to criminal court as an expert witness. They did not have a personal interaction with the victim of the crime but rather were there to serve as an expert on the subject matter of forensic nursing. Their role as an advanced forensic nurse was to evaluate the actions taken (ie, review all of the records) by the general forensic nurse of the victim and determine if the general forensic nurse acted appropriately within their guidelines. The advanced forensic nurse provided their information in the form of written and then in-person testimony. The questions that they were asked while on the stand arose from their written testimony, and the advanced forensic nurse answered objectively.

Discussion

The advanced forensic nurse provided unbiased analysis of the records and statements given to them. Utilizing their advanced training and years of experience, they were able to provide expert witness testimony without opinionated statements.

SUMMARY

Forensic nurses play a critical role in the legal system as objective medical providers at all levels of nursing – from the generalist forensic nurse at the bedside to the advanced forensic nurse leader. All forensic nurses are skilled in the evaluation of physical and emotional trauma reactions, the collection of evidence, objective documentation of findings in the medical record, and treatments of medical findings, whether directly supervised under protocols or in the independent advanced forensic nursing practice. All aspects of the forensic nursing practice are important parts of any legal case. As such, it is imperative for the forensic nurse to understand the structure of the court system, including all parties' roles. Ultimately, the unbiased testimony of a forensic nurse is regarded highly by both judges and jurors.

DISCLAIMER

Laura Zimm, JD, is considered an expert in her field, and she produced this chapter entirely based on her professional perspective and experience.

Chapter 13

PROVIDING TESTIMONY

Valerie Sievers, MSN, RN, CNS, AFN-C, SANE-A, SANE-P, DF-AFN
Jennifer L. Johnson, DNP, MSN, APRN, WHNP-BC, AFN-BC, SANE-A, SANE-P, AFN-C, DF-AFN

KEY POINTS

1. *Forensic nurses practice at the interface of health care and legal arenas.*

2. *Providing testimony during trial is an expected outcome of forensic nursing practice.*

3. *The forensic nurse provides unbiased, objective testimony, whether testifying as a fact or expert witness.*

INTRODUCTION

Forensic nurses provide medical forensic care, including evaluation of persons affected by crime and violence. After direct care of the forensic patient and when there are charges pursuant to the crime, the forensic nurse provider may receive a subpoena to testify. The **subpoena** is a written order to appear and provide testimony on a particular topic, sent by an attorney of the court (eg, prosecution or defense attorney). The derivation of the word subpoena is Latin and interpreted to mean *under penalty*.[1] In either case, the forensic nurse recognizes that their role in the courtroom is as an educator, providing objective, unbiased information related to the actual care of the patient, and an opinion for the court if qualified as an expert witness. Forensic nurses possess additional knowledge and skills through continuing education courses or college credit. Others have graduate degrees from accredited universities, schools, or colleges of nursing.

THE ROLE OF THE FORENSIC NURSE

The foundation of forensic nursing is based in nursing science, forensic science, and legal principles. Global violence and crime set the stage for forensic nursing practices, providing care and treatment at many points along a societal continuum where health and legal systems intersect. A primary focus of forensic nursing practice lies in recognizing the health consequences of trauma from violence, while promoting access to equitable health care and improving health outcomes.[2] When called to testify, the forensic nurse is a licensed health care professional serving in the role of educator to the judge and jury. The education provided in the courtroom during testimony may include explanations of medical terminology, health care procedures, anatomy and physiology, nursing standards of practice, medical diagnosis and treatment, steps in an evidentiary examination, and appropriate collection of evidence. Additionally, forensic nurses may be asked to explain injury identification, photographs of evidence, and objective documentation. Health care professionals use their knowledge and clinical experiences to inform the public about health care dynamics to provide a foundation for the fact, determined by the jury's decision about guilt or innocence.

PREPARATION FOR TESTIMONY

Forensic nurses, comfortable with the often-chaotic health care environment, may experience apprehension at the thought of being in an unfamiliar courtroom providing testimony. The novice forensic nurse without testimony experience may find it beneficial to observe criminal trial proceedings and expert testimony offered by health care providers, forensic nurses, law enforcement, and other forensic scientists.

The clinical opportunity to visit a courtroom during a trial proceeding, when the nurse is not a witness, exposes the forensic nurse to information about the structure and process of a trial, as well as observation of both positive and negative attributes of fact and expert witnesses.

In criminal trials, the subpoenaing attorney is a prosecutor or an attorney for the defense. Usually, the prosecutor represents the state and the defense represents the accused. All criminal defendants are guaranteed the right to an attorney in a criminal trial. When a health care professional receives a subpoena, the first step is to review the subpoena for details such as the date of the trial, jurisdiction, name of the prosecutor or defense attorney, and case number. Contacting the subpoenaing attorney is important to facilitate communication about the referenced trial information, specifically scheduling the testimony.

When preparing for testimony and the anticipated ***voir dire*** (ie, examination of the witness), the forensic nurse must share a current curriculum vitae (CV) in advance of trial. The CV is not merely a resume or job history. The CV is a detailed review of professional accomplishments and includes professional education and degrees, employment experiences, scholarly or organizational memberships, publications, presentations, certifications, and any grants, awards, or honors. Nursing credentials (eg, licenses) are listed along with degrees earned and board certifications. A CV is considered a "living document" that needs to be updated frequently.[3,4] A variety of templates for a professional CV are available online and included in word processing programs.

In advance of trial, the forensic nurse reviews any health care documentation (eg, written and electronic medical records, treatment records, diagrams, and photography) associated with the patient care encounter. The forensic nurse then schedules a time to meet with the subpoenaing attorney. In a criminal case, the prosecutor typically represents the district attorney's office. In all cases, the forensic nurse educates the court about the forensic nursing medical forensic evaluation, the findings, and the treatment protocols as well as the professional background, credentials, and expertise. The forensic nurse should also be knowledgeable about nursing policies, procedures, standards of care, or clinical pathways that support the scope of practice. **Table 13-1** defines the legal terms the forensic nurse may encounter.

Table 13-1. Legal Terms and Definitions[2]

Legal Terms	Definition
Arraignment	An initial step in the criminal justice process, where a defendant is charged and informed of constitutional rights
Trial	An examination, usually with testimony offered before a tribunal
Subpoena	A writ issued under court authority, compelling a witness to appear at a judicial proceeding
Testimony	A statement made by a witness under oath, usually related to a legal proceeding
Direct Examination	The initial questioning of a witness by the attorney who called the witness with the intent to present testimony supporting a factual argument
Cross Examination	The questioning of a witness by the opposing attorney to discredit the witness or testimony provided on direct examination
Hearsay	Evidence based not on a witness's personal knowledge but on another's statement not made under oath
Objection	A procedure whereby a party asserts that a particular witness, line of questioning, or piece of evidence is improper
Verdict	An opinion rendered by a judge or jury on a question of fact

In the courtroom, when a forensic nurse is called to the stand, the attorneys will challenge the forensic nurse during voir dire.[2] These questions lay the foundation for determining the expertise of the witness, reflecting the education, employment, scholarship, and practice experiences listed on their CV. Opposing counsel in the case is also afforded the opportunity to ask questions, specifically to determine if objections to the nurse's testimony as an expert exist. The judge determines if the questioning is adequate to allow the witness to testify as either a fact witness or an expert witness.

The *fact witness* testifies about first-person individual knowledge on a case. The fact witness relays their firsthand observations and understanding of what was said or seen in the encounter with a patient who may have been affected by violence or criminal activity.[2]

By reason of education, specialized training, or experience, an *expert witness* has specific knowledge of the subject in question. Following judicial determination, they form an opinion to assist the jury in understanding the subject matter in dispute.[5] When an attorney calls a witness for a hearing, trial, or deposition, the attorney questions the witness during a *direct examination*. During direct examination, the prosecutor introduces evidence, which may include the medical record documentation and components of an evidentiary kit completed as part of a medical forensic examination. The opposing attorney also has the opportunity to ask questions during a *cross-examination*. The purpose of cross-examination is to create doubt as to the credibility of the witness.[6]

The forensic nurse testifies as a fact witness or expert witness in criminal or civil proceedings where the goal is always to educate the judge and jury. Testimony often includes conveying complex health care concepts in clear, concise language, including defining terms and relaying factual information about forensic nursing practice and the processes of the medical forensic examination. As a health care professional, the forensic nurse must provide an objective testimony in any legal proceedings. Telling the truth and educating the trier of fact demonstrates a commitment to the ethical standards in forensic nursing practice.

CASE STUDIES

Case Study 13-1

A 34-year-old woman presented to the emergency department (ED) with a concern for sexual assault. She remembered being out with friends and meeting a man that she had only briefly met a few times prior. She had a lapse in memory from the time that she was at a local pub, drinking with friends, and then she awoke in her room. Upon waking, she realized that her bed was broken, and her room was disheveled.

While in the ED, the patient received a medical screening examination, and the ED staff contacted the forensic nurse examiner on call for a consult. Upon arrival, the forensic nurse examiner briefly talked with the patient about the process of the examination and what to expect. The patient was unsure if she wanted to report the occurrence of a potential sexual assault to law enforcement. The forensic nurse discussed her options for completing a medical forensic examination without reporting to the police. The forensic nurse also informed the patient that the crime laboratory will not complete drug toxicology testing without a police report. The forensic nurse suggested that one option would be to complete a urine drug screen in the ED and retain a urine sample for a toxicology kit should she decide to report to police in the future.

While awaiting results of the urine drug screen, the patient underwent a medical forensic evidentiary examination. During the detailed anogenital assessment, the forensic nurse identified a bleeding laceration to the posterior fourchette and bruising to her hymen. Both injuries were consistent with the patient's concern of sexual assault. After providing medication for potential exposure to sexually transmitted infections, the urine drug screen results indicated a positive finding for benzodiazepines. Based on the patient's history, the forensic nurse reviewed the information and discovered that the patient did not take any medication that would provide a false positive on the urine drug screen.

The patient was discharged with instructions for a follow-up examination in 72 hours and the sexual assault kit identification number should she decide to report to the police later.

Five days later, law enforcement contacted the forensic program and reported that the patient opted to report the sexual assault, and they wanted to arrange for recovery of the evidence collected. The detective retrieved the clothing collected, toxicology kit containing blood and urine, and the sexual assault evidentiary kit.

While the evidence was being analyzed at the crime laboratory, a man the patient remembered from the pub applied for a position in which a background check was required. He completed the background check with no negative indicators; however, the last phase of the interview process required the man to submit to a DNA test to be completed through CODIS. The man provided a buccal sample, and upon analysis, there were 5 cold case hits, including a positive identification to the sexual assault kit that was just recently analyzed in the crime lab. Law enforcement contacted the business to set up a time that they could have the man present for the final phase of his screening for employment. At this time, he was taken into custody.

Discussion

A forensic examination proved fruitful not only for this patient but also for the 5 other women that had previously completed examinations without positive identification of the male perpetrator.

The forensic nurse anticipated the opportunity to testify in court about the process of the medical forensic examination, evidence identified and collected, and injury evaluated as part of the detailed anogenital assessment. Following receipt of a subpoena, compelling the forensic nurse to testify at trial, the first step was to communicate with the prosecutor or attorney that initiated the subpoena. This initial contact provided an exchange of information about the ordered appearance of witnesses as well as the process of the medical forensic examination. The forensic nurse also discussed the potential use of photographs or drawings and diagrams during direct examination with the prosecutor.

Prior to testimony, the forensic nurse thoroughly reviewed the medical forensic records, diagrams, photographs, steps in evidence collection, and all laboratory results in this case, including toxicology. The forensic nurse, whether acting as a fact or expert witness, must be well-versed in the details of their respective curriculum vitae, as these are regularly reviewed during the process of voir dire.

On the day of testimony, the attorneys' office communicated with the forensic nurse witness about the anticipated time for responding to the court. The forensic nurse was prepared, arrived well in advance of the requested time, and dressed in business attire appropriate for the courtroom environment. Since witnesses are generally sequestered, the forensic nurse waited in an area designated and separate from the courtroom until called by the attorney to testify. While waiting, the specifics of the case were not discussed with any other personnel. When called to the stand and sworn in, the forensic nurse remembered that the continuation of practice and care involves relaying the truth.

Summary
Forensic nursing practice encompasses the intersection of nursing with legal systems and utilizes borrowed science from sociology, criminology, victimology, and forensic science. One key aspect of the forensic nursing practice is providing testimony in criminal and civil trials as a fact or expert witness. In this role, the forensic nurse provides unbiased, objective testimony, educating the judge, jury, and the public about the knowledge and skill required to practice as a generalist and advanced forensic nurse.

References
1. Gifis SH. *Barrons dictionary of legal terms.* 3rd ed. Barron's Educational Series; 1998.

2. Malmgren J, Leahy C. Overreaching issues: Testifying. In: Price B, Maguire K, eds. *Core curriculum for forensic nursing.* Wolters Kluwer; 2016:221-227.

3. Caruso C. Testifying as a forensic nurse. In: Lynch, VA, Barber-Duvall J, eds. *Forensic nursing science.* Elsevier-Mosby; 2011:544-559.

4. What's the difference between a resume and a CV? The Writing Center, University of North Carolina at Chapel Hill. Accessed January 21, 2021. https://writingcenter.unc.edu/tips-and-tools/curricula-vitae-cvs-versus-resumes/

5.   Constantino RE. The anatomy and physiology of a lawsuit for the forensic nurse. In: Constantino RE, Crane PA, Young SE, eds. *Forensic Nursing: Evidence-Based Principles and Practice.* F.A. Davis Co.; 2013:64-78.

6.   Sisko N. Glossary. In: Dickinson J, Meyer A, eds. *Legal Nurse Consulting Principles and Practices.* 4th ed. Routledge; 2019:957

Chapter 14

Forensic Nursing Documentation and Photography

Valerie Sievers, MSN, RN, CNS, AFN-C, SANE-A, SANE-P, DF-AFN
Diana K. Faugno, MSN, RN, AFN-C, CPN, SANE-A, SANE-P, FAAFS, DF-IAFN, DF-AFN
Stacey A. Mitchell, DNP, MBA, MEd, RN, AFN-C, SANE-A, SANE-P, DF-AFN, FAAN

Key Points

1. *Accurate, evidence-based documentation is an essential skill for forensic nurses.*

2. *Forensic photography is a useful tool for the medical-forensic examination.*

3. *Written and photographic documentation is valuable evidence for future legal proceedings.*

Introduction

Accurate, thorough, and consistent documentation is an essential skill for health care professionals and necessary when nurses and physicians are providing care to patients affected by interpersonal violence and crime. Poor documentation adversely affects legal outcomes in cases requiring a forensic health care response. If medical terminology is misused, normal or injury findings are misinterpreted, or documentation is noted to be absent or inconsistent in the medical record, the absence and inconsistency with standards of practice and care become the focus in adjudication. In addition to written documentation, forensic photography is a tool that supports descriptions of injury or normal findings and provides an authentic visual record of assessment findings at the time of the medical forensic examination. Body diagrams are also used in addition to photography for documentation in forensic cases. The Academy of Forensic Nursing encourages the use of standardized diagrams for documentation in forensic practice.[1]

Documentation

Forensic documentation usually takes 3 forms: written, diagram, and photograph. Each form of documentation builds upon the other.[2] When there are legal implications in patient care, more than one form is helpful for cross-reference of documentation. Records generated by the forensic nurse often enter as evidence during courtroom proceedings in criminal and civil cases. All aspects of forensic nursing documentation must be clear, accurate, detailed, and descriptive.[3] Elements of the documentation include the narrative of the events (history of injury); location of injuries; care interventions and referrals provided; any evidence identified, collected, packaged and preserved; and the documentation establishing a chain of custody.

Forensic nurses capture written accounts of the patient's history and use quotations to accurately capture their lived experience. The forensic nurse also captures objective and descriptive observations of a patient's presentation and demeanor in the narrative. For example, words to describe the patient's affect include "poor eye contact,"

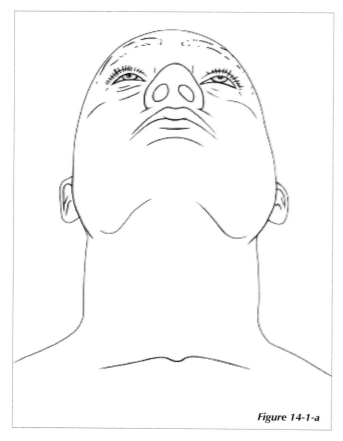

Figure 14-1-a

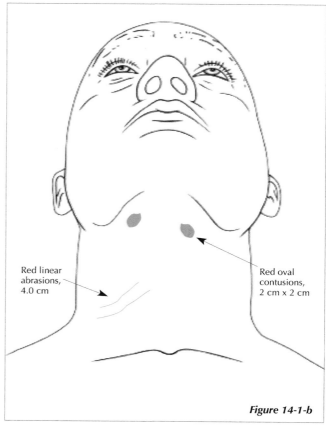

Red linear
abrasions,
4.0 cm

Red oval
contusions,
2 cm x 2 cm

Figure 14-1-b

Figure 14-1-a. *Sample neck diagram, blank.
(© AFN and ION Medical Designs, LLC, 2018.
Used with permission.)*

Figure 14-1-b. *Sample neck diagram with mark-
ups demonstrating the location of abrasions and
contusions. (© AFN and ION Medical Designs, LLC,
2018. Used with permission.)*

"crying," "yelling," or "wringing hands." The nurse thoroughly describes injuries or
the lack of injuries and normal anatomy. All evidence collected is documented, and
some evidence, such as clothing, is described and photographed. Of particular interest
are defects, such as missing buttons and tears.

Diagrams and body maps allow for a visual placement of injuries, so anyone reviewing the medical record sees the locations of any injuries or findings. Diagrams should
include the size, shape, and color of the wounds next to the drawing (**Figures 14-1-a
and b**).[4] The objective written narrative provides the foundation for the diagrams.
Photographs show the true and accurate representation of what the nurse observed
during the examination.

The saying "if it wasn't documented, then it wasn't done" applies even more to forensic nursing than other situations. Therefore, comprehensive documentation in
medical-forensic cases is necessary. The forensic nurse expects every case to have legal
implications whether is it related to criminal activity, maltreatment, or a civil issue.
Hospital departments such as risk management, patient safety, compliance, and accreditation often access forensic nursing documentation. Thorough documentation
of an event, especially if the event occurred on hospital property, provides the basis for
settlement negotiations or assists with reducing damages awarded during civil litigation. Poor documentation has the potential to negatively impact any case; therefore,
the forensic nurse must take the time necessary to meticulously document all activities and findings in medical-forensic cases.

PHOTOGRAPHIC DOCUMENTATION
Photography has been widely used in a variety of forensic practice areas including
child maltreatment, nonfatal strangulation, sexual assault, physical abuse and neglect,
interpersonal violence across the lifespan, and death investigation. Today, patients

expect photographs to be taken as part of their evidence collection.[5] Consistent photography with each forensic patient supports the comprehensive approach to the evidentiary examination.

In addition to photographing specific injuries that a person sustains, it is important to consider photographing other findings or personal effects that may help the forensic nurse to document the occurrence of trauma. Clothing is often torn, cut, blood-spattered, or contaminated with foreign materials (**Figure 14-2**). Traumatic injuries like gunshot wounds, stab wounds created by knives or sharp instruments, and lacerations following blunt force trauma require photography prior to manipulating (eg, cleaning or surgical repair). Patients seen in a variety of clinical settings as an emergency department (ED), clinic, child advocacy center, or jail also benefit from photographic documentation. Justification for photographic documentation in programs often includes[6]:

— Recording and documenting injuries and potential evidence, especially when the evidence cannot be preserved indefinitely or will be altered by treatment or repair

— Acting as a future aid to memory

— Documenting features and details that contribute to the evidentiary examination (eg, condition of clothing worn by the patient)

Patients must provide informed consent for photographs both verbally and in writing.[7] The consent form includes information on the type of photographs to be taken, who has access to the photographs, and how the images will be used, stored, and secured. Current policies that guide photographic documentation and storage are necessary for facilities and their patients, who are in need of a forensic health care response.[6]

The rule of thirds, fourths, and fifths is a standard approach to forensic photodocumentation of trauma and injury.[8] An important initial image is called a "bookend card," which includes identifiable information such as the patient's hospital wristband, a computer-generated identification label, or a commercially prepared label. ***Bookend identification*** demonstrates the first and last (ie, beginning and end) of a series of photographs taken as part of the medical forensic examination. The bookend card also contains the name of the patient, date of birth, date and time of the examination, health care provider name, credentials, and case number. The first photo is the identification photograph (eg, the patient's face and upper body). After the identification photograph, a full body photo of the front and back of the clothed patient should be taken to document the appearance of the patient.[9] These images capture the condition of clothing worn at the time, the criminal activity or episode of violence, and any visible body surface injuries. Scales and rulers provide context for measurements and should be used as a reference in the images.[10] Often, a patient may have changed clothes prior to presenting to the hospital or clinic for their examination. Prior to clothing collection, the forensic nurse determines whether the patient is wearing the same clothes that were worn at the time of the assault or injury. If not, asking about the location of that clothing is important. The activities following the assault are also important in assessing whether the clothing currently worn has body fluids, drainage, or staining that is of evidentiary value.

Sequential photos of wounds or injuries follow the standard rule of thirds, fourths, and fifths.

— The first image should include the location of the injury or wound and be photographed at a distance that provides a view of anatomic orientation (ie, far away).

— The second image should be half the distance closer than the first image (ie, mid-range).

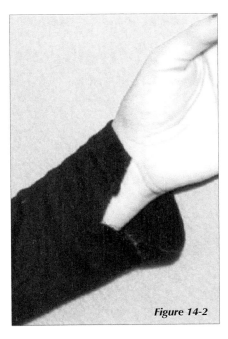

Figure 14-2. *A 23-year-old female whose partner ripped her shirt during an assault. Note the tear to the bottom of the sleeve.*

Figure 14-2

— The third image is a close-up of the injury with a standard reference scale or ruler (ie, close range).

— The fourth image is the same close-up of the wound without a scale.

— The fifth image is the closest image possible to capture the entire injury if needed.[11]

TIPS FOR PHOTOGRAPHIC DOCUMENTATION
— Prior to obtaining any photographs, obtain verbal and written consent.

— Be considerate of patient comfort and privacy.

— Be familiar with the equipment.

— Always wear gloves if your hands are in the photo.

— Be consistent. If using a measuring scale or ruler for a bruise on one part of the body, use in all areas where there is a bruise.

— Photographs and written documentation must match. The narrative description of injuries, photos, and body map should reflect the same terminology and measurements.[12]

— Peer review of medical-forensic examinations should include a review of photography.[13]

— Are photographs clear?

— Is the lighting correct?

— Are photographs taken at a 90° angle?

— Are photographs taken both with and without a scale or ruler?[14]

— Photography must follow organizational policies and procedures in the clinical area related to the storage and release of photos.[6]

— Hospital departments such as Compliance and Risk Management may assist nurses with forensic policy development.

EQUIPMENT
The forensic nurse determines the type of camera equipment necessary to meet current best practices. Camera bodies and lenses vary in cost. Budget restrictions impact purchasing quality and uses, which vary by brand. Cell phones are never appropriate for forensic photography as storage of the images is not secure.

CASE STUDIES

Case Study 14-1

The forensic nurse was called to the hospital entrance. A visitor was lying on the floor, reporting that she tripped while entering the hospital. The visitor was taken to the ED for examination and treatment. The forensic nurse photographed the hospital entrance, documenting a dry floor without any floor mats or obstructions. She then went to the ED and obtained a history from the visitor/patient. The patient told the forensic nurse that she was texting while walking and hit the sliding glass door. The forensic nurse documented no visible injuries or swelling. The patient stated that it was "her fault." The forensic nurse contacted security to preserve any video footage. She also documented the patient's history and physical examination in the forensic record and on the incident report. The photos were uploaded to a secure server that only the forensic nurses can access.

Discussion

Two weeks later, the hospital received a call from an attorney who told the hospital he was filing a lawsuit. In the lawsuit, the complainant (the visitor) reported that she tripped on a floor mat that was not flat on the floor at the entrance. The forensic nurse provided the images of the hospital entrance and her documentation to Risk Management and the hospital attorney. The lawsuit was dismissed.

Case Study 14-2

A 22-year-old woman was transported by ambulance to the local ED with injuries from what she described as a violent, physical assault by her boyfriend with multiple episodes of strangulation. She had already reported this assault to the police, who were investigating. A forensic nurse was called in to care for the patient, provide a medical forensic examination, and collect evidence. The patient signed the consent form for the evidentiary examination and photography. In addition to assessing the patient who was medically cleared in the ED, the forensic nurse documented the history provided by the patient. She reported, "We were arguing all day. I told him he needs to move out of my house and get help for his drinking and addictions. He smelled like he had been drinking. He started pushing me around, grabbing and twisting my arms and hitting me in the face and head with his open hand. I tried to lock myself in the bedroom, but he got in and pushed me on the bed. His hands were around my neck, and I couldn't breathe! I scratched at his hands and got away, but then he pushed me against the wall and started choking me again. I think I passed out because I woke up on the floor. He wasn't in the bedroom, so I slammed the bedroom door shut, grabbed my phone, and dialed 911. When the cops showed up, he was sitting on the floor in the kitchen with a crack pipe."

As part of the medical forensic examination, the forensic nurse performed a head-to-toe assessment using diagrams, written documentation, and photographs to properly document the multiple areas of injury on the patient's body. A strangulation tool was completed as part of the documentation and diagrams to correlate with photos depicting redness, abrasions, and scratches on her neck and upper chest and petechial hemorrhages in both eyes. The forensic nurse also documented that the patient described "waking up on the floor" after an episode of strangulation and that her voice was "hoarse."

Later that evening, the patient was discharged to go home with family members who remained with her and watched for the complications that can occur due to strangulation. Her boyfriend was placed in custody and faced charges of domestic violence resulting in injury, strangulation, attempted homicide, and possession of illegal substances.

Discussion

Two years later, the forensic nurse received a subpoena to testify in this case of domestic violence and strangulation. After reviewing the medical forensic examination documentation, diagrams, and photographs, the forensic nurse met with the prosecutor to review the case prior to trial. The prosecutor intended to call the forensic nurse as an expert witness. The following week, as part of the testimony, the forensic nurse was allowed to relay the history of events provided by the patient, show the diagrams and photographs of injury due to strangulation, and educate the jury about the various injuries, including their descriptions and measurements. Several days later, after deliberation, the jury returned a guilty verdict. Jury members later suggested to the prosecution team that the forensic photodocumentation and explanation of injury contributed to their decision.

Summary

The practice of forensic nursing is an evolving specialty that reflects an evidence-based response to the epidemic of interpersonal violence and trauma. Forensic nurses have a responsibility to provide a complete and comprehensive medical forensic examination that includes exquisite documentation. Best practice forensic documentation includes written, diagrammatic, and photographic records that, when done accurately, provide important, demonstrative evidence in future legal proceedings.

References

1. Academy of Forensic Nursing. Academy Package 1. Accessed December 20, 2021. https://goafn.thinkific.com/courses/anatomy1

2. Kogan AC, Rosen T, Navarro A, et al. Developing the geriatric injury documentation tool (Geri-IDT) to improve documentation of physical findings in injured older adults. *J Gen Intern Med*. 2019;34(4):567-574. doi:10.1007/s11606-019-04844-8

3. Limandri BJ. *Efficient and Effective Documentation in Nursing Care*. Oregon State Board of Nursing Sentinel. 2021;40(3):4-7. Accessed December 16, 2021. https://www.oregon.gov/osbn/Documents/Sentinel_2021_August.pdf

4. Hess CT. Understanding your documentation requirements. *Adv Skin Wound Care*. 2018;31(3):144. doi:10.1097/01.ASW.0000530374.61754.a3

5. Nittis M, Hughes R. Forensic photo-documentation in adult sexual assault—what do patients think? *J Forensic Leg Med*. 2021;77:102092. doi:10.1016/j.jflm.2020.102092

6. Office on Violence Against Women. A national protocol for sexual assault medical forensic examinations, adult/adolescents. 2nd ed. US Department of Justice; 2013. https://www.ojp.gov/pdffiles1/ovw/241903.pdf

7. Sievers V, Faugno D. Best Practice Forensic Photo-Documentation: Show me the injuries! *Leg Nurse Consul*. 2021;32(4):26-31.

8. Dunlop J. What is the rule of thirds? (And how to use it in photos!). Expert Photography. 2021. https://expertphotography.com/improve-your-composition-the-rule-of-thirds/

9. Gouse S, Karnam S, Girish HC, Murgod S. Forensic photography: Prospect through the lens. *J Forensic Dent Sci*. 2018;10(1):2-4. doi:10.4103/jfo.jfds_2_16

10. Sieberth T, Ebert LC, Gentile S, Fliss B. Clinical forensic height measurements on injured people using a multi camera device for 3D documentation. *Forensic Sci Med Pathol*. 2020;16(4):586-594. doi:10.1007/s12024-020-00282-9

11. Faugno DK, Sievers V, Shores M, Smock B, Speck PM. *Domestic Violence and Nonfatal Strangulation Assessment*. STM Learning, Inc.; 2020.

12. Ernst EJ, Speck PM, Fitzpatrick JJ. The element of naturalness when evaluating image quality of digital photo documentation after sexual assault. *Adv Emerg Nurs J*. 2012;34(3):250-258. doi:10.1097/TME.0b013e3182616eb2

13. Bloemen EM, Rosen T, Cline Schiroo JA, et al. Photographing injuries in the acute care setting: development and evaluation of a standardized protocol for research, forensics, and clinical practice. *J. Acad. Emerg. Med*. 2016;23(5):653-659. doi:10.1111/acem.12955

14. Ernst EJ, Speck PM, Fitzpatrick JJ. Usefulness: forensic photo documentation after sexual assault. *Adv Emerg Nurs J*. 2011;33(1):29-38. doi:10.1097/TME.0b013e3182083128

Chapter 15

Telehealth and Forensic Nursing

Alex L. Classen, MPS-HLS, BSN, RN, FNE A/P, CPN, GFN-C
Jessica M. Volz, DNP, CRNP, FNE A/P, FNP-BC, AFN-C, SANE-A, SANE-P, NE-BC, DM-AFN

Key Points

1. *Telehealth is an effective method for increasing access to health care due to its convenience and ease of access.*

2. *Forensic nursing models of care use telehealth technology to increase access to health care for victims in rural or underserved areas by connecting community hospitals to forensic nursing services.*

3. *Evidence supports telehealth as an effective adjunct in the nurse-patient relationship; it is just as effective as in-person health care interventions, with high patient satisfaction levels for forensic telehealth.*

Introduction

The terms *telehealth* and *telemedicine* are used interchangeably by the World Health Organization (WHO) and refer to the use of information and communication technologies (ICT) to increase access to care and medical information, therefore improving patient outcomes.[1] The WHO outlines 4 key elements of telehealth: clinical support; breaking geographical barriers to connect users who are not in the same physical location; involving various types of ICT; and improvement of health outcomes.[1]

Shifting away from the traditional in-person health care interaction, the gradual adoption of virtual interactions has gained acceptance from patients and providers alike. The COVID-19 pandemic caused a rapid surge in telehealth implementation to ensure continued health care accessibility despite universal stay-at-home orders. For victims of violence, the pandemic created many new barriers including reduced access to critical health care and community resources. Health encounters using virtual technologies are not studied; however, the pandemic required nimble adjustments in the provision of care. Early data supports specialized care and treatment for victims of violence using telehealth.[2]

Barriers and Concerns

Assault victims frequently experience systemic, logistical, and attitudinal barriers that prevent them from accessing health care after an assault.[3] Lack of childcare, transportation difficulties, limited access to services, cost, stigma, self-blame, cultural variables, and confidentiality are key barriers contributing to a limited access to health care for victims after an assault.[3,4] Telehealth technology offers the unique advantage of virtually bringing the forensic nurse's specialized care and treatment for victims of violence to the bedside, helping to mitigate some of the commonly cited barriers to accessing health care.

While access to care via telehealth might be the only or more desirable option for some patients, some logistical barriers do exist. Barriers include concerns about patient confidentiality, technology safety, and delays and interruptions with technology itself.[5] Additionally, low internet connectivity, lack of device access, and general technology difficulties also exist, particularly for older adults and those with lower incomes.[6] For forensic nurses themselves who do not have access to HIPAA compliant videoconferencing solutions, significant concerns arise around patient privacy and protection of health information.[6]

Abusers may use technology-based coercive control, so forensic nurses need to be aware that utilizing technology might be triggering for some patients.[7] Technology-based coercive control also poses certain safety risks. Forensic nurses utilizing telehealth technology should assist patients as they manage their privacy settings and explain how to turn off location sharing on their devices. E-literacy may be limited, so forensic nurses need training on how to best support patients in the safe use of assistive technology, such as securing devices with passwords and deleting electronic footprints.[4]

Regulatory barriers of telehealth imposed by state and federal regulations add an additional barricade for rapid, widespread telehealth implementation. Telehealth laws vary from state to state, with no 2 states having the same regulations when it comes to coverage and payment.[4] Federal and state licensing laws may inhibit providers from providing telehealth services across state lines.[8] While the Interstate Medical Licensure Compact aims to streamline credentialing across state lines, federal telehealth policy reform is necessary to ensure equitable care for patients.[8]

PATIENT RECEPTION OF TELEHEALTH SERVICES

Recent technological advancements have allowed for online personalized safety planning for victims through computerized systems, web-based applications, and smartphone applications to help, inform, and support victims of intimate partner violence (IPV). In the new technology-driven era, it is evident that many victims seek information and support online as a primary resource. Patients who received telehealth post-assault services from a trained forensic nurse were able to access health care while ensuring their safety by remaining in the comfort of their own home. Technology helps combat IPV by giving victims easy access to essential resources and service providers, as well as reducing their feelings of isolation through contact with their social networks. Many victims also join online support groups, equipping them with safety devices, resources to help them develop safety plans, and a place to record evidence of their abuse and find empowerment.[4]

The forensic nurse plays a key role in teaching e-literacy and online safety planning for victims. Forensic nurses can provide personalized IPV care through an intersectional lens to determine how to better tailor support for victims' individual needs. This may be achieved through crisis and counseling support via the internet, telephone, text messaging, or through a mobile application.[7] Forensic nurses can quickly build a rapport with IPV victims to facilitate supportive conversations, explain controlling behaviors, and help victims develop a support network and safety plan.[7] Safety-oriented applications and digital tools are also key for victim safety.[7] Forensic nurses can implement IPV screening tools and victim danger assessments to assess a victim's risk for IPV.[9]

IMPLEMENTING VIRTUAL RESOURCES

Since the initial creation of health care technology, there have been multiple variations of telehealth implemented to increase access to health care and support victims of assault. These include psychological counseling, interventions, coping strategies, patient education, and medical forensic examination follow-up. Telehealth videoconferencing is highly successful in providing mental health care through psychoeducation and coping strategy models to help treat symptoms of posttraumatic stress disorder and depression in assault victims.[10,11] Patients experience effective treatment outcomes, including dramatic symptom improvement, and report high levels of satisfaction for the virtual mental health services.[11] Video intervention has also proven to be a cost-effective tool to aid in the intervention and healing process after an assault.[10]

As technology continues to advance, mobile applications have become a vital virtual resource for assault victims. The implementation of mobile applications successfully provides immediate access to information.[12] Mobile applications mitigate many barriers experienced by victims attempting to access health care, such as scheduling, extensive time commitments, costs, stigma, logistics, cultural variables, and language.

FORENSIC NURSING TELEHEALTH CARE MODELS

The need for forensic nurses in every hospital is evident, but many hospitals, especially those in rural areas, do not have the funding and support to employ them. Forensic nursing telehealth provides expert consultation, rapid evaluation, evidence collection, and timely response to community needs in underserved areas.

Patients presenting for care after a recent sexual assault have unique needs that require clinicians to provide the following: emotional support and crisis intervention; assessment and treatment of injuries; administration of an emergency contraceptive, sexually transmitted infection testing, and HIV prophylaxis; and knowledge and experience to properly conduct a medical forensic examination and collect evidence.[13] The victim advocate allows for emotional care and support and connects the patient to community resources that can meet unique post-assault care needs.[13] One model of telehealth in forensic nursing care is a nurse-led model for providing comprehensive, high quality, post-assault care to rural and underserved communities. This model provides live sexual assault examination consultations with expert sexual assault nurse examiners, essential clinical precepting, peer review, quality assurance, and regular access to training and education.[14] While the initial model explicitly served sexual assault victims, the framework can be implemented for programs serving all victims of violence (ie, IPV, physical assault, child maltreatment, elder abuse/neglect, and human trafficking). The detailed description of collaborative partnership, coalition building, and program design and implementation serves as a guide for hospitals and health systems seeking to implement telehealth programs to improve the care provided to victims of violence.

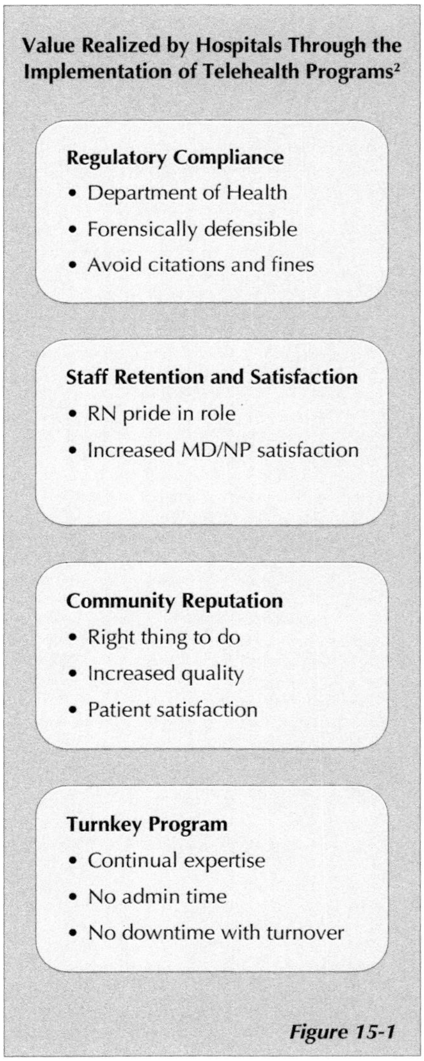

CASE STUDIES

Case Study 15-1

A 26-year-old patient was assaulted by their longtime friend the night before seeking medical care. The patient lives in a rural area of Nebraska, and the nearest hospital that provides medical forensic examinations was 4 hours away. The patient did not want to call the police and instead presented to the local community clinic. The family medicine physician at the clinic had not performed a medical forensic examination since their residency many years ago. Since the clinic was part of a sexual assault medical forensic telehealth program, the physician was able to work with a forensic telehealth nurse to provide high quality, trauma-informed care. The patient reported being unaware that access to a complete medical forensic examination would be possible because of the remote location of the clinic.

Discussion

The COVID-19 pandemic highlighted the need for remote telemedicine for rural and remote patients not wanting to report to law enforcement.[2] In this case, both the sexual assault victim and the attending physician benefited from the expansion of practices and values in hospital systems (**Figure 15-1**). Through the advent of telehealth, the forensic nurse was able to provide comprehensive care to the patient and ensure that they had a safety plan in place before discharge. At the conclusion of the examination, the patient reported feeling cared for and glad for access to expert care from the telehealth forensic nurse.

SUMMARY

The successful implementation of various technologies and telehealth models increases patients' access to health care. Virtual technologies provide immediate access

Figure 15-1. *Beneficial elements of telehealth programs, including regulatory compliance, staff retention and satisfaction, community reputation, and reduced staff turnover, saving hospitals money, time, and preserving confidence in the SANE experience.*

Value Realized by Hospitals Through the Implementation of Telehealth Programs[2]

Regulatory Compliance
- Department of Health
- Forensically defensible
- Avoid citations and fines

Staff Retention and Satisfaction
- RN pride in role
- Increased MD/NP satisfaction

Community Reputation
- Right thing to do
- Increased quality
- Patient satisfaction

Turnkey Program
- Continual expertise
- No admin time
- No downtime with turnover

Figure 15-1

to resources for victims of assault and increase communication with specialized care providers. Robust forensic nursing telehealth models not only supply medical providers with forensic nursing expertise, but they also connect victims with specialty services and community resources. These telehealth models provide the foundation for collaborative partnerships, coalition building, and program design and implementation for hospitals seeking to implement forensic nursing telehealth programs in rural and underserved areas.

REFERENCES

1. WHO Global Observatory for eHealth. *Telemedicine: opportunities and developments in Member States: report on the second global survey on eHealth.* World Health Organization; 2010. https://apps.who.int/iris/handle/10665/44497

2. Miyamoto S, Bittner C, Perkins DF, et al. The Sexual Assault Forensic Examination Telehealth (SAFE-T) Systems: Program Evaluation Final Report to the US Department of Justice, Office for Victims of Crime. The Pennsylvania State University. April 20, 2022. https://safetcenter.psu.edu/safetcenter/files/2018/01/DOJ-OVC-SAFE-T-Grant-Final-Report.pdf

3. Gilmore AK, Davidson TM, Leone RM, et al. Usability testing of a mobile health intervention to address acute care needs after sexual assault. *Int J Environ Res Public Health.* 2019;16(17):3088. doi:10.3390/ijerph16173088

4. Al-Alosi H. Fighting fire with fire: exploring the potential of technology to help victims combat intimate partner violence. *Aggress Violent Behav.* 2020;52(101376). doi:10.1016/j.avb.2020.101376

5. Wood L, Baumler E, Schrag RV, et al. "Don't know where to go for help": safety and economic needs among violence survivors during the COVID-19 pandemic. *J Fam Violence.* 2021:1-9. doi:10.1007/s10896-020-00240-7

6. Lieneck C, Garvey J, Collins C, et al. Rapid telehealth implementation during the COVID-19 global pandemic: a rapid review. *Healthcare (Basel).* 2020;8(4):517. doi:10.3390/healthcare8040517

7. Slakoff DC, Aujla W, PenzeyMoog E. The role of service providers, technology, and mass media when home isn't safe for intimate partner violence victims: best practices and recommendations in the era of COVID-19 and beyond. *Arch Sex Behav.* 2020;49(8):2779-2788. doi:10.1007/s10508-020-01820-w

8. Lee NT, Karsten J, Roberts J. Removing regulatory barriers to telehealth before and after COVID-19. Brookings. 2020. Accessed December 26, 2021. https://www.brookings.edu/research/removing-regulatory-barriers-to-telehealth-before-and-after-covid-19/

9. Kaukinen C. When stay-at-home orders leave victims unsafe at home: exploring the risk and consequences of intimate partner violence during the COVID-19 pandemic. *Am J Crim Justice.* 2020;45(4):668-679. doi:10.1007/s12103-020-09533-5

10. Miller KE, Cranston CC, Davis JL, Newman E, Resnick H. Psychological outcomes after a sexual assault video intervention: a randomized trial. *J Forensic Nurs.* 2015;11(3):129-36. doi:10.1097/jfn.0000000000000080

11. Gray MJ, Hassija CM, Jaconis M, et al. Provision of evidence-based therapies to rural survivors of domestic violence and sexual assault via telehealth: treatment outcomes and clinical training benefits. *Train Educ Prof Psych.* 2015;9(3):235-241. doi:10.1037/tep0000083

12. Hicks DLL, Patterson DPL, Resko SPL. Lessons learned from iCare: a post examination text-messaging-based program with sexual assault patients. *J Forensic Nurs.* 2017;13(4):160-167. doi:10.1097/JFN.0000000000000175

13. Meunier-Sham J, Preiss RM, Petricone R, Re C, Gillen L. Laying the foundation for the national telenursing center: integration of the quality-caring model into teleSANE practice. *J Forensic Nurs.* 2019;15(3):143-151. doi:10.1097/JFN.0000000000000252

14. Miyamoto S, Thiede E, Dorn L, Perkins DF, Bittner C, Scanlon D. The sexual assault forensic examination telehealth (SAFE T) center: A comprehensive, nurse-led telehealth model to address disparities in sexual assault care. *J Rural Health.* 2021;37(1):92-102. doi:10.1111/jrh.12474

IV

VIOLENCE ACROSS THE LIFESPAN

Chapter 16

Violence Against Children

Pamela Harris Bryant, PhD, DNP, CRNP, AC-PC
Max Veltman, PhD, RN, CPNP-PC, AFN-C
Maud D'Arcy, BSN, RN
Angela Morris, BSN, RN, CEN, SANE-A, SANE-P, EMT

Key Points

1. *Child abuse is pervasive, affecting 1 billion children globally every year, and minority children are disproportionately affected.*

2. *Child abuse can be physical, social, psychological, and spiritual in their environment (school, home, or online), and caretakers are typically the primary offenders.*

3. *Adverse childhood experiences (ACEs) cause long-lasting effects on a person's health and well-being, including length of life.*

4. *All health care providers are responsible for actively screening for child abuse.*

Introduction

It is estimated that around 1 billion children globally experienced emotional abuse, physical and sexual violence, or neglect in 2019.[1] Violence against children can occur at the hands of parents, caregivers, peers, authority figures, or strangers. Most often, maltreatment takes place in the child's home, community, school, or over the internet.[1,2] Experiencing violence during childhood impacts the victim's long-term health and well-being, leaving long-lasting physical and mental health outcomes that can lead to an early death.[3]

Child maltreatment is defined as an action or failure to act that results in harm (or the potential for harm) to a child (ie, anyone under the age of 18). ***Intentional maltreatment*** is purposefully perpetrated and often includes physical, sexual, and psychological abuse. ***Child neglect*** is another form of child maltreatment that occurs when a caregiver fails to act on behalf of the child, resulting in harm or the potential for harm to the child. Child neglect may include failing to meet a child's basic physical, emotional, medical, or educational needs, as well as failure to provide adequate supervision.[5] In cases of child maltreatment, harm to the child may not be the intended consequence but adults are responsible for their actions, or lack thereof, so by the legal definition, it is still considered maltreatment.

Adverse Childhood Experiences and the Multidisciplinary Approach

A landmark study[6] on ACEs provided the epidemiological evidence that determined that ACEs have a lasting effect on a child through adulthood and can even lead to an early death. These experiences are divided into 3 groups: abuse, neglect, and household challenges that are amenable to prevention tactics.[2] This study uncovered how ACEs are strongly associated with risk factors for disease and well-being throughout

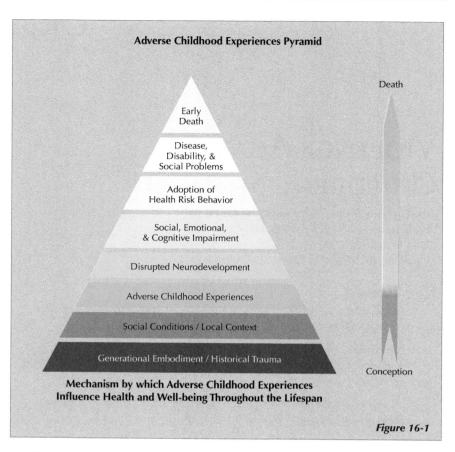

Adverse Childhood Experiences Pyramid

Death

Early
Death

Disease,
Disability, &
Social Problems

Adoption of
Health Risk Behavior

Social, Emotional,
& Cognitive Impairment

Disrupted Neurodevelopment

Adverse Childhood Experiences

Social Conditions / Local Context

Generational Embodiment / Historical Trauma

Conception

**Mechanism by which Adverse Childhood Experiences
Influence Health and Well-being Throughout the Lifespan**

Figure 16-1

Figure 16-1. Adverse childhood experiences life course. Adapted from the Centers for Disease Control and Prevention.

the life course,[6] as noted in **Figure 16-1**. Additionally, the frequency of the long-term effects of ACEs[7] are chronicled in **Figure 16-2**.

The response to ACEs is multidisciplinary. Multidisciplinary teams (MDTs) include child protection agencies, prosecuting attorneys, forensic physicians, advanced forensic nurses with pediatric specialization, registered nurses, forensic interviewers, and advocates. Advocates guide families through the interpretations and explanations of the evidence generated by the MDT supporting a charge of child abuse or neglect.[8] When there are biases, misinterpretations, or communication failures with families, the consequences are significant.[9,10] Quality and safety in child abuse evaluation are essential to ensuring a program is free of bias.[10] These processes ultimately protect children from further harm.

Forensic nurses consider many factors when working with children. In forensic nursing cases, parents are often fearful, exhibiting significant anxiety. Navigating stressful information related to the child is an important skill for the forensic nurse to master. Forensic nurses possess other skills including, using psychomotor dexterity when the child is uncooperative, evaluating genitalia, and adhering to precise protocols. After the child has a full evaluation, forensic nurses provide follow-up instructions that guide them to specialized referrals and/or consultation with the child's primary care provider.[8]

Pediatric forensic nurses work collaboratively with other disciplines participating in MDTs that meet regularly, and the members provide their vocational expertise during the case discussion, where the forensic nurse or physician comments on the medical issues involved with the cases. These teams often count on the advanced forensic nurse's expertise, relying on them to provide a differential diagnosis that eliminates all other possible causes for the findings, which guides the pathway to prosecution. Registered nurses provide information related to their evaluation, documentation,

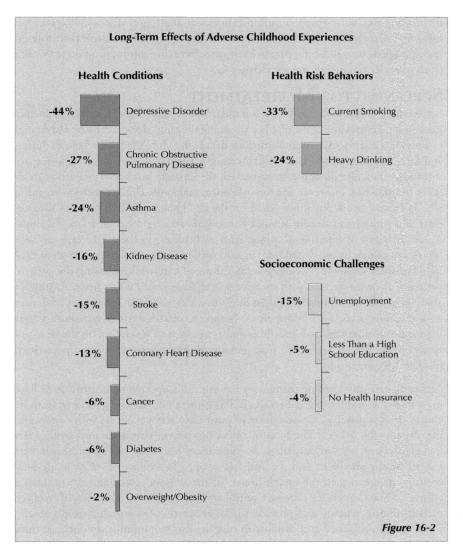

Figure 16-2

Figure 16-2. Long-term effects of adverse childhood experiences. Adapted from the Centers for Disease Control and Prevention.

and referral, but differential diagnosis is outside the scope of the registered nurse. Being able to understand the legal boundaries in one's practice and educate the jury about one's role are essential skills for all members of the MDT.

When children are maltreated, medical-legal evaluation of the child is stressful, as parents who are recently made aware of the abuse are distraught, while their children may be joyful and cooperative.[10] When the outcry is not welcome by the core family, the child may exhibit resistance during the evaluation, reflecting the anxiety projected from parents or guardians. It is an assumption that children have traumatized backgrounds when they are seen in a medical-legal evaluation by a forensic nurse. Oftentimes, the victim has positive feelings toward the offender. Regardless, the forensic nurse uses their training to create a safe environment, be transparent, and facilitate patient-centered, trauma-informed care with the following values: safety; trustworthiness and transparency; peer support; collaboration and mutuality; empowerment and choice; and sensitivity to cultural, historical, and gender issues.[11] When successful, children and parents emerge satisfied with the process, but not necessarily with the results.

Throughout this process, the forensic nurse must remain professional and able to provide person-centered, trauma-informed care. Due to this challenging environment, forensic nurses are often subject to compassion fatigue. They are responsible for making decisions about communication, conducting evidence collection, and following strict protocols, which can create stress. To deflect the stress their role can cause, forensic nurses should practice self-care. For more information on recovering from provider fatigue, please see chapter 4.

SCREENING FOR MALTREATMENT

Screening for child maltreatment is a standard of practice. This process may include screening parents without the child or screening the child alone if they are old enough to provide a history. An extensive history details the child's behavior before, during, and after any injury, which is vital to creating a linear narrative and exposing any inconsistencies. Should abuse be suspected, the separate interviews guarantee an absence of influence. However, the forensic nurse makes the clinical decision regarding who is present in the interview based on the child's age and their capacity to cooperate and understand details of what is necessary during the evaluation. All nurses screen for signs of intentional injury, such as bruising to the torso, ears, or neck, injuries to nonambulatory children, or noticeable injuries at various degrees of healing. The forensic nurse provides trauma-informed care while assessing the patient's behavior, their interaction with caregivers, and their physical condition. If physical abuse is suspected, a provider is then likely to order a skeletal survey and laboratory tests to gather additional information. Suspected sexual abuse may require screening for sexually transmitted infections and pregnancy.[12] Depending on the signs and symptoms exhibited, treatment may include prophylaxis for exposure or treatment for definitive organisms.

All health care providers are mandatory reporters of suspected maltreatment. Following a report, Child Protective Services (CPS) gathers information generated from the visit as soon as possible. Coordination of outpatient services occurs with community members of the MDT.[12] The forensic nurse also provides wrap-around services that include the provision of outpatient or community resources, crisis hotline numbers, mental health providers, and medical follow-up. The impact of ACEs is life-long, creating an urgency in the establishment of prevention, screening, and mitigation efforts.[9,13] The Centers for Disease Control and Prevention has a number of resources to help inform parents and providers alike about the dynamics of child abuse.[2,14] Developing confidence and comfort in care for this community, the forensic nurse should practice considerations that include MDT debriefing, self-care techniques, and continued education, which help grow the forensic nursing professional in ensuring the safety of the children.

CASE STUDIES

Case Study 16-1

A 2-month-old child presented to their primary care physician with bleeding gums and a torn frenulum. The patient had not met growth milestones, and the parents reported that the child was not feeding well. The mother stated that she did not know why the child's gums were bleeding. Upon evaluation of the child, a diagnosis of failure to thrive and hospitalization followed. In watching the maternal-child interaction, it was discovered that the child rejected the mother's attempts at feeding, and the mother pushed the bottle into the infant's mouth.

Discussion

In this scenario, the mother stressed that the family was unable to meet the infant's needs. This case demonstrates subtle findings that may imply a health risk to the infant. Medical-legal intervention with hospitalization and involvement of CPS may be necessary.

Case Study 16-2

A 5-year-old child presented to the emergency department with a stomach ache. When undressed and evaluated, the child had bruises at varying stages of healing. One bruise, on the upper left abdomen, had an imprint of a "boot toe." The mother stated that the child fell off of his bicycle. Magnetic resonance imaging was conducted on the child, and the diagnosis was a ruptured spleen.

Discussion

Interviewing children with parents in the room may result in children denying the information necessary to make a diagnosis regarding the cause of injury. In this case, the forensic nurse should send the parent out of the room to build trust and encourage the child to reveal how the injury occurred. Regardless, the nurse is a mandated reporter and must make a report when there is suspicion of child abuse. The nurse's suspicion that abuse had occurred was validated when the child was sent for further testing that demonstrated a ruptured spleen. Additionally, the parents' choice to delay reporting was another signal that the child may have been subjected to intentional physical harm.

SUMMARY

Violence against children, which includes physical, social, psychological, and spiritual abuse, affects 1 billion children globally. This abuse can take place in the child's home, school, orphanage, or foster home, as well as in various community settings. Abuse can cause a long-lasting negative effect on the child's health and well-being. A multidisciplinary approach must be taken when caring for the child, and the forensic nurse plays an important part on the MDT by evaluating and eliminating causes for the abuse. Screening for child maltreatment is a standard of practice, and every forensic nurse should be well-versed in the steps that should be taken when caring for victims of maltreatment.

REFERENCES

1. *Global status report on preventing violence against children 2020*. World Health Organization; 2020. Accessed November 22, 2021. www.who.int/publications/i/item/9789240004191

2. *Preventing Adverse Childhood Experiences (ACES): Leveraging the Best Available Evidence*. Centers for Disease Control and Prevention; 2019. Accessed November 22, 2021. www.cdc.gov/violenceprevention/pdf/preventingACES.pdf

3. Center on the Developing Child. In Brief: The science of early childhood development. 2007. Accessed November 22, 2021. www.developingchild. harvard.edu/resources/inbrief-science-of-ecd/

4. Anda RF, Dong M, Brown DW, et al. The relationship of adverse childhood experiences to a history of premature death of family members. *BMC Public Health*. 2009;9(106). doi:10.1186/1471-2458-9-106

5. Shipman SJ, Hankins J, Sanchez RV, Speck PM. Introduction to child maltreatment. In: Alexander R, Faugno D, Speck PM, eds. *Child Abuse Quick Reference for Health Care, Social Service and Law Enforcement Professionals*. 3rd ed. STM Learning, Inc.; 2017:1-10.

6. Felitti VJ, Anda RF, Nordenberg D, et al. Relationship of childhood abuse and household dysfunction to many of the leading causes of death in adults. The Adverse Childhood Experiences (ACE) Study. *Am J Prev Med*. 1998;14(4):245-58. doi:10.1016/s0749-3797(98)00017-8

7. Merrick MT, Ford DC, Ports KA, et al. *Vital signs:* estimated proportion of adult health problems attributable to adverse childhood experiences and implications for prevention — 25 states, 2015-2017. *MMWR Morb Mortal Wkly Rep*. 2019;68(44):999-1005. doi:10.15585/mmwr.mm6844e1

8. Meunier-Sham J, Cross TP, Zuniga L. The seven pillars of quality care in a statewide pediatric sexual assault nurse examiner program. *J Child Sex Abus*. 2013;22(7):777-95. doi:10.1080/10538712.2013.830665

9. Preer G, Sorrentino D, Ryznar E, Newton AW. Child maltreatment: promising approaches and new directions. *Curr Opin Pediatr*. 2013;25(2):268-274. doi: 10.1097/MOP.0b013e32835eb347.

10. McPeters SL, Bryant PH, Speck PM. The quagmire of social determinants of health for the legal nursing consultant: evaluating failure to thrive. *J Legal Nurse Consult.* 2021;32(3):15-25.

11. Understanding the impact of trauma. In: *A Treatment Improvement Protocol Trauma-Informed Care in Behavioral Health Services.* US Department of Health and Human Services; 2014:59-85.

12. Gonzalez D, Bethencourt Mirabal A, McCall JD. Child abuse and neglect. Stat Pearls. 2021. https://www.ncbi.nlm.nih.gov/books/NBK459146/

13. Denton J, Newton AW, Vandeven AM. Update on child maltreatment: toward refining the evidence base. *Curr Opin Pediatr.* 2011;23(2):240-8. doi:10.1097/MOP.0b013e3283446010

14. Danaher F, Vandeven A, Blanchard A, Newton AW. Recognizing, diagnosing, and preventing child maltreatment: an update for pediatric clinicians. *Curr Opin Pediatr.* 2018;30(4):582-590. doi:10.1097/MOP.0000000000000648

Chapter 17

Violence Against Adolescents and Adults

Deborah St. Germain, DNP, RN, AFN-C, SANE-A
Jaclyn Rodriguez, BSN, BS, RN, SANE-A
Heather J. Hayes, DNP, APRN, FNP-BC, AFN-C
Kimberly A. Foster, MBA, BSN, RN

Key Points

1. *Violence against adolescents and adults occurs primarily in the home.*

2. *There are 3 methods of violence – physical, psychological, and sexual.*

3. *Anyone can become a victim of violence, and each developmental stage has different, predictable risks.*

4. *Forensic nurses are frontline health care providers caring for patients who have experienced violence across the lifespan.*

Introduction

Violence—the leading cause of death, illness, and injury in adolescents and adults—is defined as intentional acts or behaviors designed to cause physical, psychological, emotional, and/or spiritual harm that is directed at oneself, another person, groups, communities, or countries. Violence can range from acts like bullying, physical fighting, and stalking to more severe forms, such as sexual assault, strangulation, human trafficking, homicide, and withholding food, water, or medical treatment. As frontline health care providers, forensic nurses care for patients who have experienced violence. Their education on the 3 pillars of forensic nursing (legal, forensic science, and nursing) promotes evidence-based, trauma-informed, and person-centered practices in the assessment, treatment, intervention, and continual evaluation of the nursing care plan. As such, the forensic nurse is a collaborator in the patient's care, focusing on their needs for support and information, all while implementing the nursing process.[1]

Types of Violence

A person may experience a single or multiple types of violence within a relationship, and it may not only be directed toward the primary victim but also to the people and animals loved by the victim. The violent behaviors are designed to control victims through ploys that use[1,2]:

— Physical abuse, such as pushing or hitting

— Sexual abuse, including forcing a person to have sex or engage in sexual activity

— Emotional abuse, such as degrading, gaslighting, and influencing/controlling their behavior

— Intentionally damaging property

— Financial abuse, including controlling bank accounts and money without consent

All forms of violence cause numerous adverse physical and psychological effects, including depression, low self-esteem, substance abuse, suicide, and increasing vulnerability to other health problems throughout victims' lifetimes. In addition, adverse events that occur in childhood are linked to future adolescent violence perpetration, chronic health problems, and mental illness in adulthood.[3] These types of violence fall into 3 broad categories, as defined in **Table 17-1**. Please refer to chapter 16 for further discussion on adverse childhood experiences.

Table 17-1. Violence Categories, Descriptions, and Motives

TYPES OF VIOLENCE	DESCRIPTIONS OF VIOLENCE	MOTIVES
Physical	— Ranges from an occasional slap to regular, life-threatening physical beatings — Strangulation increases lethality of physical assaults — May include threats against children or parents	— Promoting terror and fear of further physical violence
Psychological	— Includes isolation and academic, emotional, financial, technological, and verbal abuse	— To increase terror and fear of physical violence
Sexual	— Ranges from sexual and reproductive coercion to violent rape — Often involves drugs and alcohol to increase victim vulnerability — May include threats against children	— Misguided enhancement of sexual gratification

DATING AND FAMILY VIOLENCE

Physical and sexual violence in romantic relationships is highly prevalent in adolescence and early adulthood, but it can happen at any age. Among adolescents throughout the world, boys and girls equally suffer various forms of violence. Members of the LGBTQIA+ community experience higher rates of dating violence, often due to their overall social vulnerability. Persons with disabilities also experience higher rates of dating violence.[2,4,5]

DATING VIOLENCE

Dating violence occurs during the continuum of a romantic relationship, taking place anywhere from the introductory phase to its ending. Prevalence rates of relationship violence in adolescence and young adulthood range between 30% and 35%. In many countries, adolescent girls reported that most commonly perpetrated sexual violence was by a romantic or intimate partner. The biggest risk factor for experiencing dating violence is having previously experienced dating violence. Other factors that increase dating violence risk for adolescents and emerging adults include a history of childhood victimization, substance abuse, and having peers who participate in dating violence or aggressive behaviors.[2,4]

College students are particularly vulnerable to assault; as many as 1 in 5 women and 1 in 16 men report experiencing sexual assault while in college. Drug-facilitated or alcohol-enabled sexual assault may be used to incapacitate the person, affecting their ability to consent to sexual activity, resist the assault, and even remember the details of the assault. During their first year of college, 15% of young women experienced rape involving drugs or alcohol. Protective factors for mitigating violent outcomes include having a strong social support system and demonstrating a higher level of emotional intelligence.[6]

FAMILY VIOLENCE

Family violence, also referred to as domestic violence, occurs in any familial relationships between current or former intimate partners; married or unmarried couples; persons in heterosexual or same-sex relationships; parents or stepparents and children; or between persons with disabilities and their caregivers. It also extends to interactions with siblings, grandparents, grandchildren, and other extended family members. Family violence includes not only physical abuse, but also sexual, emotional, economic, psychological, spiritual, and financial abuse.

Violence leaves long-lasting effects on the mental and physical health of those who experience it, and adults involved in violent relationships often suffer for years.[7] Following an abusive relationship, victims may have difficulty forming satisfying relationships with others. In a violent household, the family member being abused may fear for their safety, the safety of another person (eg, a child), or an animal's safety. Legislation identifies domestic or family violence as a form of child abuse, such as when a child hears, sees, or directly experiences a violent event.

Family violence is the leading contributor to preventable death, disability, and illness among women aged 15 to 44 years.[7] Some victims of family violence are murdered or die as a result of their injuries. Between 32% and 47% of all homicides annually are domestic or family homicide victims who are intimate partners, parents, or children of the abuser. Socially, family violence weakens family and community structures. Victims of family violence may find it difficult to go to school or get a job, or they may turn to crime, alcohol, or drugs as coping mechanisms.[8]

GENDER, PREGNANCY, AND VIOLENCE

Family violence affects pregnant women at alarming rates. Twenty-two percent of women who experienced intimate partner violence by their current partner were pregnant at the time of the violence, and 25% of women who experienced intimate partner violence by a previous partner were pregnant at the time of the violence. Women aged 18 to 24 experience significantly higher rates of physical and sexual violence than women in older age groups. Additionally, there is growing evidence that women with disabilities are more likely to experience violence.[9]

OTHER FORMS OF VIOLENCE

Adolescents and adults may experience a variety of other forms of violence throughout their lifetime. Individuals that join gangs may experience gang violence. Over the past decade, gang violence has risen sharply, especially in large cities. Juvenile gang killings are now the fastest growing type of homicide. Those in gangs are also more likely to experience gun violence. Worldwide, the effects of gun violence extend not only to those who are killed but also to those who witness it, know someone who was shot, or live in fear of the next shooting in their community.

Violence can affect individuals throughout their entire life and come from anyone they interact with. While adolescents are more likely to experience sexual assault, older adults are more likely to experience financial abuse. Elders may be abused by family members, caregivers, or others they interact with. While financial abuse is more prevalent in older adults, older adults can also experience sexual and physical abuse.

THE COMPREHENSIVE ROLE OF FORENSIC NURSING

Forensic nursing continues to expand and develop from early work in sexual assault to caring for any individual who experiences violence. Forensic nurses ensure that patients who experience violence receive the highest quality of both medical and forensic nursing care. This care is framed around specific evidence-based practices, but each step must be individualized.

Individualization occurs when the forensic nurse tailors their care to meet the patient's specific needs based on physical and mental development and abilities, gender, sexual-identity, injury level, citizenship status, chronic medical conditions, and a whole host of other situations. An example of this is patient age differences in the reporting process for sexual assault. An adult patient may have a choice whether to report the crime to law enforcement, whereas for a child or adolescent, sexual abuse must be mandatorily reported in most jurisdictions.

Traumatic situations may cause a patient with previous trauma to become re-traumatized. When a patient is consciously or unconsciously reminded of past trauma, this results in a re-experiencing the initial trauma event. Triggers may include attitudes, situations, or environments that replicate the dynamics of the original trauma, such as loss of power, control, or safety. Therefore, it is crucial to give patients control over what is happening to them and their body, giving choices when appropriate. Forensic nurses are trained to listen without judgment, provide support and empowerment, and to respect the patient's autonomy to select their desired level of participation during each step in delivery of care.

These steps may involve:

— Obtaining informed consent from the patient or legal representative

— Completing a medical and forensic history using trauma-informed principles

— Performing a detailed head-to-toe assessment to determine the extent of injuries and the presence of potential evidence

— Using equipment such as an alternative light source to identify any foreign materials, substances, or bruising otherwise not visible to the naked eye

— Performing a detailed anogenital exam in the cases of sexual assault using Toluidine blue dye, the urinary catheter technique, specialized positioning for speculum insertion, and sample collection methods using appropriate swabbing techniques

Forensic nurses use forensic photography and body diagrams for thorough documentation. Throughout the process of the medical forensic examination, the forensic nurse considers potential sources of evidence transfer that occurred during the violent crime.

As health care providers, forensic nurses must continuously focus on the patient's medical needs while performing the medical forensic examination. Patients who have experienced violence may need radiographic imaging, wound care, sexually transmitted infection prophylaxis, pregnancy prevention, chronic disease management, and behavioral health interventions. The forensic nurse prioritizes the patient's medical needs over their forensic needs and ensures that the patient is provided with all treatment options necessary to begin the path to healing from the traumatic event.

Prior to discharging a patient, the forensic nurse screens for a safe environment for the patient to return to, if the patient has thoughts of hurting themselves or others, and if they have suicidal ideation. Additionally, the forensic nurse confirms that the patient understands the importance of follow-up care related to their treatment. If injuries are identified, the forensic nurse also makes sure the patient knows how to care for those injuries and why they should return for further evaluation.[1]

In addition to providing medical information, the forensic nurse encourages victims of violence to connect with community resources to provide support and aid in their recovery. Community resources may include rape crisis centers, domestic violence agencies, crime victim compensation programs, homeless shelters, trauma recovery programs, and counseling services. Many community organizations employ individuals with lived experience to discuss their trauma with others who have also experienced trauma.[1,5,7]

Although adolescents' traumatic experiences are comparable to that of adults, their psychological immaturity leaves them struggling long-term to cope and adapt. It is well known that rates of psychological trauma vary depending on type of trauma, but left untreated , trauma results in high rates of depression, anxiety, post traumatic stress disorder, and suicide in adolescents. Therefore, resources for parents and adolescents should strongly encourage engagement in therapy soon after a traumatic event.

CASE STUDIES

Case Study 17-1

This 18-year-old woman returned from her first semester at college excited for new experiences and meeting new people, including potential romantic partners. On her first day home, her ex-boyfriend from high school texted her to meet him at a local park. She refused due to family obligations. Over the next few days, she noticed him frequently driving past her home and showing up when she visited friends and shopped at the mall. He also texted her every 10 minutes asking if she was thinking of him.

On Saturday evening, she attended a party with several friends that her ex-boyfriend had prevented her from socializing with during high school. Along with her friends, she drank alcohol and smoked a bit of marijuana. Her ex-boyfriend showed up at the party and insisted she leave with him in his car. Despite her reluctance, she went with him to prevent making a scene at the party, and he took her to a nearby motel. At the motel, she told him that she did not want to continue a sexual relationship with him. He became angry and called her a vulgar name. He slapped her across her face and then forced her to have sexual intercourse with him. During the rape, he strangled her repeatedly while asking her if it felt good. He also took pictures of her while raping her and posted them to his social media account. Afterwards, he dropped her off at the party and threatened to rape her again if she told anyone what happened. As she left his car, he called out to her that he loved her. Back at the party, she told a friend what happened and allowed them to drive her to the local sexual assault center for care.

Discussion

This patient experienced many forms of dating violence. Specific laws regarding dating violence vary by state and local jurisdictions. Forensic nurses are trained in their jurisdiction and work within their state and local laws and definitions. Her ex-boyfriend's stalking included a combination of physical, emotional, and sexual violence such as strangulation, repeated surveillance, unwanted texts, sexual assault, and threats of future violence.

Commonly, patients blame themselves for actions they thought to take but did not, tried to take but could not, or did take, which resulted in more serious harm. She may have blamed herself for attending a party, drinking alcohol, smoking marijuana, leaving with him, and so on. Violence is never the patient's fault. When someone uses abuse and violence against another person, it is always part of a larger pattern of control. Her ex-boyfriend used a pattern of abusive and coercive behaviors to maintain power and control over a former or current intimate partner.

Fortunately, forensic nurses are knowledgeable, well-trained, and available to provide patient-centered and trauma-informed care, which allowed her to have choices throughout the encounter, while receiving care that was designed specifically for her needs. The forensic nurse obtained consent and a medical and forensic history using trauma-informed principles. The nurse performed a detailed head-to-toe assessment to determine the extent of injuries. Additionally, they identified and collected potential evidence that was on the body and clothing and completed documentation that included photos, body diagrams, and descriptions. While performing the examination, the nurse provided necessary medical care for her injuries.

After collecting evidence and providing care, the forensic nurse offered community resources, such as a rape crisis center, trauma recovery program, college counseling services, and crime victims' compensation program to aid in the patient's recovery. The forensic nurse provided follow-up services for her by finding resources closer to the patient's community. In the following weeks, especially once she has returned to college, the patient may have difficulty concentrating on school due to fear, depression, and low self-esteem. She may begin experiencing thoughts of suicide, engaging in substance abuse, and isolating from friends. The supportive services provided by the forensic nurse make sure that she does not travel through the recovery process alone.

Since the patient was an adult at the time of the assault, in most systems, she will choose whether to report this to law enforcement. Law enforcement would handle any charges or arrests made in this case, as well as collect any additional evidence required for their investigation.

Summary

Anyone can be affected by violence, regardless of their age, gender, sexual identity, cultural background, ability, religion, wealth, status, or location. Perpetrators of violence use methods that include physical, psychological, and sexual abuse, but their motives are varied depending on the assailant. Violence against adolescents and adults occurs primarily in the home, but there are risks at each developmental stage. The generalist forensic nursing role is useful at the bedside with acute victims of violent crimes. This role includes objective documentation of injuries, navigating the available resources both in and outside the hospital, and providing supportive information for patients' follow-up with community agencies.

References

1. Lynch V, Duval J. *Forensic Nursing.* 2nd ed. Mosby-Elsevier; 2011.

2. de Toledo Blake M, Drezett J, Vertamatti MA, et al. Characteristics of sexual violence against adolescent girls and adult women. *BMC Women's Health.* 2014;14(1). doi:10.1186/1472-6874-14-15

3. Duke NN, Pettingell SL, McMorris BJ, Borowsky IW. Adolescent violence perpetration: associations with multiple types of adverse childhood experiences. *Pediatrics.* 2010;125(4):e778-e786. doi:10.1542/peds.2009-0597

4. Teen Newsletter: January 2021 - Teen Dating Violence. Centers for Disease Control and Prevention. March 11, 2021. https://www.cdc.gov/museum/education/newsletter/2021/mar/index.html

5. Taquette S, Monterio DLM. Cause and consequences of adolescent domestic violence: A systematic review. *J Inj Violence Res.* 2019;11(2):137-147. doi:10.5249/ jivr.v11i2.1061

6. Mellins CA, Walsh K, Sarvet AL, et al. Sexual assault incidents among college undergraduates: prevalence and factors associated with risk. *PLoS ONE.* 2017;12(11):e0186471. doi:10.1371/journal.pone.0186471

7. Huecker MR, King KC, Jordan GA, Smock W. Domestic violence. StatPearls [Internet] Publishing; National Library of Medicine. 2019. Updated February 10, 2022. https://www.ncbi.nlm.nih.gov/books/NBK499891/

8. Domestic Violence and Firearms. The Educational Fund to Stop Gun Violence. Updated July 2020. https://efsgv.org/learn/type-of-gun-violence/domestic-violence-and-firearms/

9. Berhanie E, Gebregziabher D, Berihu H, Gerezgiher A, Kidane G. Intimate partner violence during pregnancy and adverse birth outcomes: a case-control study. *Reprod Health.* 2019;16(1). doi:10.1186/s12978-019-0670-4

Chapter 18

VIOLENCE AGAINST ELDERS

Amy Carney, PhD, NP, FAAFS

Debra S. Holbrook, MSN, RN, SANE A, FNE A/P, AFN-C, DF-AFN, FAAN

Patricia M. Speck, DNSc, CRNP, FNP-BC, AFN-C, DF-IAFN, FAAFS, DF-AFN, FAAN

KEY POINTS

1. *Violence against elders is common across all socioeconomic levels, both in the United States and internationally.*

2. *Violence against elders takes many forms, including physical, financial, sexual, and emotional abuse.*

3. *While elder abuse can be difficult to detect, it is imperative for health care providers and those who work with an older population to learn the indicators of abuse in order to intervene and protect this vulnerable population.*

INTRODUCTION

Elder abuse did not come to public attention until the 1970s. At that time, more established research was being conducted in the fields of child abuse and domestic violence; therefore, the study of elder abuse was slow, lagging 30 years behind the aforementioned fields. However, elder abuse is a pervasive public health problem in the United States. Types of violence against elders includes neglect and physical, sexual, financial, and emotional abuse.[1] Elder abuse is not committed against only one ethnic group or in one nation; mistreatment occurs in diverse communities, across all socio economic levels.

EPIDEMIOLOGY AND CONSEQUENCES

It has been estimated that elder abuse happens to 5% to 10% of older adults in the United States annually and is often unrecognized. While much of the abuse against elders is not reported or is under-reported, the consequences are well established, including exacerbation of chronic conditions, hospitalization, depression, an increase in nursing home placements, and a significant increase in morbidity and mortality. Furthermore, while it is not easily quantifiable, elder abuse is estimated to cost billions of dollars annually. It has also been noted that the incidence of abuse will increase as the aging population increases, further adding to both cost and illness. Therefore, it is imperative that health care providers be able to identify abuse and be willing to report. Health care workers may be hesitant to report, however, because deliberate injury in this age group can be difficult to differentiate due to polypharmacy, normal aging of the skin, and co morbid conditions. Individual states, however, have risen to the challenge of mandated reporting by developing and refining laws that encourage mandated professionals to report abuse.[2,3]

RISK FACTORS

Multiple risk factors that put an elder in danger of abuse have been identified.[4] Elders living in care facilities may be more vulnerable to physical and sexual abuse and neglect, as they are more likely to be cared for by non-family, medical caregivers. In contrast, independent elder adults may be more likely to be victimized by individuals they know, such as a non-caregiver, unrelated friend or business partner. When a family member is the caregiver of an elderly individual, the stress and burden of caregiving are associated with abuse. Additionally, reports have been made of multiple incidents of abuse occurring together, such as physical abuse reported along with financial abuse or neglect.[5]

CASE STUDIES

Case Study 18-1

This 83-year-old female patient was residing in a long-term care facility with Medicaid as the payer of first resort. She was diagnosed with dementia, osteoarthritis, and depression. When another patient who had higher-paying private funding applied to the facility, she was placed in a van with her possessions, taken to a town miles away, and left in a back alley. She was picked up by several men who kept her in a building where other men would come and pay to have sex with her. The patient was found despondent, bleeding from her vagina and rectum, and suffering from wounds to her entire body that were in various stages of healing. She was taken by emergency medical services (EMS) to a trauma center where a forensic nurse examiner (FNE) was called in to assess her and complete a medical evidentiary examination. The patient was oriented to person only (ie, only able to identify herself and close relatives) but did reveal being "left somewhere, and they all hurt me. They just kept hurting me." An evidentiary kit was completed, which included trace, biological, and photographic evidence. Thirty days later, the patient was discharged to a safe and competent long-term care facility. She died 6 months after admission.

Discussion

The patient's original long-term care facility was fined, and arrests were made, including the administrator and the van driver. These individuals pled guilty to a lesser prison sentence. The patient was never able to identify the perpetrators who held her captive; therefore, no arrests of her offenders were made.

Case Study 18-2

This 72-year-old male patient had a history of addiction to alcohol and methamphetamine. He was also a type 1 diabetic and had a physical disability with limited use of his left lower extremity secondary to a train accident. He "burned his bridges" with friends and family during his younger adult life but became sober in his 60s. The patient's cousin and her daughter permitted him to move in with them. One evening, the patient's neighbors found him screaming for help as he dragged himself to their door. EMS was called, and he was taken to a nearby hospital where he was treated for his wounds and admitted. An FNE was consulted to interview and document his wounds. The forensic medical interview revealed several years of him being forced to sit on a bench, being repeatedly beaten and kicked, burned with

Figure 18-1. Patterned wound. Photograph courtesy of Debra Holbrook.

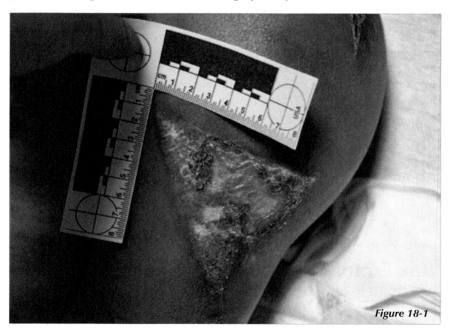

Figure 18-1

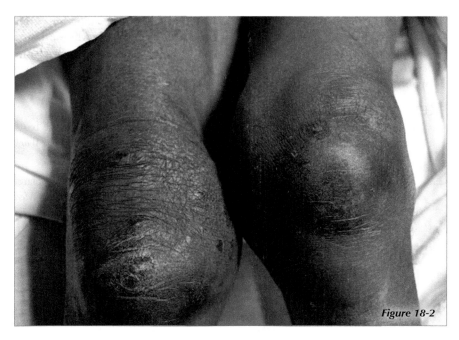

Figure 18-2

Figure 18-2. *Edema/bony deformities of bilateral knees. Photograph courtesy of Debra Holbrook.*

an iron, and verbally abused (**Figure 18-1**). On the day that he was able to leave and seek the neighbor's help, his knees had been beaten with "a baseball bat" (**Figure 18-2**). The documented wounds were consistent with his history and included a patterned burn to his left upper extremity, bruises in various stages of healing on much of his body, and abrasions and cuts. Many of these were healed by secondary intent and were in various stages of healing, including scars. His knees appeared painful and edematous, requiring surgical repair. Adult Protective Services, as well as law enforcement, were consulted by the FNE, who utilized the multidisciplinary team concept model and other available resources.

Discussion

The patient was discharged to a long-term care facility for further recovery. Mental health and advocacy counselors were brought in as part of the care team, and his discharge included therapy sessions to ensure a plan for safety and well-being. His cousin and her daughter were arrested, convicted of elder abuse, and are serving time in prison.

Case Study 18-3

This 80-year old male patient had not planned for his future life. He went to a financial planning program that was recommended by a friend in an attempt to start preparing for the future. The financial investor told the patient that they had a fund for investment and that the buy-in was half of his savings, but the man promised to double his funds every 2 years. The patient was desperate and did not consult his family, even though his family was attempting to obtain court-ordered guardianship over him due to his worsening dementia. The patient rode with the investor to his bank, and with the investor's supervision, withdrew the funds and gave them to the investor. Later, the patient used his clinic's transportation to attend a regular health care visit with an advanced forensic nurse (AFN). The AFN was treating the patient's dementia with medical therapies and behavioral modification. As part of the health assessment, the AFN used the decision matrix for elder safety (DMES)[4] to logarithmically document the patient's decline and risk for elder abuse at each visit. During the visit, the patient told the AFN about the "windfall" to solve his financial problems over the next few years of his life. Alert to financial abuse schemes targeting older adults with cognitive challenges, the AFN notified the patient's family. His family contacted the court, who granted guardianship. The family asked for the court to take legal action against the investor, and they issued a summons to the investor.

Discussion

The investor, charged with financial abuse of an elder person, denied financial manipulation of the patient for personal financial gain. The investor said the investment had not yet materialized, but it could, and the money would not be returned to the patient because it had been invested already. The court convicted the investor of misdemeanor elder abuse, and he was fined.

SUMMARY

Violence against elders is common across all socioeconomic levels, both in the United States and internationally. It takes many forms, including physical, financial, sexual, and emotional abuse. While this abuse can be difficult to detect, caring for victims of elder abuse is a necessary skill for health care providers and those who work with older populations. The key to prevention is sentinel observers who routinely contact elders in community dwellings, as when they are taught the indicators of abuse, there is opportunity to intervene and protect this vulnerable population.

REFERENCES

1. Storey J, Perka M. Reaching out for help: recommendations for practice based on an in-depth analysis of an elder abuse intervention programme. *Br J Soc Work.* 2018;48(4):1052-1070. doi:10.1093/bjsw/bcy039

2. Rosen T, LoFaso V, Bloemen E, et al. Identifying injury patterns associated with physical elder abuse: analysis of legally adjudicated cases. *Ann Emerg Med.* 2020;76:266-276.

3. Anetzberger G, Breckman R, Caccamise P, Freeman I, Nerenberg L. Building a national elder justice movement, state by state. *Am Soc Aging.* 2020;44:111-116.

4. Speck PM, Baker, N. Case study series: assessing risk for elder abuse using the decision matrix for elder safety (DMES). *J Leg Nurse Consult.* 2021; 32(2):36-42.

5. Weissberger G, Goodman M, Mosqueda L, et al. Elder abuse characteristics based on calls to the national center on elder abuse resource line. *J Appl Gerontol.* 2020;39:1078-1087.

Chapter 19

WHEN DEATH IS THE OUTCOME

Stacy A. Drake, PhD, MPH, RN, AFN-BC, D-ABMDI, FAAN
Annette Cannon, PhD, MA, MSN, RN, D-ABMDI

KEY POINTS

1. *Forensic nurses have skills and knowledge that are transferable to medicolegal death investigation roles, either as an elected official or forensic fatality team member.*

2. *The generalist forensic nurse can ideally fill medicolegal death investigator roles.*

3. *The advanced forensic nursing practitioner provides valuable insight in medicolegal death investigations.*

INTRODUCTION

Forensic nurses have a variety of career opportunities within the medicolegal death investigation setting. Forensic nurses must understand the medicolegal death investigation systems, cause and manner of death, and the roles of various nurses and consultants within the system. The forensic nurse can translate traditional roles in nursing into the medicolegal death investigation setting.

MEDICOLEGAL DEATH INVESTIGATION OVERVIEW

In the United States, the 2 main systems of death investigation are the coroner and the medical examiner (ME) systems, but some states may have a combination of these systems. The system used is largely dependent upon state laws.[1] As of 2022, no uniform system of death investigation is prevalent in the United States. Regardless, the systems of death investigation work with other professionals, including those with investigation agencies, hospitals, laboratories, media, and families surviving the decedent.

Health care providers are often challenged when dealing with medicolegal death investigation as system types and titles are frequently used synonymously. Both the ME and coroner systems in the United States perform the same functions; however, the structure of the agency (ie, elected or appointed), are often the distinguishing differences of system types. Additionally, death investigation, as carried out in medicolegal death investigation through the office of the coroner or ME, is distinct from that performed by law enforcement.[2] Although the 2 entities work collaboratively, their roles have different outcomes. The ME or coroner is responsible for determining cause and manner of death, whereas law enforcement determines crime occurrence, seeks the assailant, and prepares the evidence of the death and person of interest for litigation. Both death investigators and law enforcement use laboratory results and radiology to assist in the unique role processes and determination for action.

CAUSE AND MANNER OF DEATH

The terms "cause of death" and "manner of death" are often misunderstood. The distinction between them is based on category, description and/or mechanism, and medical opinion. The cause and manner of death are often decided by a combination of medical opinion, information gathered within a comprehensive death investigation that includes interviews and law enforcement reports, and physical examinations that include autopsy reports, laboratory results, and radiology. The interpretations about cause and manner of death, made from the records of the interprofessional teams identified above, are important to families, public health, and the criminal justice system.

The *cause of death* is the condition, disease, or trauma that led to the death (eg, drug toxicity, stab wound), while the *manner of death* is a description of how the death occurred. The manner of death has 5 classifications: natural, accident, homicide, suicide, and undetermined. Determining the manner of death necessitates consideration of all evidence, which often creates a puzzle requiring logic to uncover the ultimate manner of death. Natural deaths are due primarily to disease or conditions.[3] Accident deaths are from unintentional injury or poisoning. A homicide death is due to an intentional act by another person (not necessarily implying criminal intent), while a suicide death is from self-inflicted acts with the intent to harm oneself. A death is classified as undetermined when determination of the manner is not possible or when there are 2 or more competing possibilities and no manner is more convincing than another. The *mechanism of death* is what occurred physiologically to cause the person to die. For example, with a stab wound of the chest, the person dies from sharp force injuries (cause) puncturing the lung and causing hemorrhage (mechanism). Therefore, the cause of death would be sharp force injuries, the mechanism of death would be hemorrhage, and the manner is determined by circumstances surrounding the injuries (eg, homicide).

When cause and manner of death are not straightforward, the determination requires logic related to the objective findings and death investigation criteria. Often, pressure from the community may influence the determination. However, the objective and unbiased final determination should base its conclusion on scientific evidence rather than on appeasing any members of the public, political constituents, legal or law entities, or personal preferences.

ROLES IN DEATH INVESTIGATION

MEs are often physicians; however, they may be nurses, who are often appointed by a local or state governmental body in larger jurisdictions. Their duties include overseeing medicolegal death investigations (eg, postmortem examinations), ensuring identification of the decedent, and certifying the cause and manner of death on the legal death certificate.[1]

Forensic pathologists are physicians who are board-certified in anatomic pathology and/or clinical pathology as well as forensic pathology. In large jurisdictions, forensic pathologists serve as MEs. In other locales, the chief medicolegal officer, who is an ME or coroner, employs forensic pathologists to conduct postmortem examinations and provide professional assessment of cause and manner of death.[4] The collection of data includes conducting an external examination of the decedent and an internal examination of their organs, as well as performing an autopsy. Autopsy results and ancillary testing, which includes toxicology, chemistry, blood cultures, and histology, combine with other findings from the death investigation to accurately identify the cause, manner, and mechanism of the death. Typically, cases referred for autopsy are those deemed suspicious, unexpected, and unnatural.[4]

Coroners are elected or appointed officials whose duties include oversight of medicolegal death investigations for a given geographical jurisdiction. Coroners may also be forensic pathologists. Their duties are similar to those of MEs.[1] Their jurisdictions may have large or small populations and are often spread over a wide geographical area. In states where a coroner requirement does not include a medical degree, there is opportunity for nurses to run for election and serve in the coroner role.

The field of forensic anthropology includes a multitude of sub-disciplines, including cultural anthropology, archaeology, linguistics, and physical (biological) anthropology. *Forensic anthropologists* typically specialize in physical anthropology and archeology (ie, the study of human osteology and skeleton interpretation). As such, forensic anthropologists serve as specialists in the identification of skeletal remains and trauma analysis of the found parts of the skeletal system.[5] Similarly, *forensic odontologists* focus on the identification of human remains by using the maxillofacial remains. The discipline of forensic odontology offers expertise in bite mark analysis through analysis of dentition impressions.[5]

Forensic nurses are ideal candidates for the role of *medicolegal death investigator (MDI)* with their academic preparation in forensic-related knowledge and skills.[6] The training required for forensic nurses includes legal principles (ie, knowledge of federal and state laws and governing practices) and forensic science (ie, recognizing and collecting forensic evidence). Their training also includes forensic nursing that spans the lifetime through death, giving them the skills to identify postmortem changes and interact with grieving families after a sudden unexpected death. Additionally, forensic nurses who are experienced in case management and quality assurance make ideal candidates for similar roles within the medicolegal death investigation setting.[7] Advanced practice forensic nurses with a specialty in pediatrics or geriatrics can also provide oversight for fatality review teams when suspicious circumstances have contributing factors to a death.

Although an MDI may hold titles such as death investigator, coroner, ME, deputy coroner, or coroner investigator,[1] they are generally responsible for examining bodies, assessing scenes, and assisting in autopsies. MDIs also serve as liaisons between the multiple disciplines involved in death investigation, assist surviving family members, collect medical and/or social history information on the deceased, and aid in determining the cause and manner of death.[2]

SUMMARY

Forensic nurses have the prerequisite baseline education in nursing and associated sciences, and with the added knowledge in medicolegal death investigation, they are ideal candidates for the role of MDI. The forensic nurse's education and ability to work, collaborate, and communicate with an interprofessional team promises success in the medicolegal death investigation system.

REFERENCES

1. Centers for Disease Control and Prevention. Coroner/medical examiner laws, by state. 2015. Updated October 26, 2016. Accessed December 9, 2021. https://www.cdc.gov/phlp/publications/topic/coroner.html

2. National Institute of Justice. Death investigation: A guide for the scene investigator. 2011. Accessed December 9, 2021. https://www.ncjrs.gov/pdffiles1/nij/234457.pdf

3. Hanzlick R, Hunsaker III JC, Davis GJ. *Guide for Manner of Death Classification*. 1st ed. National Association of Medical Examiners; 2002.

4. National Association of Medical Examiners. So you want to be a medical detective. Published date unknown. Accessed December 9, 2021. https://www.thename.org/assets/docs/2f8ae9c9-39b0-49d2-a10f-5980e0770526.pdf

5. American Academy of Forensic Sciences. Careers in Forensic Science. Accessed December 9, 2021. https://www.aafs.org/careers-forensic-science

6. Drake S, Tabor P, Hamilton H, Cannon A. Nurses and medicolegal death investigation. *J Forensic Nurs.* 2020;16(4):207-214. doi:10.1097/JFN.0000000000000310

7. Drake SA, Harper S, Wolf DA. Medicolegal death investigation and hospital patient safety and quality outcomes: a naturally synergistic collaboration. J Forensic Nurs. 2016;12(4):183-188. doi:10.1097/JFN.0000000000000128

Section  V

SPECIAL POPULATIONS

Chapter 20

FAMILY VIOLENCE

Michelle Patch, PhD, MSN, APRN-CNS, ACNS-BC, AFN-C
Kathy Bell, MS, RN, AFN-C, SANE-A, SANE-P, DF-AFN
Loretta Tsu, MA, BSN, RN, SANE-A, SCRN

KEY POINTS

1. *Biological and sociocultural constructs of a family are nuanced and complex, but they are fundamentally intended to be beneficial, supportive, and protective. Violence, whether physical, emotional, or sexual, produces a damaging ripple effect in families that can span generations.*

2. *The social-ecological model serves as a violence prevention framework. Individual factors such as financial and/or housing instability, lower levels of education, substance use disorders, and adverse childhood experiences can directly impact family dynamics and risk for violence.*

3. *The connection between animal abuse and family violence has been researched for many years, suggesting an escalation in violence and an increased risk of interpersonal assaults when the perpetrator first abuses animals.*

INTRODUCTION

For many, the idea of "family" evokes thoughts of warm, caring, and close relationships with those that they trust. These close bonds can be formed through a common ancestor (eg, blood relative), marriage, or adoption. More broadly, they may also include distant relatives, beloved friends, or pets. Legal definitions of what constitutes a family can vary based on state laws. While the biological and sociocultural constructs of a family are nuanced and complex, they are fundamentally intended to be beneficial, supportive, and protective.

Yet, idealized family bliss is far from the reality in many cases. Most families experience friction or tension from time to time, but not violence. For those experiencing violence within the family, however, these relationships can breed deep-seated fear, anxiety, self-loathing, and anger. There can also be unique concerns for families in regards to reporting or seeking care from abuse, like the fear of separating the family unit or loss of income due to the incarceration of the perpetrating "breadwinner." Family violence, whether physical, emotional, or sexual, produces a damaging ripple effect that can span generations.

THE SOCIAL-ECOLOGICAL MODEL

Forensic nurses care for individuals and families across the lifespan, as well as engage in and lead important violence prevention activities. The Social-Ecological Model[1] provides a theoretical understanding of the effect of violence within and across systems and has served as a violence prevention framework for organizations like the Centers for Disease Control and Prevention (**Figure 20-1**).

This model includes individual factors such as financial and housing instability, lower levels of education, substance use disorders, and adverse childhood experiences (including witnessing abuse), which can directly impact family dynamics and the risk for violence.

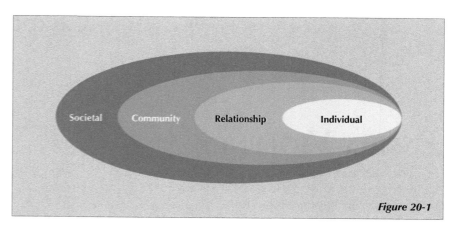

Figure 20-1.[1] The Social-Ecological Model. Adapted from the Centers for Disease Control and Prevention.

The second level of this model, "Relationship," recognizes that close-knit groups, like families, influence individuals' behaviors and experiences; thus, they also influence risk of violence victimization or perpetration.[1] In the following case studies, the diverse roles of forensic nurses as they work to respond to and prevent family violence are presented.

CASE STUDIES

Case Study 20-1

This 42-year-old woman presented to the emergency department (ED) with her 11-year-old son after they were assaulted by her husband who is the children's stepfather. She reported that she and her husband had a disagreement at the dinner table that later escalated to a physical assault in their bedroom. She stated that her husband pushed her several times and then manually strangled her with both hands. She saw her 5-year-old son come into the room, and she yelled at her husband to stop and not do this in front of him. The couple fell on the bed with him on top of her, and she felt her vision going black. At this point, the older son came into the room, jumped on top of his stepfather's back, and placed him into a chokehold. The stepfather then stood, walked backwards with the child still on his back, and slammed him into the wall. When the child released his hold on his stepfather, he was manually strangled by his stepfather with 1 hand. When she "came to," the mother screamed for her husband to stop. She pulled her older son away from him, picked up her younger son before running to a neighbor's house to call 911. Her husband drove away before law enforcement arrived. The neighbor agreed to watch the younger son while the mother and older son were taken to the hospital.

At the hospital, a forensic nurse evaluated both of them separately, approximately 4 hours after the assault. The examination included documenting the history of the assault, a physical examination and strangulation evaluation, and photodocumentation of injuries. Together, the forensic nurse and the mother created a personalized safety plan and then collaborated with the physician, a social worker, and a law enforcement advocate for a safe discharge plan.

The mother's physical examination showed only a linear abrasion to her midline neck, and she reported neck pain and dizziness. Using validated instruments (eg, the Danger Assessment tool and the Power and Control Wheel), the forensic nurse worked with her to assess the abuse she experienced and her future risk. Her resulting Danger Assessment[2] score was a 12, which means she was at an increased risk of lethal violence in her relationship with her husband. She reported that the violence had been escalating from verbal to physical violence in the past year. She expressed concern for how he behaved toward the children, although she had previously never witnessed him physically harming them. The mother also discovered that multiple items on the Power and Control Wheel[3] were what she was experiencing in her relationship, and she did not realize they were abuse until she discussed them with the forensic nurse.

The older son did not appear to have any injuries, but upon further examination, the forensic nurse found diffuse petechiae to his soft palate and uvula (**Figure 20-2**). He complained of coughing and odynophagia. He reported that he was afraid of his stepfather and felt that he had to "be vigilant" to protect his mom and brother. He stated that his stepfather would wrestle them sometimes but would get serious about it very quickly. He had not told his mother about this before. With this disclosure and the information discussed with the forensic nurse, his mother expressed that her main concern was their safety. Because she was not sure if her husband had been arrested, she was unsure of if they should go home or to a shelter.

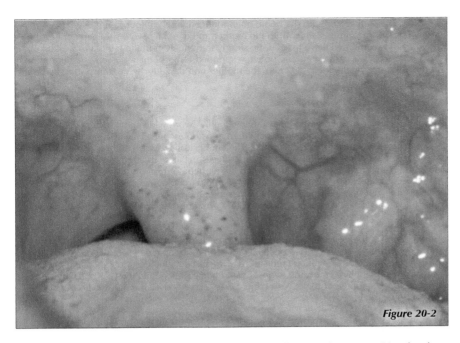

Figure 20-2

Figure 20-2. *Petechial hemorrhages of uvula, found during the forensic nurse's assessment.*

These findings were then discussed with the ED team. No further orders were initiated at that time, and recommendations included post-discharge follow-up with the family's primary care provider and return to the ED for any emergent symptoms. The social worker and forensic nurse explained their mandatory reporting responsibilities to child protective services (CPS) with the mother present. Once her questions and concerns about that process had been answered, she said that she felt less apprehensive and that she appreciated their candidness. The social worker assisted with calling CPS while the forensic nurse worked with her for discharge planning.

The forensic nurse explored options with the mother, considering her physical safety, the desire to keep her and the children together, and the need for her and her son to be monitored for any post-strangulation sequelae. When the victim advocate informed her that her husband had been arrested, she decided to pick up her younger son from the neighbor's home and stay with another family member for a few days. To supplement teaching, the forensic nurse provided the mother with written resources on discharge, including strangulation signs and symptoms and when to return to the hospital, and recommended sharing this information with the family member with whom she was staying so that they could monitor for any changes as well.

Discussion

Working in a team environment is crucial to improved patient outcomes. Close collaboration of the forensic nurse with the physician, social worker, and victim advocate provided the family with options for a personalized discharge plan. Educating the patient about strangulation while completing a thorough assessment empowers the patient to engage in the monitoring of their health after discharge. While it is not uncommon for patients to have few injuries after experiencing strangulation, there is still an elevated concern for internal injuries and increasing symptoms for hours and days after the assault.

Using validated instruments to collaboratively assess a patient's relationship supports the forensic nurse's ability to have candid conversations with patients about their safety. Many patients do not realize that facets of their relationship are abusive and can lead to an increased risk of danger. Each patient's needs are different, and they are the expert on their safety; therefore, the forensic nurse should work closely with them to examine their family relationships and develop personalized safety plans.

Case Study 20-2

This woman and her 10-year-old daughter presented to a Family Safety Center (FSC) for assistance. The woman reported that the child's father had recently become more aggressive and violent. The physical violence was primarily aimed at the mother. The most recent act occurred the day prior, resulting in injuries to her face and knee. The woman noted that her husband became increasingly irritated and was calling her names, stating that she was "lazy" and "no good." She said she asked him why he was so mad, and he responded by punching her in the face, knocking her to her knees. Their daughter witnessed the assault and ran with her mother to her room, where she then shut and locked the door. After the incident, the husband left and did not return that night. The next day, while at home with their dog, her husband walked into the home unannounced and, without saying a word, shot the family dog, killing him instantly. Both the mother and daughter were shocked and terrified that they too would be killed. Instead, he simply laid the gun on the table and walked out of the house. 911 was called, and the police responded. After being assessed and determined medically stable by the local ED team, the mother and daughter were transported by police to the FSC.

Discussion

Animals (ie, pets) are a common part of many families worldwide and can benefit the emotional growth and development of children and adolescents. Having a pet also provides psychological and social support to adults. The connection between animal abuse and family violence has been researched for many years, suggesting an escalation in violence and an increased risk of interpersonal assaults when the perpetrator first abuses animals. The abuse of family pets has deleterious effects on emotional and psychological well-being,[4] with common feelings of anger, sadness, and anxiety. Furthermore, the effects of animal abuse coupled with other effects of domestic violence, such as PTSD symptoms, low self-esteem, guilt, shame, and depression, magnifies the trauma.

After explaining the examination process, the forensic nurse obtained consent from mother and assent from her daughter to proceed. Placing them in separate examination rooms, the forensic nurse carefully obtained medical histories and detailed descriptions of the events, as well as individual physical examinations. Due to being punched in the face and exhibiting visible trauma, a full neurological assessment was completed for the mother. Proper documentation included a written description and photographs of each injury.

The forensic nurse also performed a trauma-informed assessment of both individual's emotional states while completing their history and physical examinations, paying close attention to their ability to focus and respond to their current situation. Interventions to address the physical and emotional responses included non-pharmacologic comfort measures for the injury and sharing ways to self-soothe when feeling anxious. A Danger Assessment[2] was also completed with the mother to help inform her decisions in planning for safety.

A report to CPS was also made, as the daughter witnessed both her mother's assault and her dog's death. Forensic nurses are well-versed in local child abuse reporting laws and report accordingly. Often, mothers fear that CPS is intent on removing children from homes where violence is occurring, which causes them to hesitate making a report. The forensic nurse explained the reporting process to the mother and supported her as they called CPS together. Based on an assessment of the daughter's developmental stage, the forensic nurse also worked with her to develop a safety plan.

The forensic nurse's goal in this case was to empower the patients through collaboration, an identification of their strengths, and a building on strategies that have worked for them in the past. Educating families on the long-term effects of witnessing violence is an important role of the forensic nurse. The forensic nurse provided a referral to a community-based child counselor along with follow-up guidance and connections to a local advocacy system, thus supporting their ongoing evaluation and a continual update of their safety plans.

SUMMARY

Whether narrowly or broadly defined, families experiencing violence have unique needs for assessment, safety planning, and care intervention. Frameworks like the Social-Ecological Model are helpful in holistically understanding the impact of violence within the family unit as well as how that violence both affects and is affected by other systems. Forensic nurses are well-positioned to develop and lead violence prevention and response efforts, providing compassionate and high-quality care to families in the midst of healing.

REFERENCES

1. Centers for Disease Control and Prevention. The social-ecological model: a framework for prevention. Updated January 28, 2021. Accessed 2021. https://www.cdc.gov/violenceprevention/about/social-ecologicalmodel.html

2. Campbell JC, Webster DW, Glass N. The danger assessment: validation of a lethality risk assessment instrument for intimate partner femicide. *J Interpers Violence.* 2009;24(4):653-674.

3. Domestic Abuse Intervention Programs. The Duluth model wheel gallery. 2017. http://www.theduluthmodel.org/training/wheels.html

4. Collins EA, Cody AM, McDonald SE, Nicotera N, Ascione FR, Williams JH. A template analysis of intimate partner violence survivors' experiences of animal maltreatment: implications for safety planning and intervention. *Violence Against Women*. 2018;24(4):452-476. doi:10.1177/1077801217697266

MINORITY HEALTH

Kimberly Foster, MBA, BSN, RN
Sarah L. Pederson, BSN, RN, AFN-C, SANE-A, SANE-P

KEY POINTS

1. *Analysis of social determinants of health data shows that minority populations experience adverse health impacts, including early death, disproportionate to their representation in the community.*

2. *Disproportionate poor health outcomes in minority communities often result from systemic discrimination.*

3. *The quality of health outcomes of vulnerable persons is correlated to whether they receive coordinated support from community stakeholders.*

INTRODUCTION

The terms "minority health" and "health disparities," once frequently intertwined, assumed that minorities always experienced health disparities.[1] The National Institute of Minority Health Disparities separated the definitions of minority health and health disparities across the National Institute of Health during the 2015 and 2016 fiscal year, believing that separation may allow for research advances within the field.[2] These newer definitions primarily distinguished the science behind the 2 terms. *Minority health* refers to the various health characteristics of racial and/or ethnic minorities who may be socially disadvantaged due to potential discriminatory acts within the health care system.[1-3] The science of *health disparities*, on the other hand, categorizes racial or ethnic groups (ie, American Indian or Alaska Native, Asian, Black or African American, and Native Hawaiian or other Pacific Islander) and focuses on the differences in their health outcomes.[2] Disadvantaged populations are adversely affected based on 1 or more of the following health outcomes, as seen in **Table 21-1**. Health disparities affect racial and ethnic minorities, people with lower socioeconomic statuses (SES), rural residents, and sexual and gender minorities.[2,4]

MINORITY HEALTH

Throughout the world, members of minority groups, primarily Black and Indigenous people of color (BIPOC), experience health statuses and health care that do not compare to that of the dominant cultures within which they live.[5] Much of what they experience may occur due to their country's societal structure and health care system. For example, research studies to approve treatments for illnesses frequently do not include enough BIPOC participants to determine whether they experience different effects from the medications. Using reasoning that certain choices are made for safety, research programs recruit healthy participants who are usually White and male. Recruitment efforts for these types of research have often excluded minorities and women either due to logistics or location. However, even when minority populations receive targeted invitations to participate in research studies, such as with the research for the COVID-19 vaccine, their participation lags behind that of white males.[5] Many African Americans refer to the legacy of adverse treatment during previous research studies, (eg, US Public Health Service Syphilis Study at Tuskegee, in

Table 21-1. Impact of Health Disparities
A Health Disparity (HD) is a Health Difference that Adversely Affects Disadvantaged Populations, Based on One or More of the Following Health Outcomes.
— Higher incidence and/or prevalence and earlier onset of disease
— Higher prevalence of risk factors, unhealthy behaviors, or clinical measures in the causal pathway of a disease outcome
— Higher rates of condition-specific symptoms, reduced global daily functioning, or self-reported health-related quality of life using standardized measures
— Premature and/or excessive mortality from diseases where population rates differ
— Greater global burden of disease using a standardized metric

which participants were infected with syphilis and then denied health care services), as reasons to refuse participation in modern research.

HEALTH DISPARITIES

Health disparities exist in different populations' morbidity and mortality from injury or illness, life expectancy, disease burden, ability to pay for health care, treatments, and access to care, as seen in **Table 21-1**. The Institute of Medicine, Unequal Treatment cited differences in health care and outcomes for minorities in the areas of[6]:

— Asthma

— Cancer, including breast, lung, and colorectal

— Cardiovascular diseases, including myocardial infarction and heart attack

— HIV/AIDS

— Mental health

— Screening and preventive services

The COVID-19 pandemic revealed that many of these disparities continue. For example, early in the pandemic, it became apparent that African Americans were more likely to require hospitalization and to die from the disease. Another distressing example of health care disparities is the maternal mortality rate or the number of pregnancy-related deaths. The United States ranks 55th globally for maternal mortality, with Black non-Hispanic mothers twice as likely to die from pregnancy-related reasons.[7] The life expectancy of African Americans remains lower than that of non-Hispanic Whites. Addressing health disparities within a community requires focusing on equity and social justice in research and health care delivery.

SOCIAL DETERMINANTS OF HEALTH

Social determinants of health (SDOH) are defined by the Centers for Disease Control and Prevention (CDC) as conditions in the places where people live, learn, work, and play that affect a wide range of health risks and outcomes.[1] Over the last 30 years, health care professionals discovered evidence that many factors beyond the efficacy of medical care impact health outcomes on individual and population levels. Nonmedical factors such as economic stability, education level, neighborhood, and social community context affect a person's wellness (**Figure 21-1**).[3] In addition, structural factors including national wealth, income inequality, and access to health and education create barriers that prevent certain groups from achieving health outcomes comparable to others.

Figure 21-1. Social Determinants of Health (Source: Healthy People 2030, US Department of Health and Human Services, Office of Disease Prevention and Health Promotion[3])

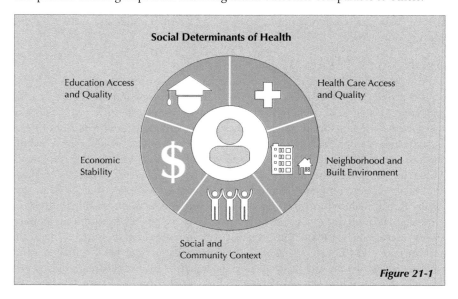

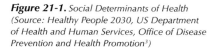

LEGISLATION AND HEALTH DISPARITIES

Discrimination against specific groups of people creates health disparities. Groups historically targeted with discriminatory practices are less healthy than those who have escaped such treatment. The legislative tools used to combat discriminatory practices often positively impact minority health. The determination of whether discrimination has occurred under most legislation depends on disparate treatment or disparate impact.[8] The Health Resources and Services Administration Office for Civil Rights enforces laws related to discrimination in health care. Over the last century, the United States has increasingly enacted laws prohibiting discrimination and enhancing health care access (**Figure 21-2**).[8] These key legislative milestones, along with continuing work by social justice proponents for equitable health care, have played a role in improved health outcomes for minority groups who experience health disparities.

Figure 21-2. Timeline of Laws Prohibiting Discrimination and Health Care Access (©Foster, K. (2021) Used with permission.)

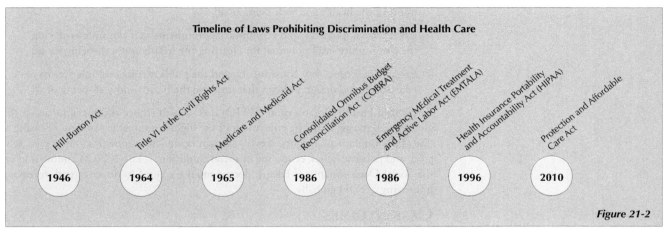

Figure 21-2

STRUCTURAL INTERSECTIONALITY AND FORENSIC NURSING PRACTICE

Racial and ethnic minority attributions impact the treatment received from professionals within the medical, educational, social, and/or criminal justice settings. Historically, underprivileged communities have a much higher rate of adverse health outcomes because of the unequal distribution of resources.[2-4] When a person's identity, ethnicity, or race affects how they are treated in health care settings, they may experience negative health outcomes.[3] ***Structural intersectionality*** provides an approach to population health research, combining the study of structural racism, structural sexism, and intersectionality. As an intersectional practice, forensic nursing offers opportunities to impact structural violence, social justice, and equity concerns. Therefore, forensic nurses who understand these intersectional issues can shift their care to better address the impact of violence and trauma on patients from groups experiencing inequality.

The forensic nurse must be aware of personal prejudices and biases to avoid discrimination and strive to facilitate interactions that mitigate health disparities experienced by minorities. In forensic nursing, the patient typically presents for care in a crisis state or has undergone a traumatic experience that makes trust and communication difficult. A patient with a history of health disparities related to race or ethnicity may present challenges in creating rapport and trust during the patient-nurse encounter, requiring the forensic nurse to incorporate trauma-informed care principles into the patient encounter. Research has identified that SDOH are more important than health care or lifestyle choices in influencing health.[1] Addressing SDOH is necessary for improving minority health and reducing longstanding inequities in health outcomes.[1] The forensic nurse must identify gaps in their patients' conditions and collaborate with the interdisciplinary team to ensure that patients have connections to community resources that help shape their daily life.

PROMOTION OF MINORITY HEALTH FOLLOWING VIOLENCE: HEALTH EQUALITY

Health equity exists when the same opportunities are available to all individuals to reach their full health potential.[4] The CDC's National Center for Chronic Disease Prevention and Health Promotion ensures that all citizens in the United States have access to the best health care possible.[4] Healthy People 2030, the US Department of Health and Human Services' national health objectives initiative, includes overarching goals to achieve health equity[2]:

— Eliminate health disparities, achieve health equity, and attain health literacy to improve the health and well-being of all

— Create social, physical, and economic environments that promote achieving the community's full potential for ensuring the health and well-being for all

— Engage leadership, key constituents, and the public across multiple sectors to take action and design policies that improve the health and well-being of all

The World Health Organization (WHO) links health equity and social justice at the global level, stating that "the enjoyment of the highest attainable standard of health is one of the fundamental rights of every human being without distinction of race, religion, and political belief, economic or social condition."[1] The WHO Commission on the Social Determinants of Health documented the need to direct attention toward improving SDOH globally.

CASE STUDIES

Case Study 21-1

This patient, a 40-year-old Black woman, lived in a neighborhood that 3 waves of gentrification have bypassed. She dropped out of school in 10th grade to help her father support the family's 3 younger children after their mother died in childbirth. With her support, the patient's 3 younger siblings graduated from high school and eventually college. They live in other states, and she rarely sees them. She later raised 2 children of her own who also live far away.

Before the COVID-19 pandemic began, the patient had a stable job at a warehouse. In February 2020, she evicted her abusive live-in boyfriend. When the warehouse shut down a month later due to the pandemic, the isolation instigated the patient's depression. Her depression worsened even as panic about the disease calmed down. Her enhanced unemployment benefits did not make up for her previous income with regular overtime. She earned gig income from delivering food and providing rides, yet she could not make ends meet. The patient did not refill her high blood pressure medications for several months due to the cost, and her landlord threatened eviction as soon as the moratorium was lifted. Her dire financial situation caused her to reconsider her abuser's offer to move in with him.

Once her boyfriend returned, the abuse began again in earnest. Although he kept the patient isolated, he did take her for an annual checkup. During the exam, he stayed in the room hovering over the patient. With the patient's permission, the nurse practitioner informed the patient in front of her boyfriend that she was pregnant. She also stated the patient was prediabetic. The nurse practitioner asked her boyfriend to leave the room for a few moments, she then conducted a screen for domestic abuse The patient admitted that her current home situation included physical, emotional, and also sexual abuse in which her boyfriend refused to use a condom despite her protests.

The treatment plan offered included a referral to a domestic violence program as well as an obstetrician. The nurse practitioner gave the patient a hotline number to call and helped her install an innocuous app on her phone that dialed 911 or the hotline in case of emergency. The nurse practitioner also suggested that the patient get a COVID-19 vaccination. She declined the vaccine because of fear and skepticism regarding its development. Ultimately, the patient declined much of the care offered by the nurse practitioner due to fear of consequences from her boyfriend. She did agree to follow up with an obstetrician.

Discussion

This patient's story illustrates the structural challenges many minorities and women face regarding their health. Her challenges in many nonmedical areas (SDOH) impact her ability to manage her hypertension. Societal structures (eg, health care costs, economy, etc.) have created an environment that makes patients like this one more vulnerable to violence. The abuse the patient is experiencing will also impact her unborn child. Although legislation has reduced blatant discrimination against minorities, less attention has been paid to underlying impediments to optimal health care outcomes. This case furthermore illustrates that forensic nurses must remain sensitive to patients past and current situations that impact their health and treatment plans. Forensic nurses should also understand their state laws and internal protocols as they relate to disclosures of abuse.

Case Study 21-2

This patient, a 34-year-old Hispanic woman, relocated to the United States from Mexico with her family when she was an infant. She was raised in a low-income family and had limited access to health care throughout her life. Her father died suddenly at the age of 37 due to a myocardial infarction when she was 15 years old, leading her to drop out of high school and get a job to help with the family bills. She eventually obtained her GED, completed her undergraduate degree, and began working a new job that provided health insurance. She presented to the nurse practitioner for a physical and complains of frequent headaches and fatigue. She told the nurse practitioner, "I have not felt well for about a year, but I did not have the resources or time to see a doctor. I was trying to finish school and wanted to wait for my benefits at my new job to be active." Her blood pressure on intake was 168/98, and her blood pressure was retaken 30 minutes later and was 156/92. The nurse practitioner created a care plan to address her complaints and elevated blood pressure.

The patient was provided with discharge planning and health education, and a follow-up appointment was made.

Discussion

Minority health classifies ethnic groups to include Latino or Hispanic; therefore, minority groups within this definition can experience social disadvantage and face potential discriminatory acts. Medical professionals should be aware of the "health characteristics and attributes of minority racial and ethnic groups who are usually underrepresented in biomedical research to understand health outcomes in these populations."[2] This results in increased barriers to medical professionals' access to evidence-based research specific to their patients from minority populations.

Based on this patient's family and personal history, the nurse practitioner understood that she faced a higher risk for condition-specific syndromes and earlier disease onset. In addition, the nurse practitioner recognized that premature mortality rates are influenced by ethnicity and race. This woman was a high-risk patient with a family history of cardiac disease in conjunction with her current health presentation. By understanding the dynamics of health disparities that minority populations may face, the nurse practitioner was able to create a patient-centered care plan and will continue to monitor the patient.

SUMMARY

Forensic nursing aligns with nursing practices globally with a specialty that focuses on patients with specialized needs following violence and trauma. The definition of violence and trauma remains the same regardless of race, ethnicity, or socioeconomic status.[9] As noted with health disparities and SDOH, the recovery trajectory is determined by access to the necessary health services to mitigate the adverse outcomes of trauma. The forensic nurse must understand the relationship between minority patients and health disparities and the resulting health consequences. Forensic nursing requires respect for the patient's culture, beliefs, and lifestyle, and avoidance of further alienation of an already marginalized population.[10] Forensic nurses have an essential role in caring for minority populations and have the opportunity to interrupt the cycle that leads to health disparities. Promoting an environment of safety, caring and healing is essential for all patients, especially those that face inequities in the health care system.

REFERENCES

1. World Health Organization. Accessed December 8, 2021. https://www.who.int/health-topics/social-determinants-of-health#tab=tab_1

2. National Institute on Minority Health and Health Disparities. Minority Health and Health Disparities: Definitions and Parameters. Updated March 31, 2021. https://www.nimhd.nih.gov/about/strategic-plan/nih-strategic-plan-definitions-and-parameters.html

3. Healthy People 2030. Social Determinants of Health. US Department of Health and Human Services, Office of Disease Prevention and Health Promotion. https://health.gov/healthypeople/objectives-and-data/social-determinants-health

4. Centers for Disease Control and Prevention. Social Determinants of Health: Know what affects health. Updated March 10, 2021. https://www.cdc.gov/socialdeterminants/about.html

5. Flores LE, Frontera WR, Andrasik MP, et al. Assessment of the inclusion of racial/ethnic minority, female, and older individuals in vaccine clinical trials. *JAMA Netw. Open.* 2021;e2037640. doi: 10.1001/jamanetworkopen.2020.37640

6. Smedley BD, Stith AY, Nelson AR. *Unequal Treatment: Confronting Racial and Ethnic Disparities in Health Care.* National Academies Press (US); 2003.

7. Hoyert DL, Miniño AM. Maternal Mortality in the United States: Changes in Coding, Publication, and Data Release, 2018. *National Vital Statistics Reports.* 2020;69(2):1-18.

8. Health Disparities: Nondiscriminatory Quality Healthcare Services. US Department of Health and Human Services. Updated July 26, 2013. https://www.hhs.gov/civil-rights/for-individuals/special-topics/health-disparities/index.html

9. Quaile HC. Trauma-Informed Care for the Primary Care Provider. Women's Healthcare. August 5, 2020. https://www.npwomenshealthcare.com/trauma-informed-care-for-the-primary-care-provider/

10. Hammer RM, Moynihan B, Pagliaro EM. *Forensic Nursing: A handbook for practice.* 2nd ed. Jones & Bartlett Learning; 2013.

Chapter 22

NATIVE AMERICAN POPULATIONS, HISTORICAL TRAUMA, AND ROLE OF THE FORENSIC NURSE

Jeneile Luebke, (Bad River Band of Lake Superior Chippewa) PhD, RN
Barb Blackdeer-Mackenzie, (Ho-Chunk Nation) Community Healer, Author, Artist, and Consultant
Patricia M. Speck, DNSc, CRNP, FNP-BC, AFN-C, DF-IAFN, FAAFS, DF-AFN, FAAN

The authors of this chapter are committed to using terminology that respects and honors the individuals to whom this chapter refers. Currently, there are over 570 federally recognized American Indian and Alaskan Native Indian tribes in the United States. While no single term is universally accepted by all Indigenous peoples in the United States, the terms "American Indian, Alaskan Native, Indigenous, and Native American," are used for data reporting purposes only and appear in the form the terminology was originally published. It is not meant to minimize, exclude, or generalize the individuals involved, nor endorse one form of terminology over the other. Further, we are choosing the term "survivors" rather than "victims" to honor the strength and resiliency of the Indigenous people.

KEY POINTS

1. *The Native American/American Indian (NA/AI) population migrated to the American continent over 40 000 years ago. Approximately 500 years ago, European colonization led to disease exposure, death, cultural genocide, eugenic policies, and legislative divestment of treaties between sovereign nations, leading to historical trauma and the dilution of Native oral traditions and history.*

2. *The NA/AI population experiences higher rates of rape and disappearance among women, increased drug and alcohol abuse, and jurisdictional mazes between reservation, local, and federal authorities, resulting in high incarceration rates.*

3. *Today, NA/AI women and their children bear the burden of continued structural racism in federal and local legislation that, without stakeholder engagement, denies justice to the sovereign nations and Native peoples.*

4. *Forensic nurses have a responsibility to use trauma-informed care to create safe spaces for NA/AI patients.*

INTRODUCTION

Indigenous history transcends millennia, and over 40 000 years ago, the people migrated freely over the lands. Established trade routes across Asia and the Americas existed for centuries and supported common tribal nations' ethnobotany and therapeutic recipes that included certain teas, tinctures, poultices, salves, and balms, which contained ingredients unavailable in all tribal nations' climates. In addition, the American Indian, Alaskan Native, Indigenous, and Native American cultures had dominant views of women as sacred and complete, able to transmogrify a spirit or soul into a physical state of being in a child. Women were contributors and active partners in the survival of a tribe, whether it be making a support system and community for children and elders or completing any task that might be considered traditionally men's work, including farming, fishing, trapping, and hunting as needed. Women were respected for being able to do anything—fill in as needed anywhere—and revered for the ability to grow a baby in their body. Children were gifts of the Creator that were given to parents for a short time. For all time, *supportive kinship* care systems help women who were widowed or divorced and children who were orphaned, and they include Native families' structures, clans, nations, and tribal alliances. These supportive kinships are able to help individuals as they process and heal from various traumas.

The earliest traumas, known as historical trauma, have an epigenetic influence on health, even when a person knows nothing about their past.[1] ***Historical trauma*** is defined as "the cumulative emotional and psychological wounding over one's lifetime and from generation to generation following loss of lives, land and vital aspects of culture."[1] Historical trauma greatly impacts the health outcomes of contemporary Indigenous populations.

COLONIZATION AND ITS EFFECTS ON INDIGENOUS POPULATIONS

The Oxford dictionary defines ***colonization*** as "the act of taking control of an area or a country that is not your own, especially using force, and sending people from your own country to live there."[2] Colonialism established colonies with the aim of occupation and ownership, and early colonists not only enslaved native inhabitants, they displaced them as well.[3] Colonization and colonialism as historical constructs in Europe and the Middle East date back to Hammurabi, Persia, and Asia, where colonization imposed religion, language, economics, and other cultural practices. As archeologists discover artifacts of these human ancestors, DNA provides an insight into the tribal migratory nature of the world's populations.[4]

The Eurasian continent has the largest land mass on earth and has been artificially divided into various communities, countries, and cultures.[5] By the time Europeans traveled to North and South America, there were already thriving Indigenous populations. Today's evidence supports that there had been approximately 40 000 years of Indigenous occupation in the Americas by the time of discovery. Objectification—focusing on gender, skin color, and heritage—became a hierarchical tool that colonizers wielded to promote their beliefs of superiority. Over time, this tool helped reinforce stereotypes, justifying their implicit and explicit biases and supporting an ongoing racist and sexist view of the people around them. Outgrowths of objectification and dehumanization include war, genocide, eugenics, slavery, and sex trafficking. **Table 22-1** distinguishes some of the primary differences between the cultures of European colonizers and NA/AI populations.

Table 22-1. Cultural Differences Between European (colonizer) Culture and American Indian, Alaskan Native, Indigenous, and Native American Culture in the 15th through 20th Centuries

INDIVIDUALS/GROUPS	EUROPEAN CULTURE	AMERICAN INDIAN, ALASKAN NATIVE, INDIGENOUS, AND NATIVE AMERICAN CULTURES
Women	—Private property (Hammurabi Code) —Virginal status valued as property	—Sacred and complete
Children	—Property —Often used as extensions of family for labor	—Gifts of the Creator —Given to parents for a short time

(continued)

Table 22-1. Cultural Differences Between European (colonizer) Culture and American Indian, Alaskan Native, Indigenous, and Native American Culture in the 15th through 20th Centuries *(continued)*

INDIVIDUALS/ GROUPS	EUROPEAN CULTURE	AMERICAN INDIAN, ALASKAN NATIVE, INDIGENOUS, AND NATIVE AMERICAN CULTURES
Family	—Nuclear family —Independent with individual efforts	—Supportive kinship care
Divorced/widowed women and their children	—Property rights denied —Single status is God's punishment —Support through prostitution or indentured servitude; poor houses	—Support from native families' structures, clans, nations, and tribal alliances

ASSIMILATION AND RECULTURALIZATION

Due to colonization, the NA/AI population suffered from forced migration, disease exposure and death, massacres, and slavery. Pre-European contact, it is estimated that up to 100 million Indigenous people existed throughout the Americas.[6-8] By 1920, there were approximately 100 000 Native Americans left in North America; of those remaining, 60 000 were part of an active prison camp-school system known as Indian Boarding Schools.[9,10] The assimilation and reculturalization efforts of the United States under law required enrolling NA/AI children 3 to 17 years of age in mandatory secular or religious Indian schools.[11] The intent was to *"kill the Indian, save the man."*[11] This concept of reculturalization is attributed to United States Army Cavalry Captain Richard Pratt,[11] who started Carlisle Indian School in 1879. Eventually, there were 350 federally funded schools that housed thousands of NA/AI children with the intent of assimilation into mainstream American ways using various methods of discipline and punishment (eg, beatings, isolation in cages, rape, electric chairs, deadly physical punishments, imprisonment).[12] These punishments were used to encourage compliance with learning the English language and basic apprentice/life skills, such as farming and other trades. Non-Native descendants of the boarding schools thought their families did charitable work, but the historical memory is different for persons affected, as the NA/AI view was that their children were stolen from their families.[13] Many of these schools remained operational until 1970 in the United States, with the last school in Canada closing in 1996.[11]

The historical impact of boarding schools such as Carlisle was a loss of the diverse Native oral history, which included cultural narratives with stories, songs, poetry, values, and worldviews. Many believe that the NA/AI language was a gift from the Creator, and that *the words are sacred*. Another impact was siblings' separation (eg, forced adoptions with non-NA/AI families).[14] As children were taken away, the first-language Native speakers (grandparents) were dying without being able to pass on their Native languages and customs to next generations. Another phenomenon is the influence of non-Native environments that dilute traditional tribal knowledge among youth through current technology all while the pool of elders with Native knowledge and traditions grow smaller with the passing of each generation. The end result of colonization is that many Native groups know little to nothing about their long history.

VIOLENCE AGAINST VULNERABLE POPULATIONS

Throughout United States history, the subjugation of women and dehumanization of people of color has been systemic, as largely reflected in laws and policies enacted over time. For example, in 1830, the *Indian Removal Act* moved native people from their homelands east of the Mississippi River basin to the west. When it comes to Indigenous women and girls, these systemic issues can include sex trafficking and mass sexual exploitation. Missing or Murdered Indigenous Women (MMIW),

Missing or Murdered Indigenous Women/Girls/Two-spirits (MMIWG2S), and Missing or Murdered Indigenous Relatives (MMIR) are phrases used to describe the horrific treatment of NA/AI people. In some areas, Indigenous women living on tribal lands are murdered at 10 times the national average; murder is the third leading cause of death for NA/AI people.[15] The crisis of MMIWG2S has deep roots in historical and contemporary settler colonial influence and injustice. NA/AI women have been sexualized and objectified since the earliest colonial contact. For example, Christopher Columbus wrote in his journal about violating tribal girls and women as young as 9 years old. This sexualization of NA/AI women has continued through today, and it has led to them being significantly more likely to experience sexual assault during their lifetimes in comparison to women of other races.[16] At any stage, an Indigenous person may all too easily become a part of MMIWG2S.

Forced sterilization was another violent method used to control the growth of NA/AI communities. Sterilization of NA/AI women was performed by Indian Health Services (IHS) from 1970 to 1976, where up to 25% to 50% of NA/AI women were sterilized using coercive and deceitful tactics by IHS professionals.[17,18] The United Nations considered the eugenics a genocidal practice, and forced sterilization by the IHS implicated the United States government.[19] Family destruction has resulted in NA/AI woman experiencing higher rates of sex trafficking, abuse, and disappearance than any other group of women. Up to 25% of all NA/AI children are still being removed from their homes and placed into foster care. Many of these children are placed in non-Native homes because of a lack of NA/AI families with the state-implemented *appropriate* certification. NA/AI women are also disproportionately incarcerated, representing 2.5% of the prison population but only 0.7% of the total United States female population.[20] The impact of the government's structural actions is destruction of the NA/AI family.

In Indigenous culture, NA/AI women transmogrify a soul into physical existence. As a part of Indigenous worldview, Mother Earth is yet another woman experiencing violations. **Figure 22-1** represents the identified areas of violence against NA/AI women.

Figure 22-1. Native view of violence against American Indian women, illustrating the intersecting systems of oppression fueling the crisis of gender-based violence against NA/AI women[20] © Dr. Jeneile Luebke (2020) Used with permission.

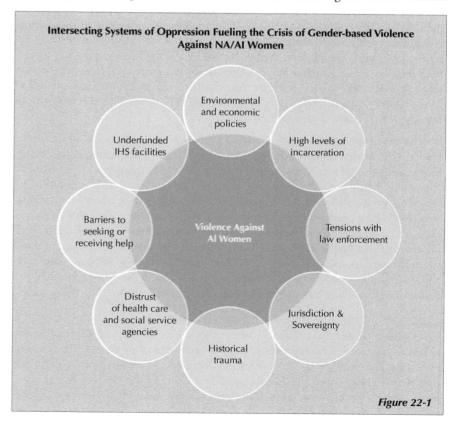

FORENSIC NURSING ROLE

Forensic nurses have a special interest in ensuring trauma-informed and survivor-led care for patients intersecting with legal systems. For NA/AI women who have no reason to trust structurally racist health care and legal systems, the forensic nurse has ethical tenets to guide their practices. Forensic nurses should also have respect for the human dignity and the lived experiences of a vulnerable population desiring to reclaim their lost culture and traditions.

NA/AI patients have voices that are informational, providing a path toward *respect for the culture* and *acceptance without judgement* of the NA/AI journey, encouraging *supportive kinship* care. The *supportive kinship care practices* exist to reunite NA/AI to Indigenous communities formerly separated during colonization. Today, the federal Indian Child Welfare Act says that if a NA child is being treated at a health care facility, the provider is responsible for reporting the child's possible affiliation with a tribe (and if possible, identifying the tribal nation to which the child belongs) to social services.

Forensic nurses often encounter NA/AI women when there is a complaint of a sexual assault. However, forensic nurses need to provide holistic care that is not just focused on the collection of forensic evidence. Forensic nurses also should work to provide support and advocacy for survivors of violence. The *jurisdictional maze* between federal and tribal authorities reduces the chance for prosecution when the crime occurs on tribal land. During the nurse-patient encounter, the forensic nurse must implement trauma-informed care principles. Providers may unintentionally perpetuate oppression and create barriers to care for survivors of violence. Examples of this behavior are described below in **Table 22-2**.

Table 22-2. Testimonials from NA/AI Survivors of Violence[20]

MISTAKES	NA/AI VOICES
Invalidating their experiences	"I was turned away from a shelter because I had been drinking, and they didn't believe me that I was abused."
Having a paternalistic attitude	"My sister was living with me, and I was just kind of helping her get through high school. My mom had moved in with me too, and I had a lot going on. And the counselor basically was like, 'You're 26, why don't you just go out and get your own apartment and let them deal with what they have going on?' ... the counselor had no understandings around kinship and relationships and family... she had a very individualistic sense of what was right, and it did not fit very well and made me feel ashamed. So, I never went back to counseling there, anywhere."
Victim shaming/ blaming	"I was referred a legal advocate for low-income people to help me file a restraining order and build a case. And then at the same time, she was one of the people that made me feel really terrible about the fact that I had been in a relationship like this for so long. She was helpful, and was mostly pretty kind and everything, and she really did work hard... but I remember her getting very upset and she was like, 'Well, you're the one that chose to be with him. You're the one that kept going back to him'... I was totally shocked by that. I didn't know what to say, I didn't know how to feel. I just remember that I did feel really weird and bad. I was like, 'Oh that doesn't feel good.' And it made me feel like I was being re-traumatized or reliving the situation by the fact that I was trying to get help and trying to get out of this situation, and she was just sort of like, 'well, you're the one that chose.'"
Ignoring their need for safety	"Let us know we're safe. Take us to a safe place. If they see what's happening, bring us somewhere. Try to get us away from the abuser, even if they're sitting right outside. Let them know that it's okay, [and] we can get you out safely."

(continued)

Table 22-2. Testimonials from NA/AI Survivors of Violence[20] *(continued)*

MISTAKES	NA/AI VOICES
Not respecting their autonomy/ self-sovereignty	"I actually wanted to report the abuse, but they didn't take me seriously. The police saw that there was drinking going on and judged me. They didn't take my injuries or anything seriously. They would make me leave for the night and cool down and let my abuser stay, and they never arrested him because I would fight back, or they didn't believe me. I didn't get justice."
Trivializing and minimizing abuse	"I did call the police a few times after abuse. A lot of it was when I was intoxicated. They didn't take my injuries or anything seriously. They would make me leave for the night and cool down and let my abuser stay, and they never arrested him because I would fight back, or they didn't believe me."
Missed opportunities for screening or provide resources	"Try to get us away from the abuser, even if they're sitting right outside. The nurse asked me if I felt safe while my abuser was sitting next to me. I couldn't say no, and I wanted to."

© *Dr. Jeneile Luebke (2020) Used with permission*

Providing survivor-led care means that forensic nurses acknowledge that survivors are the experts in what they need. Forensic nurses can do this by:

— Offering culturally specific resources when available, especially advocacy services

— Providing humanistic care (respect and non-judgement)

— Listening attentively

— Respecting confidentiality

— Promoting access to needed services for common health issues, such as mental health disorders or substance misuse

— Helping in safety planning

— Respecting autonomy (self-sovereignty)

— Believing and validating survivor experiences

— Acknowledging the injustice of what happened

To further advocate for this population, nurses and other health care providers can contact their legislators to include tribal nation jurisdiction in the Violence Against Women Act. While the Act was reauthorized on March 16, 2022, the current iteration of the legislation only covers cases of rape, and it does not include Alaska Native or Inuit people. The 2022 VAWA authorization contains a provision to establish a pilot program for NA/AI tribes to exercise "Special Domestic Violence Criminal Jurisdiction," which recognizes the authority of tribes to exercise criminal jurisdiction over non-Natives who commit certain crimes (stalking, domestic violence, and sexual assault) against a Native victim on tribal land. The pilot is limited to five tribes initially, with additional five tribes added each year.[21] Health care providers do not need to wait for federal legislation to be more compassionate. Better state and local policies are a means of providing better care, and having culturally-responsive Brown, Black, or Indigenous People of Color (BIPOC) advocates helps ensure ongoing communication and collaborative partnerships with local tribes. Navigating local systems with this lens will benefit all communities without compromising the ethics of the forensic nurse as a witness.

CASE STUDIES

Case Study 22-1

A teenage NA/AI girl and her aunt fought, so the girl left the house in a huff. A truck of non-Native men stopped and pulled the girl into their truck. She fought but was held down and raped. The men later discarded her in a ditch, where she was found by her brothers, who brought her to the IHS for post-rape care. The forensic nurse asked the teen if she wanted her aunt in the room with them. She shook her head "no," but her aunt stated loudly that she wanted her to take pills to avoid pregnancy. The forensic nurse explained that with the teen's permission, she would share information after the evaluation, and the aunt was asked to leave. When they were alone, the forensic nurse asked the girl about her desire to participate in the medical-forensic evaluation. When she said yes, the forensic nurse explained the evaluation process and gave her permission to decline any service. The teen said she understood. Understanding the need for *kinship practices,* the forensic nurse confirmed that the teen did not want her aunt in the room, but the teen changed her mind, asking for her aunt as her support person. The forensic nurse then invited the aunt to return.

Discussion

The initial establishment of safety and trust allowed the patient to direct her own care. This set the stage for the teen to return to her cultural kinship beliefs and invite her aunt back in on the process. The key is for forensic nurses to respect the patient's lived experience and personal interpretation of *kinship practices* without judgement. In any forensic nurse/patient relationship, special care is taken to respect all cultures without judgement and begin the medical forensic evaluation by implementing trauma-informed care. The time taken to establish aunt-niece connections will have benefits long after the survivor returns home.

SUMMARY

Centuries of European colonialization in the Americas resulted in a number of detriments for the NA/AI population, including disease exposure, forced termination and assimilation, eugenic reproductive policies, and legislative divestment of treaties between sovereign nations. Today, the NA/AI population continues to experience higher rates of rape and disappearance among women, drug and alcohol abuse, and issues with reservation, local, and federal jurisdictions. Forensic nurses have a responsibility to listen to NA/AI voices, recognize their historical and current traumas, and use trauma-informed care to create safe spaces for expressing traumatic experiences and facilitating kinship practices.

REFERENCES

1. Brave Heart MYH. The return to the sacred path: reflections on the development of historical trauma healing. Indian Health Service. Accessed February 2, 2022. https://www.ihs.gov/sites/telebehavioral/themes/responsive2017/display_objects/documents/slides/historicaltrauma/htreturnsacredpath0513.pdf

2. Dictionary: Colonization. Oxford University Press. Accessed February 2, 2022. https://www.oxfordlearnersdictionaries.com/us/definition/english/colonization

3. Hixson WL. American settler colonialism: a history. *J Am Hist.* 2015;101(4): 1227-1228. doi:10.1093/jahist/jav042

4. Yu H, Spyrou MA, Karapetian M, et al. Paleolithic to Bronze Age Siberians reveal connections with first Americans and across Eurasia. *Cell.* 2020;181(6):1232-1245.e20. doi:10.1016/j.cell.2020.04.037

5. Dunn MG. Exploring your world: the adventure of geography. National Geographic Society. Updated September 20, 2011. Accessed February 2, 2022. https://web.archive.org/web/20190716045120/https://www.nationalgeographic.org/encyclopedia/continent/

6. Denevan WM. *The Native Population of the Americas in 1492.* 2nd ed. University of Wisconsin Press; 1992.

7. Estimated Indigenous populations of the Americas at the time of European contact, beginning in 1492. Statista. January 1, 1983. Accessed June 9, 2022. https://www.statista.com/statistics/1171896/pre-colonization-population-americas/

8. Dunbar-Ortiz R. *An Indigenous Peoples' History of the United States*. Beacon Press; 2015.

9. Smith DM. Counting the dead: estimating the loss of life in the Indigenous Holocaust, 1492-present. 2017. Accessed June 9, 2022. https://www.se.edu/native-american/wp-content/uploads/sites/49/2019/09/A-NAS-2017-Proceedings-Smith.pdf

10. Carlisle Indian School Digital Resource Center. Dickinson College. Accessed June 9, 2022. https://carlisleindian.dickinson.edu/

11. Mejia M. The US history of Native American boarding schools. The Indigenous Foundation. Accessed June 9, 2022. https://www.theindigenousfoundation.org/articles/us-residential-schools

12. 1897: Indian boarding schools teach manual labor. National Library of Medicine. Accessed June 9, 2022. https://www.nlm.nih.gov/nativevoices/timeline/385.html

13. Rykken P. Bridging the divide: First Nations history at Black River Falls High School. Wisconsin First Nations. Accessed June 9, 2022. https://wisconsinfirstnations.org/wp-content/uploads/2017/08/Rykken-Bridging-the-Divide.pdf

14. Greensmith H. Best interests: how child welfare serves as a tool of white supremacy. Public Eye. Updated November 26, 2019. Accessed February 2, 2022. https://politicalresearch.org/2019/11/26/best-interests-how-child-welfare-serves-tool-white-supremacy

15. Missing and murdered Indigenous people US Department of the Interior Indian Affairs. Accessed June 9, 2022. https://www.bia.gov/service/mmu/missing-and-murdered-indigenous-people-crisis

16. Rosay A. Violence against American Indian and Alaska Native women and men. *NIJ*. 2016;(277):38-45.

17. Rutecki GW. Forced sterilization of Native Americans: later twentieth century cooperation with national eugenic policies. *Ethics Med*. 2011;27(1):33-42.

18. Kennedy EJ. On Indigenous Peoples Day, recalling forced sterilizations of Native American women. MinnPost Newsroom. Updated October 14, 2019. Accessed February 2, 2022. https://www.minnpost.com/community-voices/2019/10/on-indigenous-peoples-day-recalling-forced-sterilizations-of-native-american-women/

19. Daniel R. Since you asked: what data exists about Native American people in the criminal justice system? Prison Policy Initiative. April 22, 2020. Accessed February 2, 2022. https://www.prisonpolicy.org/blog/2020/04/22/native/

20. Luebke JM. Intimate Partner Violence in the Lives of Urban American Indian Women: A Continuation of Colonial Injustice. Theses and Dissertations. University of Wisconsin; 2020. https://dc.uwm.edu/etd/2554

21. Hagen D. New provision of Violence Against Women Act empowers tribal jurisdiction. Alaska Public Media. March 28, 2022. Accessed August 2, 2022. https://alaskapublic.org/2022/03/28/new-provision-of-violence-against-women-act-empowers-tribal-jurisdiction/

Chapter 23

Sexual and Gender Diversity in Patients

Ecoee Rooney, DNP, RN, AFN-C, SANE-A, DF-AFN
Diana K. Faugno, MSN, RN, CPN, AFN-C, SANE-A, SANE-P, FAAFS, DF-IAFN, DF-AFN

Key Points

1. *Trauma-informed care principles actively create safe environments for sexually and gender diverse (SGD) patients, with transparent processes that allow for the development of trustworthiness, peer support, and mutual self-help.*

2. *Health care providers must maintain unconditional positive regard for SGD patients and their health care needs by using trauma-informed principles to establish a positive healing environment.*

3. *Recognize that persons who identify as SGD who are victims of sexual violence or intimate partner violence (IPV) often hesitate to access survivor resources due to negative historical encounters with professionals, lack of services sensitive to their identities, and out of fear of revictimization due to heterocentric structures.*

Introduction

Sexuality is a part of being human. ***Sexual orientation*** is an enduring emotional, romantic, sexual, or affectional attraction to another person. Sexual orientation can be a fluid concept, and people may use a variety of terms to describe their sexual orientation.[1] Sexuality refers to the combination of one's biological sex, sexual orientation, sexual practices, and gender identity.[2] Historically, the sexes were socially controlled through various institutions in efforts to "protect" individuals and society from the perils of sexual variety and expression. Religion characterizes some forms of sexuality as sinful, the legal system has criminalized certain sexual behaviors, and the medical community medicalized certain forms of sexual variety and expression, namely homosexuality,[3] as a disease or an illness.[2] However, social attitudes recently changed to encompass a wider range of sexual diversity. For example, the American Psychiatric Association removed the diagnosis of homosexuality as a mental disorder from its manual in 1973.[1]

Sexual identity politics exposed the social and political inequalities of a heterosexist society by focusing on equality rights for LGBTQIA+ individuals (ie, those that identify as lesbian, gay, bisexual, transgender, queer, or another gender or sexual identity). The civil rights movement for LGBTQIA+ rights experienced success over the past 70 years in mobilizing efforts to change discrimination on the basis of sexual orientation and gender diversity, deem sodomy laws unconstitutional, ensure domestic partner benefits, and obtain civil unions and same-sex marriage rights. Such political and social success, in part, is through the community-wide efforts of the LGTBQIA+ population, their allies, and organizations such as the American Civil Liberties Union and the Human Rights Campaign. In this chapter, the authors will refer to the LGBTQIA+ population by using the term ***sexually and gender diverse (SGD)***.

In 2015, the US Supreme Court ruling in Obergefell v Hodges[4] extended marriage equality for same-sex couples in the United States. In 2020, the Supreme Court ruled in Bostock v Clayton County[5] that the prohibition of sex discrimination in Title VII of the Civil Rights Act protects people from discrimination based on sexual orientation and gender identity in employment. Many states, local governments, and private organizations expanded protections in workplaces, health care settings, and schools to include sexual orientation and gender identity as protected statuses.[1]

An overwhelming amount of sexual assault research focuses on heterosexual victims (usually female) and heterosexual perpetrators (usually male).[2,6] Yet, studies indicate that SGD individuals report significantly higher lifetime rates of sexual victimization than heterosexual persons.[6] There are 2 main issues to address in terms of sexual assault and violence within a SGD context. First, sexual assault continues to be the most underreported of all violent crimes, and this is even truer for SGD victims given the social stigma surrounding their identities.[6] Second, the justice and service structures designed to address sexual crimes are heterocentric structures. Many patients report experiencing judgment, hostility, or prejudice from service providers and legal representatives.[7] Moreover, the failure of the legal system to prosecute crime in the SGD community creates doubt and lowers expectations about justice being served for this population.[7]

Sexual assault has become a more prominent concern for health care professionals to address over the past several decades. In 2006, Tarana Burke,[8] an Alabama activist, first used the phrase "Me Too" in regards to surviving sexual violence. This phrase was popularized in 2017 with the emergence of the #MeToo movement among primarily cisgender women. However, discussion regarding sexual violence within SGD communities remains relatively misunderstood.[2,3,6] This is due, in part, to the marginalization of SGD communities in general, the history of SGD criminal justice suppression, and the result of misconceptions about prevalence and lack of information and resources for SGD victims.

Trauma-Informed Care

When providing care to SGD populations, the nurse should focus on recognizing the context of the patient's experience, as SGD persons may have experienced previous sexual trauma.[6] Trauma as a universal experience is the underpinning concept for trauma-informed care; trauma informs all future experiences. There are 6 overriding principles that frame trauma-informed care: safety; trustworthiness and transparency; peer support; collaboration and mutuality; empowerment and choice; and sensitivity to cultural, historical, and gender issues.[9]

Health care practitioners also need to be mindful of the possibility that members of the SGD community have previously experienced trauma by other medical or law enforcement professionals. This may include the patient being judged, labeled, misunderstood, misheard, "othered," or having their lived experiences diminished or ridiculed within the health care or justice systems. Ensuring that all patients receive trauma-informed care that is specifically focused on their needs and perceptions is essential. Depending on the SGD patient experience, nurses can begin building trust by trying to understand their patients better and providing unconditional positive regard to each person they serve. This practice creates a safe environment wherein the nurse can facilitate rapport with patients, allowing them to feel more comfortable sharing difficult information that is necessary for them to receive services and care.

Case Studies

Case Study 23-1

This 18-year-old man, recently came out as gay to his family and friends. They have all been loving and supportive of him since coming out. He worked the night shift at his father's manufacturing business. One night, 4 of his classmates from high school were driving by and recognized him while he was walking to work. One guy yelled "Hey, faggot," as the car went by. Shortly after, the car turned around and the group backtracked toward him. All 4 men got out of the car, grabbed him, and dragged him behind a secluded row of trees near the factory. They took turns repeatedly sexually assaulting him, both orally and anally, before leaving him semi-conscious in the grass, naked and bleeding from his anus. A jogger found him a few hours later and called the police. The officers who arrived on the scene talked back and forth in low tones, and one officer said to the other, "Looks like what happened here is this one got taught a lesson."

Discussion

In this scenario, the patient experienced extreme trauma but received a non-trauma-informed and judgmental response from the first responders. He should have received trauma-informed and compassionate care from the first responders before being brought to the designated location for medical forensic examinations in the town. With the patient's consent, the sexual assault nurse examiner would have provided the forensic examination and treatment for his injuries, including relevant prophylaxis for sexually transmitted infections (depending on his risk and current recommendations from the Centers for Disease Control and Prevention). A medical advocate, trained in providing supportive mental health first aid to patients who have been sexually assaulted, would respond to the hospital as well. This advocate would have connected the patient with support in navigating the legal system so he did not become revictimized in the process of receiving services. He then would have been given a case number in order to work with the district attorney assigned to his case, as he would most likely want to press charges against his perpetrators since he had the full support of his family. The first responders (in this case, law enforcement) were judgmental, which made the patient feel unsafe in disclosing the details of the assault. If the patient were to be revictimized in the future, he would unlikely to disclose his assault due to negative experience with the justice system.

Case Study 23-2

This 35-year-old lesbian woman, had been living with her 37-year-old partner of 7 years, in a small Florida community. When the couple first started going out, they frequently engaged in sex with one another until around 5 years ago, when their sexual activity began to taper off. The younger woman was a local musician who played guitar at area coffee shops on the evenings and weekends, and lately had become more occupied with her music and spent less time with her partner. One night, her partner had a few glasses of wine while out with her friends and came home late to find her asleep in their bed. The partner undressed, got under the covers, and began to put her hand in between the younger woman's legs. She awoke and told her partner that she was not in the mood and encouraged her to sleep on the sofa instead. Her partner continued to move her hand up towards her vagina before holding her down while she penetrated her with her fingers. She cried out in pain and begged her partner to stop, yelling "no," several times, but her partner pushed harder. She tried to get out from under her partner, but she could not free herself from her hold. She stopped resisting and laid there, waiting until her partner pulled out her hand and passed out next to her. The next morning, she felt like what had happened was wrong, but did not know what to do or who to talk with. Since the two had been together, nothing like that had happened, and she had only ever heard of sexual assault happening with men as perpetrators.

Discussion

She knew she had experienced something traumatic and wished to report her experience, but she was unsure of where to go. Due to the heteronormative response to sexual assault and biases in many health care services, she was unsure if she would be taken seriously if she disclosed her assault. She also worried that if she was believed, her partner could potentially be sent to jail. Additionally, she did not even know what resources were available to her and did not identify herself as being a victim of IPV. If she were to present for a forensic evaluation, a trauma-informed response would be necessary during her examination. An advocate could support her in understanding IPV in the context of her relationship and inform her of her rights and available services. If she wanted to quickly exit the relationship by moving into a domestic violence shelter, she could also be at risk of being placed in a location where her partner, another woman, could ostensibly pose as a victim to gain access to her. The shelter would need to understand her circumstances and be equipped to keep patients safe in all types of circumstances. Overall, her experience illustrates the isolation many members of the LGBTQIA+ community experience when they need to intersect with the medical, law enforcement, and legal systems.

Case Study 23-3

This 22-year-old pansexual person, met a 23-year-old on an online dating site. Both individuals are nonbinary. On their second date, the older of the two suggested they go to a local bar for a few drinks before heading back to their place. After the bar, the two were lying on the bed, holding hands and kissing, when the date unbuttoned their jeans before moving their head down to perform oral sex. They tried to pull away from their date, insisting they were not ready for sex and just wanted to keep making out. Their date said they did not believe them because their penis was clearly erect. They firmly said "no," but their date held their waist down and placed their mouth on their penis. They pushed their date away, quickly grabbed their clothing, and then left. They were frustrated, angry, and visibly upset as they felt violated but did not know what to do. They thought, "If I tell my friends, they are going to assume I wanted it."

Discussion

They felt unsure about how to handle being assaulted by their date. They were afraid that they would not be taken seriously due to biases surrounding nonbinary identities and stereotypes about pansexual people having a high drive for sexual interaction. They could have contacted the local authorities to report their date, but they were concerned about facing potential bias from law enforcement and receiving limited support from health care providers, as reporting the assault would require describing the details of their sexual encounter. They also assumed the police probably would not understand their nonbinary identity and would misgender them. A trauma-informed response is needed to support them in navigating the medicolegal system and in receiving a nonjudgmental post-assault evaluation and follow-up services.

SUMMARY

Sexuality includes a diverse array of orientations, desires, behaviors, identities, and genders. To provide trauma-informed care, health care professionals must understand the SGD community's mistrust of heterocentric systems and that sex crimes in these populations are systematically underreported, misunderstood, and judged. Providing open, unconditional positive regard for each patient allows for a constructive partnership that promotes the SGD patient's understanding of their care and options. The forensic nurse must ensure a strong, positive, and caring relationship that results in positive outcomes for all persons in their care.

REFERENCES

1. National Academies of Sciences, Engineering, and Medicine. Understanding the Well-Being of LGBTQI+ Populations. The National Academies Press. 2020. https://www.nationalacademies.org/news/2020/07/understanding-the-well-being-of-lgbtqi-populations

2. Ison J. It's not just men and women: LGBTQIA people and #MeToo. In: Fileborn B, Loney-Howes R, eds. *#MeToo and the Politics of Social Change.* Palgrave Macmillan; 2019.

3. Young E, Salton R, Estes H. Public Perceptions of #MeToo Gay Male Sexual Assault Disclosure: A Qualitative Content Analysis of Facebook Comments. Western Libraries Undergraduate Research Award. 2020. https://cedar.wwu.edu/library_researchaward/21

4. Obergefell v Hodges, 576 US 544, 665-70 (2015).

5. Bostock v Clayton County, Georgia, 140 S Ct 1731, 17-1618 (2020).

6. Calton JM, Cattaneo LB, Gebhard KT. Barriers to help seeking for lesbian, gay, bisexual, transgender, and queer survivors of intimate partner violence. *Trauma Violence Abuse.* 2016;17(5):585-600. doi:10.1177/1524838015585318

7. Ronan W. New FBI Hate Crimes Report Shows Increases in Anti-LGBTQ Attacks. Human Rights Campaign. 2020. https://www.hrc.org/press-releases/new-fbi-hate-crimes-report-shows-increases-in-anti-lgbtq-attacks

8. Garcia SE. The Woman Who Created #MeToo Long before Hashtags. The New York Times. October 20, 2017. Accessed May 9, 2022. https://www.nytimes.com/2017/10/20/us/me-too-movement-tarana-burke.html

9. Substance Abuse and Mental Health Services Administration. SAMHSA's Concept of Trauma and Guidance for a Trauma-Informed Approach. Substance Abuse and Mental Health Services Administration. July 2014. https://scholarworks.boisestate.edu/cgi/viewcontent.cgi?article=1006&context=covid

ADDITIONAL RESOURCES

The following are resources that can be helpful to individuals seeking to learn more about the LGBTQIA+ populations through understanding terms, definitions, and context:

— University of Florida, LGBTQ+ Affairs. LGBTQ Terms and Definitions. Available at: https://lgbtq.multicultural.ufl.edu/programs/speakersbureau/lgbtq-terms-definitions/

— UC Berkeley Gender Equity Resource Center. Definition of Terms. Available at: https://cejce.berkeley.edu/geneq/resources/lgbtq-resources/definition-terms

Chapter 24

PERSONS WITH DISABILITIES

Ruth Downing, MSN, RN, CNP, SANE-A
Laura Kaiser, MBA, BSN, RN, SANE-A

KEY POINTS

1. *Trauma-informed care is a core competency for all forensic nurses, requiring implementation with persons who experience ability challenges.*

2. *Person-first language (PFL) is a core competency for forensic nurses when referring to all people, especially persons experiencing challenging disabilities.*

3. *People are not their diagnosis, nor do they need to be objectified by their condition or assistive devices.*

4. *Providers should encourage people with disabilities to play an active role in their care, to their ability.*

INTRODUCTION

When discussing disabilities, it is important to note that placing people into separate categories is not always an easy task. This is due to the complexities and co-existences within each type of disability. Patients with disabilities experience violent victimization at twice the rate of those without a disability.[1] This is due to increased dependability on internal and external resources to meet ongoing personal needs. This chapter will briefly review several types of disabilities and how to apply nursing practice in providing appropriate holistic care.

LEGISLATION: AMERICANS WITH DISABILITIES ACT

The Americans with Disabilities Act (ADA) is a civil rights act that went into effect in 1990 and prohibits discrimination against individuals with disabilities in all areas of public life. This includes jobs, schools, transportation, and all public and privately owned places that are available to the public. To be protected by the ADA, a person must have a disability, which is defined by the ADA as a physical or mental impairment that substantially limits one or more major life activities, a person who has a history or record of such an impairment, or a person who is perceived by others as having such an impairment.[2]

TYPES OF DISABILITIES

DEVELOPMENTAL

A ***developmental disability*** is a severe, chronic disability that is attributable to a mental or physical impairment or a combination of mental and physical impairments of an individual 5 years of age or older.[1] Ability deficits are usually manifested before age 22 and are likely to continue indefinitely. However, older adults with medical conditions experience reduction in developmental abilities as they age.[3] There must be a substantial functional limitation in at least 3 of the following areas of major life activity, as appropriate for the person's age: self-care, receptive and expressive language, learning, mobility, self-direction, capacity for independent living, and capacity for economic self-sufficiency. Examples of a developmental disability include, but are not limited to, autism, spina bifida, cerebral palsy, hearing loss, fetal alcohol syndrome, and dementia. Patients across the lifespan may have speech and language issues that require the use of communication devices. Some orthopedic impairments include the absence of limbs, paralysis, and spinal cord damage.

INTELLECTUAL

The World Health Organization defines ***intellectual disabilities*** as conditions that start prior to adulthood and significantly decrease the person's ability to comprehend new or complex information, with reduced ability to learn or apply new skills.[4] Patients will have significantly subaverage intellectual functioning existing concurrently with deficiencies in adaptive behavior. These are manifested during the developmental period and across the lifespan, and the decline may be progressive. Some examples of congenital intellectual disabilities include Down syndrome, Fragile X syndrome, speech, and language problems. Some extend into aging populations and worsen as disease progresses.[3] Patients tend to know their own abilities, so avoid statements like "He functions at the level of a 5-year-old," as there is variation with 5-year-old children's developmental abilities. Patients may have issues with social skills, including interpersonal skills, social problem-solving abilities, and following rules.

PHYSICAL

A ***physical disability*** is a condition that affects a person's mobility, physical capacity, stamina, or dexterity.[1] A physical disability may include structural or functional impairments. Examples of a physical disability include brain or spinal cord injuries, amputations, and arthritis.

Accommodations may be needed when conducting an examination on a patient with a physical disability. Additional space is necessary to accommodate assistive devices such as walkers, splints, and artificial limbs. If the patient requires the use of a wheelchair, an adjustable table allows for transfer from their wheelchair to the examination table. A wheelchair or assistive device is a part of the person, so ask the patient's permission prior to touching or moving the devices. The forensic nursing lens considers that evidence may exist on accessibility devices or prosthetics worn by the patient. Obtain permission to swab devices from the patient prior to collecting evidence.

SENSORY

Sensory impairments affect one or more senses. They occur across the lifespan and may also affect how a person gathers information because a reduction or loss of one or more senses may result in communication difficulties. Examples of sensory impairments include blindness, sensory processing disorder, hearing impairment or loss, macular degeneration, and nystagmus. When an individual has a visual impairment or is blind, avoid flickering lights, as they can be distracting. During introductions, describe your appearance as well as those present for the examination, and provide a description of the examination room. Communication in discharge paperwork must include all accommodations such as large print and plain language or pictures.

Persons who are congenitally deaf consider their experience a culture with a unique language. When communicating with a patient who is deaf, the use of an interpreter that communicates using sign language is essential.[5] For those who are hard of hearing, always face and speak to the patient, not the interpreter. Lip reading will be impossible if the nurse is wearing a mask. Speak slowly and clearly without background noise. Communicate using plain language and known terms to ensure understanding. It may be necessary to repeat and rephrase statements. Use written communication if preferred by the patient, but validate that the patient can read, realizing that many develop considerable skills at hiding their ability deficits.

MENTAL HEALTH

Mental illness is a substantial disorder of thought, mood, perception, orientation, or memory that grossly impairs judgment, behavior, and capacity to recognize reality or ability to meet the ordinary demands of life. Some examples are attention deficit disorder, anxiety disorder, depression, obsessive compulsive disorder, bipolar disorder, and schizophrenia.

Patients with adverse childhood experiences may develop mental health disorders. When exposed to violence, mental health problems persist. The long-term effects include substance abuse, anxiety disorder, suicidal behavior, posttraumatic stress disorder, and other disabilities.[6] When assessing the patient's ability to complete an evaluation when they have mental health sequelae, it is important to implement trauma-informed care, which includes creating a safe environment and continually seeking permission to proceed. The patient's baseline should be assessed at every visit as the environment or life changes may affect the patient's needs. Is the patient able to relay information? Is the patient able to make decisions? If the answer is yes, continue with that portion of the evaluation. If the answer is no, discuss concerns with the patient and inform their treatment team. If the patient is displaying an elevated level of anxiety, the generalist forensic nurse should refer to the emergency department physician, as a medical intervention may be necessary.

MEDICAL FORENSIC CONSIDERATIONS

COMMUNICATION

Forensic nurses need to use trauma-informed care principles in all communication forms. Patients with disabilities may not identify as having a disability due to the stigma from society. Like other oppressed groups, those with disabilities have a long history of being pitied and feared by the dominating society.[7] When caring for a patient with disabilities, the generalist forensic nurse should assess for health literacy and use plain language when conversing with the patient. The nurse completing the evaluation should be identified as a "forensic nurse," not "a SANE," as those unfamiliar with the acronym may mistake it as an implication of stigmatization, indicating an assessment of mental health stability.[1]

PERSON-FIRST LANGUAGE

PFL is a core competency for forensic nurses, measurable in practices. PFL focuses on the person over the disability. When determining how to address patients, it is best to ask them how they identify and prefer to be addressed. Patients with ability challenges know that their disability does not control or define them. PFL examples include stating, "Jane has a mental health condition" or "Tony has a disability." On the other hand, identity-first language (IFL) emphasizes the person's disability or condition first (eg, "the crippled person" or "the CABG in room 6"). Practicing PFL includes stating the name of the person first, and then if necessary, describe their ability. For instance: "Steven is deaf," "Sara is blind," or "Tommy has autism." **Table 24-1** contains examples of PFL and IFL that forensic nurses may encounter.[1]

Table 24-1. Tips and Examples of Person-First Language and Identity-First Language[8]		
TIPS	USE	AVOID
Emphasize abilities, not limitations.	Person who uses a wheelchair	Confined or restricted to a wheelchair, wheelchair bound
	Person who uses a device to speak	Can't talk, mute
Do not use language that suggests the lack of something.	Person with a disability	Disabled, handicapped
	Person of short stature	Midget
	Person with cerebral palsy	Cerebral palsy victim *(continued)*

Table 24-1. Tips and Examples of Person-First Language and Identity-First Language[8] *(continued)*

Tips	Use	Avoid
Do not use language that suggests the lack of something. *(continued)*	Person with epilepsy or seizure disorder	Epileptic
	Person with multiple sclerosis	Afflicted by multiple sclerosis
Emphasize the need for accessibility, not the disability.	Accessible parking or bathroom	Handicapped parking or bathroom
Do not use offensive language.	Person with a physical disability	Crippled, lame, deformed, invalid, spastic
	Person with an intellectual, cognitive or developmental disability	Slow, simple, moronic, defective, afflicted, special person
	Person with an emotional or behavioral disability, a mental health impairment, or a psychiatric disability	Insane, crazy, psycho, maniac, nuts
Avoid language that implies negative stereotypes.	Person without a disability	Normal, healthy person
Do not portray people with disabilities as inspirational only because of their disability.	Person who is successful, productive	Has overcome their disability, is courageous

ADAPTIVE TECHNIQUES

Persons with disabilities use adaptive techniques to provide developmentally specific care or assistance, such as wheelchairs, lifts, standing frames, gait trainers, augmentative communication devices, bath chairs, and recreational items such as swings or tricycles. Ask the patient or their support person about the use of any communication device. There are several forms of communicative options, and forensic nurses may use an interpreter service according to facility policies. Communication devices include voice output devices, electronic communication devices, augmentative devices, alternative communication devices, letter boards, hearing aids, facial expressions, hand, or body gestures, use of pictures, picture exchange communication systems, handwritten communication, large print, and braille. Due to the length of time needed to conduct medical forensic evaluations, provide the patient access to charging outlets for their communication devices.

Often, including patients in a medical forensic evaluation, such as allowing them to explore the equipment that will be used, is the first step to establishing a safe environment. Adaptation with continual validation for consent during the medical forensic examination provides trauma-informed care, allowing the patient to direct activities after validation. Oftentimes, a person with significant communication ability challenges uses their facial expressions to communicate through their guardian. These are complex situations that require the forensic nurse to explain to the guardian and then turn to the patient to seek permission to proceed. Forensic nurses use ethics to ensure autonomy in decision-making and ongoing consent during the examination.

OBTAINING CONSENT FOR THE MEDICAL FORENSIC EXAMINATION

Generalist forensic nurses are not qualified to determine if a patient is competent to provide consent for a medical forensic evaluation because "competency" is a legal definition established by the courts. If not revoked by a court proceeding, the law presumes a person has the competence for self-determination. Advanced forensic nursing providers, after extensive assessments and considering co-morbidities, make recommendations to the court to inform their final ruling determining competency. "Capacity," on the other hand, is fluid and fluctuates with factors such as change in medication, illness, or infection.[3] A patient's capacity to consent for the medical forensic examination is determined by a clinician. This is based on the patient's ability to demonstrate specific knowledge of the tasks to be completed and their understanding of the risks and benefits, which are discussed with the patient before signatures. Communication needs should not be mistaken for diminished capacity.[1] The forensic nurse needs to locate the patient's power of attorney (POA) or guardian if the person lacks capacity. People with disabilities have a right to decline any portion of an examination even if a POA or guardian is involved.

DISCHARGE INSTRUCTIONS

A coordinated community response to crime includes wraparound services for the patient. The generalist forensic nurse coordinates discharge and communicates directly with the patient as well as with any agencies providing ongoing care. An analysis using a standardized tool to determine the patient's risk of further abuse is necessary before discharge.[9] Questions to consider include: Will the patient be returning home with family or friends? Is this a safe environment? Further considerations include whether the patient has access to appropriate community resources, transportation to see their current mental health provider, and community advocacy. Access to ongoing medical and mental health care is necessary, and seeking permission for referrals creates a warm handoff, ensuring care for mental health issues.

REPORTING

Forensic nurses are mandated reporters and cannot refer to the provider with a 'suspicion' of abuse. Another aspect of abuse evaluation requires following state and local mandatory reporting laws when vulnerable adults are in danger or a danger to themselves (eg, suicide or homicide ideation). Health care facilities have policies related to reporting to law enforcement, child protective services, adult protective services, and state or county disability services. For the purposes of this chapter, a list of state organizations can be found on the National Association of State Directors of Developmental Disabilities Services website.[10]

CASE STUDIES

Case Study 24-1

A 26-year-old patient with Down syndrome arrived to a facility with her caregiver. She reported that she had been sexually assaulted. She sat on an examination table and began watching cartoons while holding a teddy bear. She was talking to the teddy bear about the cartoon. Meanwhile, a victim advocate was also sitting in the room. The advocate spoke to the forensic nurse about having difficulty communicating with the patient, and she stated that she tried to explain the examination process without success.

Discussion

The forensic nurse completing the patient's sexual assault examination spoke to the caregiver that arrived with the patient. They discussed the patient's abilities, including the best way to communicate, how prior successful medical examinations were conducted, and any additional information that may be helpful when planning for the examination. The forensic nurse made sure to communicate using language that was familiar to the patient. The forensic nurse explained the use of equipment and allowed the patient to hold the swabs and use them on her teddy bear. The patient wanted her caregiver to hold her hand during the anogenital exam. The accommodation was made as requested, giving her control of her environment, and the forensic nurse made sure to frequently check back with her about the process. The sexual assault was reported to law enforcement as well as other required organizations.

SUMMARY

People with disabilities have increased vulnerability to victimization due to their dependence on others for physical care, financial support, communication, or protection. Forensic nurses have an opportunity to understand the diverse types of disabilities, accommodations, and modes of communication available. In doing so, the forensic nurse will be able to provide trauma-informed care to this patient population, according to the patient's unique needs and abilities.

REFERENCES

1. Downing R, Kaiser L. A forensic nurse examiner's guide to caring for patients with disabilities. Adult Advocacy Centers. 2020. https://www.adultadvocacycenters. org/assets/documents/aacs_forensic_nurse_examiner_guide.pdf

2. Americans with Disabilities Act of 1990. Accessed May 5, 2022. https://www. ada.gov/

3. Speck PM, Baker N. Case series for the LNC: Assessing risk for elder abuse using the decision matrix for elder safety (DMES). *J Leg Nurs Consul.* 2021;32(2): 36-42. https://view.flipdocs.com/?ID=10004296_437846

4. Fisher K, Robichaux C, Sauerland J, Stokes F. A nurses' ethical commitment to people with intellectual and developmental disabilities. *Nurs Ethics.* 2020;27(4):1066-1076. doi:10.1177/0969733019900310

5. Admire A, Ramirez B. Violence and disability: Experiences and perceptions of victimization among deaf people. *J Interpers Violence.* 2021;36(1-2):NP1-NP25. doi:10.1177/0886260517730564

6. Curry SJ, Krist AH, Owens DK, et al. Screening for intimate partner violence, elder abuse, and abuse of vulnerable adults. *JAMA.* 2018;320(16):1678-1687. doi:10.1001/jama.2018.14741

7. Dosch R. Resisting normal: Questioning media depictions of autistic youth and their families. *Scand J Disabil Res.* 2019;21(1):150-157. doi:10.16993/sjdr.56

8. People First Language. Office of Disability Rights. July 2006. Accessed May 5, 2022. https://odr.dc.gov/page/people-first-language

9. Okoro CA, Hollis ND, Cyrus AC, Griffin-Blake S. Prevalence of disabilities and health care access by disability status and type among adults—United States, 2016. *Morb Mortal Wkly Rep.* 2018;67:882-887. doi:10.15585/mmwr. mm6732a3l

10. State agencies. National Association of State Directors of Developmental Disabilities Services (NASDDDS). Updated February 16, 2022. https://www. nasddds.org/state-agencies/

Chapter 25

MALE SEXUAL ASSAULT

Diana K. Faugno, MSN, RN, CPN, AFN-C, SANE-A, SANE-P, FAAFS, DF-IAN, DF-AFN
Stacey A. Mitchell, DNP, MBA, MEd, RN, AFN-C, SANE-A, SANE-P, DF-AFN, FAAN

KEY POINTS

1. *Nearly 1 in 4 men in the United States experience sexual violence, typically at the age of 18 or younger.*

2. *Male victims are less likely than other assault victims to seek care within 24 hours of the assault, leading to a delay in care and reporting.*

3. *Forensic nurses should understand the common barriers to reporting, the best medical practices for male assault victims, and the trauma-informed approach to care.*

INTRODUCTION

According to the National Sexual Violence Resource Center,[1] 1 in 4 men will be sexually assaulted during his lifetime. It is difficult to accurately ascertain statistics about male sexual violence, as it is vastly underreported. Until 2012, the legal definition of rape applied only to females. With the definition's expansion to include men, it is anticipated the number of reports of sexual assault and rape will increase.

Men who experience sexual violence have specific needs related to medical care, evidence collection, follow-up, and referrals. Unfortunately, health care providers are often unaware of these needs, resulting in the provision of fewer services and a general lack of knowledge about the issue. Forensic nurses should understand the intricacies of male sexual assault, including barriers to reporting and methods to ensure comprehensive and compassionate care.

FACTORS AND BARRIERS IMPACTING REPORTING

Male sexual assault often goes unreported, due in part to a stereotypical belief that men cannot be victims of sexual violence.[2] Other barriers to reporting include:

— Shame

— Guilt

— Embarrassment

— Concerns over confidentiality

— Fear of unsuccessful prosecution

— Fear of being perceived as homosexual

Men who are sexually assaulted may experience erections and ejaculation during the forced sexual contact and may believe they unconsciously enjoyed the assault. Others may struggle with the belief that reporting is "unmasculine" and the myth that "real men" cannot be raped. Some believe that males cannot be raped by females, another myth that feeds into barriers to reporting.

Men are vulnerable to assault by both men and women. In 2015, Williams and Bierie[3] studied the differences between male and female sex offenders; unfortunately, data regarding females assaulting males is limited as male victims may not report that an offender was female. However, information related to females victimizing males is beginning to become more available. Female-perpetrated assault against males is often dismissed and thought of as being just a sexual experience. The shame the victim experiences adversely impacts their decision to report to law enforcement. Drug and alcohol consumption also influences reporting, as those impaired at the time of the assault do not tend to report to law enforcement out of shame and guilt.[4]

Additionally, the underreporting of male sexual assault affects post-assault medical care. Males may not seek medical attention after being sexually assaulted, or they may hesitate to do so. When they do present for health care, they find that professionals working with victims often hold negative attitudes about assault, thus impacting the quality of care delivered.[5] These harmful attitudes further traumatize the patient. Therefore, it is imperative that health care providers put aside any bias and encourage disclosure to provide appropriate care.[6]

CHARACTERISTICS OF MALE SEXUAL ASSAULT

SEXUAL ASSAULT IN CORRECTIONAL FACILITIES

As with females who are sexually assaulted, males who are sexually assaulted typically know their perpetrators, if only for a brief period of time. Studies have found that the most common victim-offender relationship is as acquaintances or friends, and males are most often—though not exclusively—assaulted in a residence. While physical injury may be less severe, health care providers must not discount the emotional trauma and should treat both accordingly. The US Department of Justice reports that approximately 1.5 million individuals are incarcerated in either state or federal correctional facilities. In general, inmates are vulnerable to sexual victimization. The National Prison Rape Elimination Commission specifically notes that inmates with mental illness and disabilities are at risk for sexual assault. In 2003, the US Congress passed the Prison Rape Elimination Act, which created a zero-tolerance standard for sexual assault in correctional facilities and mandated data collection for sexual violence in the corrections system. In 2018, correctional administrators reported 27 826 allegations of sexual victimization, a 14% increase from the 24 514 reported in 2015. Of the 1673 substantiated incidents in 2018, approximately 58% were perpetrated by other inmates and 42% by staff.[7] The consequences of male-on-male prisoner sexual assault are both psychological and physical. While safety measures for staff and other patients should be taken when examining and collecting evidence from inmates, health care providers should not allow bias against inmates to affect the provision of quality care.

The types of assault that men experience largely differ by age group. In college-aged males, Budd et al[8] identify forcible fondling as the most common assaultive act, with forcible sodomy, rape, and sexual assault with an inanimate object following in order of highest rates of occurrence. Over half of the males in this study reported that hands, feet, or physical restraints were also used. The amount of injury suffered by males is inconsistently reported in the literature. Males who experience sexual violence may or may not have nongenital physical injuries or anogenital injuries, and the degree of trauma varies from case to case. Therefore, a thorough physical assessment is warranted, as well as screening for strangulation.

THE MEDICAL-FORENSIC EXAMINATION

People seeking medical-forensic care after experiencing sexual violence should receive consistent, compassionate, patient-centered, and trauma-informed care regardless of their gender. **Table 25-1** provides an overview of the examination process. The examination and evidence collection processes for male survivors should deviate very little from what is typically conducted for female patients. The physical examination should be thorough, assessing for signs of trauma, strangulation, general physiologic changes, and foreign materials (eg, debris or fibers). For patients who report forced receptive oral copulation (ie, the patient's mouth to the

---

Table 25-1. Examination Components*

HISTORY

— Medical/surgical
— Social
— Current medications
— Circumstances of the event/assault

GENERAL PHYSICAL EXAMINATION

— Vital signs
— Physical appearance (including appearance of clothing)
— Demeanor
— Behavior and orientation
— Head-to-toe assessment
— Assessment for possible strangulation
— Injury and trauma identification
— Physiologic changes

ORAL EXAMINATION (IF INDICATED)

— In case of forced receptive oral copulation, assessment for injury
   (eg, frenulum tears, palatal bruising, petechiae)

ANOGENITAL EXAMINATION

— External genitalia and perineal area (injury identification, physical
   evidence collection)
   — Abdomen
   — Buttocks
   — Thighs
   — Foreskin
   — Urethral meatus
   — Penile shaft
   — Scrotum
   — Perineum
   — Glans
   — Testes
— Anal examination
   — Anoscope to view rectum (if indicated)

* Physical evidence collection, including collection of possible foreign materials and fluids, should be completed per community standard or agency protocol. A standard victim sexual assault evidence collection kit should be used.
Adapted from US Department of Justice, Office on Violence Against Women.[9]

---

perpetrator's genitals), a detailed inspection and documentation of the oral cavity is critical. Residual signs of oral penetration such as frenal tears, palatal contusions, and petechiae should be described and photographed in accordance with local jurisdictional policies.

Patients who experience forced anal penetration may be offered anoscopy as another component of the examination for evidence collection. Health care providers should follow the scope of practice and licensure guidelines for anoscope insertion.

CASE STUDIES

Case Study 25-1

An 18-year-old man presented to the emergency department after being "fisted" by another man in the front seat of his car. He had blood dripping down his leg. "It really hurt," he later reported. "I told him to get out." He went home and called his mother, who was a nurse, and she told him to go to the hospital. The police were called, as this crime required mandated reporting in the state. The forensic nurse noted a large laceration on his anus with frank blood present and bruising. The physician performed a medical screening examination and did not identify any life-threatening injuries. The patient consented to the medical-forensic examination and evidence collection. He was treated prophylactically for sexually transmitted infections (STIs) according to the Centers for Disease Control and Prevention (CDC) guidelines.[10] He was discharged home with follow-up instructions and referrals. The evidence collection kit was released to law enforcement per protocol.

Discussion

In this case, the medical clearance was important due to the bleeding and bruising noted by the forensic nurse. Comprehensive discharge instructions were necessary due to the laceration of the patient's anal area. Post-assault, it may be painful when defecating; therefore, having a proper diet and consuming fluids are important. This information should be included in the discharge teaching.

All patients should be offered prophylaxis for STIs before discharge. Information regarding post-exposure prophylaxis for Hepatitis B should be provided with clear guidelines given to patients about the importance of receiving treatment within 14 days of exposure. HIV prophylaxis (HIV nPEP) should be offered based upon the type of sexual contact experienced by the patient. Risks and benefits must be discussed with the patient prior to initiating HIV nPEP. More information regarding prophylaxis may be found through the CDC website.[10]

The emotional trauma experienced during a sexual assault may lead to serious, long-term consequences, especially if not treated. Health care providers should assess every patient's emotional wellbeing for signs of low self-esteem, depression, substance abuse, risk-taking behavior, and self-harming behavior. A psychiatric consult should be obtained if the patient displays or expresses suicidal ideation or planning.

Male patients may benefit from a sexual assault advocate being present during the medical-forensic examination. Some states require that health care providers offer this resource, but not all patients wish to have an advocate present at the time of the examination. Regardless, safety planning must be a component of the discharge process. This includes either the forensic nurse or the advocate providing the patient with information about shelters, protective orders, and other community resources (eg, faith-based or LGBTQ+ organizations). Concerns will differ from patient to patient. A multidisciplinary approach to discharge and safety planning ensures that an appropriate and comprehensive plan is put in place.

Follow-up care is an integral part of the discharge planning process. Individualized discharge plans are essential and must be based upon individual patients' health and safety needs. Patients who are sexually assaulted by an intimate partner, for instance, will require very different discharge instructions than patients who are assaulted by a stranger.

SUMMARY

Though strides have been made in understanding male sexual assault, more research is needed to better identify strategies for delivering high quality, patient-centered, trauma-informed care. Forensic nurses should provide consistent, comprehensive, and non-biased care during the medical-forensic examination and evidence collection process. A multidisciplinary approach provides the much-needed support this population requires. Survivors of male sexual assault will feel empowered to report and seek treatment if they perceive the health care response as one that will meet their needs.

REFERENCES

1. Smith SG, Zhang X, Basile KC, et al. The national intimate partner and sexual violence survey: 2015 data brief – updated release. Centers for Disease Control and Prevention. 2018. https://www.cdc.gov/violenceprevention/pdf/2015data-brief508.pdf

2. Sadler AG, Cheney AM, Mengeling MA, Booth BM, Torner JC, Young LB. Servicemen's perceptions of male sexual assault and barriers to reporting during active component and reserve/national guard military service. *J Interpers Violence.* 2021;36(7-8):3596-3623. doi:10.1177/0886260518780407

3. Williams KS, Bierie DM. An incident-based comparison of female and male sexual offenders. *Sex Abuse.* 2015;27(3):235-257. doi:10.1177/1079063214544333

4. Busardò FP, Varì MR, di Trana A, Malaca S, Carlier J, di Luca NM. Drug-facilitated sexual assaults (DFSA): a serious underestimated issue. *Eur Rev Med Pharmacol Sci.* 2019;23(24):10577-10587. doi:10.26355/eurrev_201912_19753

5. Nielson MH, Strong L, Stewart JG. Does sexual assault nurse examiner (SANE) training affect attitudes of emergency department nurses toward sexual assault survivors? *J Forensic Nurs.* 2015;11(3):137-143. doi:10.1097/JFN.0000000000000081

6. Holland KJ, Cipriano AE. Bystander response to sexual assault disclosures in the US military: encouraging survivors to use formal resources. *Am J Community Psychol.* 2019;64(1-2):202-217. doi:10.1002/ajcp.12333

7. Buehler, Emily D. *Sexual victimization reported by adult correctional authorities, 2016-18.* US Department of Justice; 2021.

8. Budd, KM, Rocque M, Bierie DM. Deconstructing incidents of campus sexual assault: comparing male and female victimizations. *Sexual Abuse.* 2019;31(3):296-317. doi:10.1177/1079063217706708

9. Office on Violence Against Women. *A National Protocol for Sexual Assault Medical Forensic Examinations: Adults/Adolescents.* US Department of Justice; 2013.

10. Sexually Transmitted Infections Treatment Guidelines, 2021. Centers for Disease Control and Prevention. 2021. Updated July 22, 2021. https://www.cdc.gov/std/treatment-guidelines/default.htm

Chapter 26

SUSPECT EVIDENCE COLLECTION

Diana K. Faugno, MSN, RN, CPN, AFN-C ,SANE-A, SANE-P, FAAFS, DF-IAFN, DF-AFN
Stacey A. Mitchell, DNP, MBA, MEd, RN, AFN-C, SANE-A, SANE-P, DF-AFN, FAAN

KEY POINTS

1. *Forensic evidence collected from suspects is as valuable as forensic evidence collected from victims.*

2. *Suspect evidence collection requires strict adherence to legal requirements such as search warrants.*

INTRODUCTION

Forensic evidence collection from suspects is vital for effectively investigating and prosecuting cases; however, there is little consistency from jurisdiction to jurisdiction in approaches to suspect evidentiary evaluations. Only a few states have standardized protocols and procedures for the process. Some jurisdictions do not regularly request or perform suspect examinations at all.

Suspect evidentiary examinations are routinely performed in a variety of cases, such as sexual assault, child abuse, robberies, burglaries, homicides, and other interpersonal crimes. Many forensic nursing programs, either in the hospital or community-based, incorporate the suspect forensic examination as a service offered to law enforcement. This examination is important for many reasons:

— Evidence collection aids in a more thorough and successful investigation of a case by law enforcement professionals.

— Discovery of compelling evidence may contribute to a guilty plea before trial, thus sparing the victim from testifying at the trial.

— Evidence collection may result in the exoneration of a suspect who has been falsely accused or misidentified.

— The addition of suspect evidence collection services is an ideal presentation of objectivity in forensic medical examiners, particularly when qualifying as an expert witness in the courtroom.

— Offering suspect examination services may be an additional benefit to the community and a potential source of revenue for programs.[1]

CONSENT FROM A SUSPECT

While it is necessary to obtain consent for the medical forensic examination for a victim, a suspect examination may not require consent (eg, if the court compels a suspect to provide samples for testing under subpoena). Evidence collection from a suspect may be initiated in 2 ways:

— Signed consent from the suspect

— Search warrant or court order provided by law enforcement to a health care provider

Search warrants and court orders define the items to collect. These items are specifically named on the legal documents.[2] Failure to comply with the search warrant or court order has legal implications for the suspect. If the suspect first consents to the evidentiary examination and then revokes consent, the examination immediately ceases. A search warrant or court order must then be obtained by law enforcement for the provider to complete any remaining collections.

FORENSIC EXAMINATION

The suspect examination follows a similar process as the victim medical forensic examination. However, a history of the assault is not typically garnered from the suspect by the health care provider conducting the examination.[3] Law enforcement is responsible for obtaining the assault history or interview from the suspect. Suspects often make spontaneous statements, and the health care provider records these statements using quotation marks in the medical forensic record. The only information that the health care provider obtains from the suspect is a health history.[4] If the suspect declines to answer questions, the provider immediately stops asking anything further and documents declining information in the records (eg, "Patient declined to answer any further questions.").[3,5]

Evidence collection follows the health history. Local protocols guide health care providers who adhere to the guidances concerning the suspect examination. If local protocols do not exist, the local multidisciplinary team provides guidance and assists with protocol development. Most states do not have special suspect-specific evidence collection kits, often leaving the health care provider to adapt kits used for victim evidentiary examinations. However, some commercial forensic supply companies do manufacture and sell suspect evidence collection kits. Regardless, physical evidence is collected from the suspect according to state or local protocols using an appropriate evidence collection kit. For general guidelines, refer to the US Department of Justice's *National Protocol for Sexual Assault Medical Forensic Examinations*.[4] Although the protocol is written for the care of victims, the sections related to evidence collection remain relevant for victims and suspects.[3]

Occasionally, locations outside the hospital are used for evidence collection. Jails, prisons, or police stations may serve as alternate locations. When traveling to a non-health care provider location, packing a travel bag with barrier sheets, sharps containers, and other equipment is necessary. Provider safety is important during evidence collection from a suspect. At least 1 officer should remain with the suspect in the room at all times during the forensic nursing process. Reference samples are often collected from suspects during this process. Law enforcement agencies may contract with health care providers or independent laboratories to collect these, or they may choose to obtain samples themselves. Each jurisdiction is different, so providers need to be familiar with local protocols.

While completing the suspect examination, health care providers document injury commonly associated with signs of a struggle or use of force. All injuries and findings should be photographed according to program or agency policy or within the limitations of the search warrant or court order. An anogenital examination may identify indicators of sexually transmitted diseases (STIs), including lesions or discharge. When an STI is a critical component of the investigation (eg, in cases of child sexual abuse), the health care provider collaborates with law enforcement, ensuring the correct testing methodology is requested and documented on the search warrant or court order.

Basic evidence collection varies based on jurisdictional protocols, policies, and procedures. **Table 26-1** reviews the various types of evidence that may need to be collected when working with suspects.

Table 26-1. Evidence Collection Procedures[4]

— Oral swabs

— Perioral swabs

— Genital swabs

— Buccal swab

— Fingernail scrapings, swabs, or clippings

— Hair samples (pulling or cutting)

— Dried fluid samples

— Urine sample

— Blood sample

— Debris collection

— Clothing collection

Clothing provides evidence when there are defects such as rips, missing buttons or pockets, and stains that could be relevant to the ongoing investigation.[2] The forensic nurse must photograph and document any defects in the forensic record.[4] It is also important to collect undergarments even though the suspect may have changed since the assault. The following considerations should be made when collecting a suspect's clothing:

— Avoid cutting through defects such as bullet holes or tears.

— Dry wet clothing when possible, hanging in plain view. Notify law enforcement of the wet clothing, as they have specialized drying cabinets.

— Package each piece of clothing separately in paper bags.

When appropriate, provide medical treatment for injuries during the examination process.

BARRIERS TO SUSPECT EXAMINATIONS
Suspect examinations are not routinely completed in many jurisdictions for a variety of reasons[5]:

— ***Lack of knowledge:*** Some law enforcement agencies and prosecutors are not aware of the benefits of collecting evidence from suspects.

— ***Lack of kit standardization:*** Few states have suspect-specific evidence collection kits and documentation forms.

— ***Lack of training:*** Few health care providers receive specific education related to suspect examinations.

— ***Lack of funding:*** Law enforcement agencies may lack funds to pay for the examination.

— ***Disinclination of health care providers to perform examinations:*** Health care personnel may be reluctant to work with suspects based upon safety concerns or role confusion.

Agreed-upon jurisdictional polices aid in mitigating barriers. Coordinated community response teams work collaboratively to agree upon processes and address concerns.

CASE STUDIES

Case Study 26-1

A 29-year-old man grabbed a woman in a park and threw her down behind the bushes. He attempted to put his penis in her mouth several times. When he finally penetrated her mouth, she bit his penis, breaking the skin. He pulled out and ran away. Later, he sought treatment for the penile injury at a local hospital. Police had already notified emergency rooms to call if this type of injury presented, and the triage nurse called law enforcement after the suspect entered the facility for treatment.

The suspect was arrested at the hospital and charged with sexual assault. After his arrest, he had a suspect examination and complained of pain with his penile injury. He did not voluntarily disclose anything. He was cooperative with the nurse examiner and voluntarily consented to the examination. The sheriff's officers remained on site for the entirety of the suspect's examination. Handcuffs had to be removed to swab the suspect's hands and for the nurse to note any injuries on the hands relating to the history given to her by law enforcement. The suspect was also examined by an emergency room physician due to the nature of the bite mark on his penis. Follow-up treatment instructions and medical referrals were given to the sheriff for the jail medical staff.

Discussion

Several weeks later, the DNA from the victim's mouth (obtained during her evidentiary examination) positively identified the suspect. The suspect pleaded guilty to the charge and is currently serving time in state prison.

Disclosure from a suspect is rare given their constitutional protections. During the medical forensic examination, law enforcement is present in the room to implement safety measures should something occur to escalate combative or elopement behaviors. The forensic nurse's assessment should include observations with objective documentation and photography. After evidence is collected and packaged according to the evidence management guidelines, the totality of the collection is given to law enforcement after taking signatures and noting the officer's identification to complete the chain of custody. The suspect is then discharged to a destination determined by law enforcement.

SUMMARY

Suspect examinations are a means for law enforcement to gather evidence in ongoing cases. Health care providers should ensure that suspects have both the capacity and the competence to consent to an examination. If there is any question regarding their ability to provide consent, the forensic nurse should request a search warrant or court order. Included in this are intoxicated suspects or those with a cognitive impairment. The provider must stay within the parameters of the warrant or court order. The evidence collection process and chain of custody should also follow established protocols. Health care providers are an important part of the investigative process and should complete these examinations with appropriate training and protocol support.

REFERENCES

1. SANE program development and operation guide: Suspect Examinations. Office for Victims of Crime. Accessed October 31, 2021. https://www.ovcttac.gov/saneguide/expanding-forensic-nursing-practice/suspect-examinations/

2. Investigating sexual assault: model policy. Mark Wynn Consulting. 2005. Accessed October 31, 2021. http://www.markwynn.com/wp-content/uploads/investigating-sexual-assaults-model-policy.pdf

3. Faugno D, Johnson C, Waszak D. Forensic examination of the sexual assault suspect. In: Giardino, AP, Faugno DK, Spencer MJ, Weaver ML, Speck PM, eds. *Sexual Assault Victimization Across the Life Span: Investigation, Diagnosis, and the Multidisciplinary Team.* 2nd ed. STM Learning, Inc; 2017:335-354.

4. A national protocol for sexual assault medical forensic examinations: adults/adolescents. 2nd ed. Office on Violence Against Women. April 2013. Accessed October 31, 2021. https://www.ncjrs.gov/pdffiles1/ovw/241903.pdf

5. Archambault J. Forensic exams for the sexual assault suspect. End Violence Against Women. October 2013. Updated May 2021. Accessed October 31, 2021. https://evawintl.org/wp-content/uploads/2013-10_TB-Suspect-Exams.pdf

Chapter 27

HUMAN TRAFFICKING

Rosario V. Sanchez, PhD, MSN, RN, CCRN, SANE-A
Karen B. Silva, PhD, MSN, MFN, PMHRN-BC
Laurie Charles, MSN, RN, CA-CP, SANE, AFN-C, SANE-A, SANE-P, CHSE
Patricia M. Speck, DNSc, CRNP, FNP-BC, AFN-C, DF-IAFN, FAAFS, DF-AFN, FAAN

KEY POINTS

1. *Human trafficking is a complex crime, primarily involving sex and/or labor trafficking.*

2. *Persons committing the crimes use a variety of techniques to capture and exploit an individual for their own benefit, including financial gains.*

3. *Person-centered approaches require comprehensive, wraparound services to persons experiencing human trafficking, which include a forensic nursing healthcare response.*

INTRODUCTION

Human trafficking is a business, and it is the fastest growing crime in the world, lagging just behind transnational drug cartels.[1] Declared a leading public health issue, human trafficking affects more than 12.3 million people worldwide.[2,3] Twenty-five types of human trafficking exist, and they take several forms.[4] The primary legislation in the United States, *The Trafficking Victims Protection Act of 2000* and its subsequent reauthorizations,[5] defines human trafficking as "severe forms of trafficking in persons." **Human trafficking** involves "the recruitment, harboring, transportation, provision, obtaining, soliciting, or patronizing of a person for the purpose of sex exploitation, forced labor, and/or debt bondage."[5] While sex trafficking and labor trafficking are predominant, several other forms exist.[6] **Sex trafficking** refers to the recruitment, harboring, transportation, provision, obtaining, patronizing, or soliciting of a person for the purposes of a commercial sex act, in which a commercial sex act is induced by force, fraud, or coercion, or in which the person induced to perform such act has not attained 18 years of age. **Labor trafficking** is the recruitment, harboring, transportation, provision, or obtaining of a person through the use of force, fraud, or coercion for the purpose of subjection to involuntary servitude, peonage, debt bondage, or slavery.[5]

Recognized today as an emerging health care priority worldwide, human trafficking requires the involvement and collaboration of professionals in public health, social work, health care, and direct medical forensic services, as well as members of the legal and law enforcement communities.[3,7,8] Oftentimes, entrapment occurs through a non-violent grooming process where perpetrators exert control over the trafficked persons' activities for the purposes of exploitation.[9] A broader definition of human trafficking is a violation of essential human rights and enslavement.[10] Using common language in reference to human trafficking helps to improve research, affecting legislation, regulations, and response practices globally in turn.

Human trafficking is commonly confused with other crimes and forms of violence, such as smuggling, adult sex industry (consensual), kidnapping or hostage-taking, domestic violence, child abuse, sexual assault/rape, and wage diversion.[11] Under federal law, any minor engaged in commercial sex is a victim of child abuse; therefore, health care providers are mandated reporters.[12]

IDENTIFYING TRAFFICKING

Professionals and organizations use the Action-Means-Purpose (A-M-P) model to help identify potential victims of human trafficking in their settings.[13] The A-M-P Model defines the various elements related to the acts, means, and purpose of human trafficking, as reflected in **Figure 27-1**.

Figure 27-1. *The Action-Means-Purpose (A-M-P) model.*

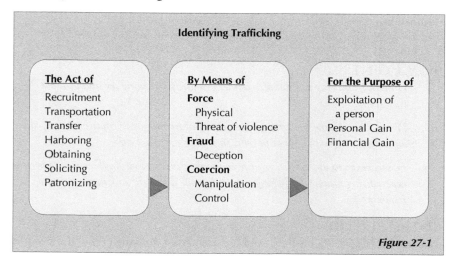

Identifying Trafficking

The Act of
Recruitment
Transportation
Transfer
Harboring
Obtaining
Soliciting
Patronizing

By Means of
Force
  Physical
  Threat of violence
Fraud
  Deception
Coercion
  Manipulation
  Control

For the Purpose of
Exploitation of
  a person
Personal Gain
Financial Gain

Figure 27-1

TRAFFICKER PROFILE

Buyers and sellers in the human trafficking industry may be of any gender, age, or socioeconomic status. Traffickers may be anyone in the victim's community, such as religious leaders, neighbors, law enforcement, and even family or friends. They may be known or unknown to the victim. The traffickers take opportunities to use power, monetary advantages, or relationships to control the victim and others. Traffickers exploit the fact that all people have minimal needs of safety, shelter, clothing, food, and water, and they manipulate victims' vulnerabilities to lure them into trafficking situations.

VICTIM PROFILE

Victims often have a relationship with the offender, who identifies their vulnerabilities for exploitation and entrapment. Victims can be of any age, nationality, gender, and socioeconomic level. Minors are often vulnerable to exploitation just by the nature of their age and development. Children who experience abuse, neglect, or rejection from family dynamics (such as sexual or gender minorities) are at higher risk for human trafficking.[9,10,14] Whether a family is loving or neglectful and/or abusive, the child's *perception* of acceptance by family or personal self-acceptance are driving factors in their decision to run away or enter high-risk situations.[14]

Minor victims may experience trafficking by strangers, acquaintances, their families, or schoolmates. Younger minors are more often trafficked by their families.[8,14] Non-familial trafficking of adolescents is similar to the trafficking of adults, as trackers often befriend adolescents through social media and online gaming. The trafficker lures the adolescent with false promises of an independent lifestyle outside the home. When situations like this occur, children tend to blame themselves for their choices, even though they were manipulated by the trafficker.[9,14] Those who experience trafficking may require mental health treatment, treatment for substance use and dependence, and a supportive environment to overcome their vulnerabilities without emotional strings or judgment.

SIGNS AND MYTHS

When working with patients, forensic nurses must have a strong understanding of the signs of human trafficking as well as the myths that surround perpetrators and victims of trafficking. Several troubling myths exist in regards to human trafficking that inhibit the delivery of justice. These myths are outlined in **Table 27-1**.

Table 27-1. Myths about Human Trafficking[11,13]
— Human trafficking is always or usually a violent crime
— All forms of human trafficking involve sex
— Traffickers only target victims they do not know
— Only undocumented foreign nationals get trafficked in the United States
— Only women and girls can be victims of human trafficking
— Human trafficking only happens in illegal or underground industries
— Human trafficking only involves moving, traveling, or transporting a person across the state or national borders
— All commercial sex is human trafficking
— People in active trafficking situations always want help getting out
— Labor trafficking is only or primarily a problem in developing countries

As one of the first lines of defense against trafficking, forensic nurses look for and recognize the signs of trafficking in their patients. Common signs of human trafficking are outlined in **Table 27-2**.

Table 27-2. Signs of Human Trafficking	
SIGNS	EXAMPLES
Physical Signs	Late presentation for an advanced illness or injury; injuries caused by violence or by lack of safety equipment
Behavioral Signs	Lack of trust in law enforcement or health care workers; vague or inconsistent explanation of injuries
Emotional & Psychological Signs	Anxiety, depression, irritability; substance abuse
Spiritual Signs	Feelings of worthlessness, self-blame, hopelessness

RESOURCES FOR RECOVERY

As demonstrated in **Figure 27-2**, persons who leave trafficking life need victim-centered wrap-around services. Forensic nurses work in multidisciplinary teams to ensure trafficking victims receive the necessary support to recover from their experiences. Additional information on trauma-informed care can be found in chapter 5.

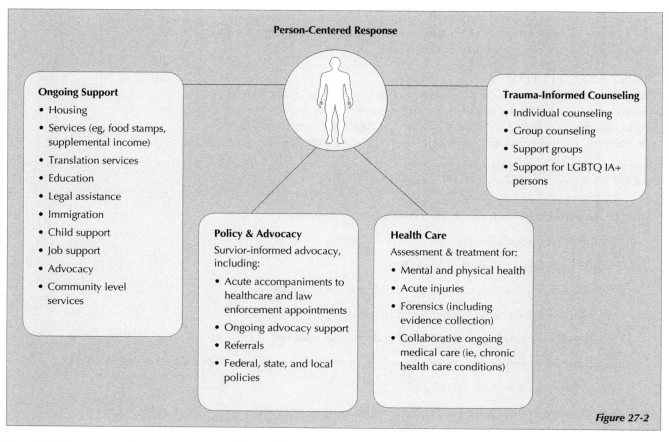

Person-Centered Response

Ongoing Support
- Housing
- Services (eg, food stamps, supplemental income)
- Translation services
- Education
- Legal assistance
- Immigration
- Child support
- Job support
- Advocacy
- Community level services

Policy & Advocacy
Survior-informed advocacy, including:
- Acute accompaniments to healthcare and law enforcement appointments
- Ongoing advocacy support
- Referrals
- Federal, state, and local policies

Health Care
Assessment & treatment for:
- Mental and physical health
- Acute injuries
- Forensics (including evidence collection)
- Collaborative ongoing medical care (ie, chronic health care conditions)

Trauma-Informed Counseling
- Individual counseling
- Group counseling
- Support groups
- Support for LGBTQ IA+ persons

Figure 27-2

Figure 27-2. *Person-centered response to trauma.*

CASE STUDIES

Case Study 27-1

An adolescent girl presented to the emergency department (ED) for acute sexual assault by 2 men. She was accompanied by her mother and a family member and reported no prior consensual sexual activity. The forensic nurse provided medical and forensic health care and completed appropriate mandatory reporting. The patient was discharged home with her mother. While she did not disclose to the nurse what happened, she did disclose to law enforcement and Child Protective Services (CPS) that her mother was selling her, along with her adolescent and pre-pubertal siblings, for drugs. However, the investigators of the case stated it was "too fantastical to be believed," and no further investigation was completed.

Two years later, this same patient returned to the ED after a police raid, during which she was found naked in a room full of adult males. She reported that she was forced to perform sexual acts on everyone in the room. She was accompanied by law enforcement to the hospital for a medical forensic examination and was immediately identified as a trafficking victim. Based on the recent findings, the forensic team became concerned and conducted an inquiry on prior forensic visits. Sadly, they realized she had been seen for sexual assault before. It was noted that a thorough initial investigation was not completed.

Discussion

In this situation, a thorough investigation would have alerted the forensic nurse, CPS, and law enforcement of the red flags of familial human trafficking. Familial trafficking does occur, and those who are victimized are often very young when the trafficking begins. If the nurse had been able to recognize the red flags of human trafficking during the patient's first visit to the ED, they could have approached the patient with their concerns. Saying things like, "I just want you to know that you are in a safe place," or "I am concerned about your safety. Is it okay if I ask a few questions about what brought you here today?" helps to establish a safe environment and begin that conversation.

Since victims of trafficking experience significant trauma, it is essential for health care providers to practice trauma-informed care. Trauma-informed care requires that health care providers focus on creating a safe environment for their patients. Once established, being transparent and fully supportive of the patient's choices is essential. When the patient is a minor, there is a mandatory reporting situation. Trauma-informed care requires the assent of the child in mandatory reporting; when there is no assent, the child is informed of the mandatory reporting law and offered the choice to be involved.

Case Study 27-2

A 65-year-old Iranian woman was brought into the ED by law enforcement after being found lying down on a sidewalk with a left-side weakness. The patient had no documents with her and did not speak English at all. Later, they realized the patient spoke Farsi, and the hospital provided an interpreter.

Upon interviewing her, the nurse found out that the patient did not know her address but was able to describe the house in an "affluent" neighborhood. She said that her bosses kept her passport since they came to the United States from Iran in 1996. She was never given the chance or means to go back home, and she has been unable to contact her family since then. She reported that her room was in the garage outside the house. She was not allowed to eat with them and worked from 5:30 AM to 11:00 PM every day, including weekends. She never received any salary, and her "bosses" told her that she was expensive to keep because she did not pay for food, shelter, or supplies for personal hygiene.

The patient reported that she had been experiencing frequent headaches and occasionally nose bleeds for many years, but she was never taken to a doctor. The night before she was found, she had a huge headache that made her cry, and she suddenly could not feel her left side or walk straight. Her "boss" told her that she was no good for them anymore and dropped her off a few blocks from a local hospital. She could not walk and did not know where she was. Someone saw her sobbing and unable to get up and called 911. She was diagnosed to have a hemorrhagic cerebral vascular accident secondary to untreated hypertension.

Discussion

Often, the identification of human trafficking patients is difficult. Some indicators that this patient was a victim of human trafficking include her late presentation for medical care, a lack of access to her own documents, and her inability to contact her family. Her descriptions of her precarious living conditions, despite living in an affluent neighborhood, and her complete lack of salary indicate that she is at risk for human trafficking. If trust develops and the patient discloses the experience was human trafficking, the plan of care begins with support for disclosure of her situation, and explanation of the next steps necessary to protect her from the trafficker. The interventions require a team effort to serve the survivor's self-identified needs and continue until independent life is attained.

Summary

The United States government provides resources to guide forensic nursing practices by defining the different types of human trafficking, explaining mimics of trafficking, and describing the primary methods of trafficking. Several forensic nursing professional organizations provide training in the identification and treatment of common presentations, beginning with recognition of the psychological outcomes of human trafficking. A person-centered approach by forensic nurses, in collaboration with community-based wrap-around services, promises to mitigate the long-term effects of the human trafficking experience.

References

1. Human trafficking task force. United States Attorney's Office, Middle District of Alabama. Updated May 2021. Accessed December 18, 2021. https://www. justice.gov/usao-mdal/human-trafficking-task-force

2. Chohaney ML. Minor and adult domestic sex trafficking risk factors in Ohio. *J Soc Soc Work Res*. 2015;7(1):117-141. doi:10.1086/685108

3. Trafficking in Persons Report 2017. US Department of State. 2017. https:// www.state.gov/wp-content/uploads/2019/02/271339.pdf

4. The typology of modern slavery: defining sex and labor trafficking in the United States. Polaris. 2017. https://polarisproject.org/wp-content/uploads/2019/09/ Polaris-Typology-of-Modern-Slavery-1.pdf

5. 22 USC § 17401 — purposes and findings. 2000. Accessed April 18, 2022. https://www.law.cornell.edu/uscode/text/22/7101

6. Types of human trafficking. Interpol. 2021. https://www.interpol.int/en/Crimes/Human-trafficking/Types-of-human-trafficking

7. Byrne M, Parsh S, Parsh B. Human trafficking: impact, identification, and intervention. *J Nurs Manag.* 2019;50(8):18-24. doi:10.1097/01.NUMA.0000575304.15432.07

8. Schwarz C. Human trafficking and meaning making: the role of definitions in antitrafficking frontline work. *Soc Serv Rev.* 2019;93(3):484-523. doi:10.1086/705237

9. Fedina L, Williamson C, Perdue T. Risk factors for domestic child sex trafficking in the United States. *J Interpers Violence.* 2016;34(13):2653-2673. doi:10.1177/0886260516662306

10. Greenbaum VJ. Child sex trafficking in the United States: challenges for the healthcare provider. *PLoS Med.* 2017;14(11):1-8. doi:10.1371/journal.pmed.1002439

11. Myths, facts, and statistics. Polaris. 2021. Accessed December 15, 2021. https://polarisproject.org/myths-facts-and-statistics/

12. Speck PM, Mitchell SA, Ekroos RA, Sanchez RV, Hilfinger Messias DK. Policy brief on the nursing response to human trafficking. *Nurs Outlook.* 2018;66(4):407-411. doi:10.1016/j.outlook.2018.06.004

13. Burt I. Modern-day slavery in the U.S.: human trafficking and counselor awareness. *Int J Adv Couns.* 2019;41(2):187-200. doi:10.1007/s10447-018-9366-7

14. Reed SM, Kennedy MA, Decker MR, Cimino AN. Friends, family, and boyfriends: an analysis of relationship pathways into commercial sexual exploitation. *Child Abuse Negl.* 2019;90:1-12. doi:10.1016/j.chiabu.2019.01.016

Chapter 28

GANG VIOLENCE

Sarah L. Pederson, BSN, RN, AFN-C, SANE-A, SANE-P
Heather Quaile, DNP, WHNP-BC, AFN-C, CSC, IF, FAANP
Rosario V. Sanchez, PhD, MSN, RN, CCRN, SANE-A
Patricia M. Speck, DNSc, CRNP, FNP-BC, AFN-C, DF-IAFN, FAAFS, DF-AFN, FAAN

KEY POINTS

1. *Gang identity is associated with criminal activity, and symbols are used among gang members to distinguish themselves from other groups.*

2. *Gangs engage in criminal activity such as drug dealing, trafficking, or selling illegal firearms to support business enterprises.*

3. *Health care facilities and professionals should be aware of symbols that suggest gang affiliation to promote safety for the facility, staff, and other persons.*

4. *Health care professionals should be cognizant of the gang types in their communities and understand the structure of membership and behaviors related to the types of gangs.*

BACKGROUND INFORMATION ON GANGS

Gangs exist in all 50 of the United States and are loosely formed groups of 3 or more individuals that exist for the purpose of criminal enterprise.[1] Gangs are commonly structured by racial, ethnic, or political lines and have growing membership and satellites that employ a level of organization and permanence. Features of gangs include unique names, symbols, colors, hand signals, slogans, aliases, tattoos, styles of clothing, hairstyles, or graffiti.[1] Gangs engage in criminal activity and employ threats, intimidation, or violence to further their criminal objectives and enhance or preserve the association's power, reputation, or economic resources. Gangs are also organized to defend their members and interests from rival criminal organizations or to control a particular location or region. Gangs develop and maintain perpetuating characteristics, including manifestos, constitutions, and codes of conduct, providing an identifiable structure and rules for initiation and advancement within the association.[2] "Through their use of open intimidation and identifiable insignia, gangs may be distinguished from other organized criminal groups such as La Cosa Nostra and other transnational criminal organizations who rely on secrecy and clandestine control of legitimate businesses and governments to advance their criminal aims."[1] With more profits, gangs gather greater power and influence in all levels of society.

Gangs are highly organized business enterprises of multiple people, often in multiple places, with organizational structures that facilitate the sustainability of the parent gang. The business enterprise of gangs allows for wealth accumulation and is typically associated with crimes involving drugs, prostitution, human trafficking, kidnapping, ransom, destruction of property, terrorism in neighborhoods, and extortion. Gang-related crimes are tracked by the federal government at the national level and include other major crimes such as firearm assault, robbery, homicide, and aggravated assault. **Table 28-1** outlines the types of gangs identified by the federal government.

Table 28-1. Violent Gangs and Organized Crime[1]

	TYPE	ORGANIZATION	DESCRIPTION
VIOLENT GANGS	Outlaw Motorcycle Gangs (OMGs)	— Bandidos — Black Pistons — Hells Angels — Mongols — Outlaws or the American Outlaws Association (AOA) — Pagans — Sons of Silence	These groups use their motorcycles to run illicit operations. OMGs are highly organized criminal groups that smuggle in drugs and firearms and commit other violent crimes. The United States has over 300 active OMGs, ranging in size from a few individuals to hundreds of chapters with thousands of members worldwide.
	Prison Gangs	— Aryan Brothers — Barrio Azteca — Black Guerilla Family — Dead Man Incorporated (DMI) — The Hermanos de Pistoleros Latinos (HPL) — Mexican Mafia (Le Eme) — Nuestro Familia	Prison gangs are criminal organizations that form within the penitentiary system and now span the country's prisons. Prison gangs are self-sustaining criminal organizations that operate outside the penal system. They often make up a select group of inmates that follow a strict hierarchy and code of conduct. Prison gangs frequently act as a conduit between drug trafficking organizations (DTOs), street gangs, and organized crime groups like OMGs, moving drugs from DTOs to gangs across the country. State prison gangs outnumber federal prison gangs.
	Street Gangs	— 18th Street — Almighty Latin King and Queen Nation (ALKQN) — Bloodline — Bloods — Crips — Gangster Disciples — Latin Kings — MS-13	Street gangs operate throughout the United States and vary in terms of membership size, racial and ethnic makeup, and organizational structure. The largest threat comes from major street gangs that smuggle, transport, and distribute large quantities of illicit drugs and rely on violence to maintain power. Local street gangs typically mimic larger, more powerful gangs in order to earn the respect of their rivals.
ORGANIZED CRIME	International Crime	— Blood clans — Networks — Cells	The term ***international organized crime*** refers to groups who work to gain power, influence, money, and more through illegal means while protecting their activities through a pattern of corruption or violence. No single structure exists for international organized crime groups to follow. There is variation between strict hierarchies, blood clans, networks, and cells.
	Infiltrated Labor Unions	— International Brotherhood of Teamsters (IBT) — La Cosa Nostra — Mafia	Historically, organized criminal groups have had significant influence and control over labor unions by instilling fear and intimidating employers and union members. The Organized Crime and Gang Section's (OCGS) Labor Management Racketeering Unit has worked with the United States Attorney's Offices to prosecute criminals by utilizing the Racketeer Influenced and Corrupt Organizations Act (RICO) to bring civil actions against labor unions and their affiliates.

Many risk factors can increase the likelihood of being recruited by gangs. Gangs seek membership from at-risk youth and recruit them through individuals, families, schools, peers, or neighborhood community domains. Gangs socialize adolescents with behaviors necessary to sustain their activities.[3] This behavior is persistent into adulthood.[3] Socialization of members encourages specific behaviors and utilizing other gang-related identifications, leading to subsequent violent crimes.

Push-pull factors encourage decisions to join or not join gangs.[4] Gang members enjoy the protection offered in groups. Even if the gang environment is toxic, gang members seek what they perceive as predictable and manageable, thus making the lifestyle preferable to unknown networks outside the gang.[6] When gang members have alcohol or drug dependence, it prohibits rational thought and the maturity necessary to leave gang life.[5] The long-term consequences of drug and alcohol dependence of gang members are poor health outcomes and shortened lives. Despite these factors, the probability of members leaving and having a successful life outside the gang improves with age as many become weary of the lifestyle or experience drastic changes in their lives, like becoming parents.[6]

Gangs historically exercise lifelong membership, yet *desistance,* the process by which gang members grow out of gang life or abstain from crime, does occur. Often, reasons for leaving are akin to the elopement process in human trafficking. These include disillusionment, job stability, family needs, the unanticipated parts of gang life, violence perpetrated against the individual or someone close to them, and a constant threat of victimization.[6,7] The forensic nurse's intervention is essential to help the patient share their experiences and understand their perceived risk for their future, which influences behavioral choices that the member makes through desistance.[6-8]

People leave a gang similarly to how they joined. When coming in, members have to give up all of their previous life associations; to leave, the member gives up their personal gang associations.[9] Risks to the member with desistance and gang de-affiliation includes the perceptions of betrayal by other gang members. Additionally, law enforcement professionals often continue to associate the individual with their history of gang membership and past criminal activity.

HEALTH CARE FACILITIES AND GANGS

Health care facilities and medical professionals provide trauma-informed care to members in their community affiliated with gang activity, and any place where gang members present for services increases the risk for gang violence.[10,11] Hospitals, parking lots, waiting areas, and out-patient care facilities are often places where long-running feuds, tensions between gangs, and increasingly violent acts of retaliation unfold.[10] Some signs that a patient may have be involved with a gang include[10,11]:

— A patient or visitor displaying obvious signs of agitation or looking like they just came from a fight

— A patient or visitor staring down (eg, "Mad Dogging") other visitors or staff members, which is a tactic often used between rival gang members

— Gang indicators (eg, gang colors, identical clothing or sports attire, tattoos, hand signs)

— A patient suffering trauma arriving with a group (eg, a shooting, stabbing, or assault victim being dropped off at the hospital entrance)

— A patient refusing to give up clothing or packages, which could indicate that those items contain weapons or illegal drugs

With gang involvement, injury often occurs, leading to the members going to the emergency department (ED) for help. Rival gang members may then try to find them. Hospitals and health care institutions can prepare for the potential escalation of gang violence by using the National Gang Center suggested protocol for medical facilities. The components of a prepared health care organization include[10]:

— Annual training from law enforcement for ED personnel, including receptionists and security officers, on gang identification (eg, providing visuals and descriptions of local gang tattoos, clothing, and existing rivalries).

— Annual review of protocols that work with local gang unit administrators; this should include requests for dispatcher notification when victims of a gang conflict are transported to the ED

— In emerging situations, policies that allow ED personnel to request further information, including the names/identifiers of the gangs involved and descriptions of suspects and vehicles, to share with security and reception personnel through a notification process

— In emerging situations, policies that limit the number of visitors who can accompany patients into waiting and treatment areas

— Policies to help hospital security address rival gang members waiting outside facilities (eg, in parking areas using Crime Prevention Through Environmental Design strategies from law enforcement and city planning agencies

— Improved awareness of the possibility of treating rival gang members at the same time (eg, implementing policies to separate patients and visitors)

— In the event of a serious community gang incident, policies to escalate security protocols that include locking down the ED and waiting area

CASE STUDIES

Case Study 28-1

This 16-year-old girl ran away from home with some friends. Within 42 hours of being gone from home, she met a man who offered to give her a ride to a local grocery store to get something to eat. She agreed to get in the car, as she was starving and had no money. Instead of being taken to the grocery store, he took her to an abandoned home and told her she could be part of a gang that would offer her protection for the "rest of her life." To be a gang member, she would need to be "jumped in," which would determine the level of respect she would possess once she became a full member. The following night, she was dropped off alone in the middle of a park. In the dark, she saw 5 gang members proceed towards her. She stated that she was kicked and punched all over her body, including her arms, back, stomach, hands, and legs. This was a customary initiation into this particular gang.

Discussion

Forensic nurses are aware of the experiences of gang members and understand that the overall picture of the average female gang member has drastically changed over the years. The modern views of female gang members have also been substantially reformed. Initiation into a gang is often a painful and humiliating experience. Initiation rituals vary by gang, and how the person enters determines the level of respect they will possess once they become a member. Getting "jumped in" is considered a form of gang initiation used by both men and women. It is regarded as the most common method of gang initiation. The process of getting "jumped in" involves receiving a moderate to a severe beating from other fellow gang members, often without fighting back.

Female gang life is often an attempt by young women to manage bleak and harsh circumstances in their life. Female motivations for joining gangs vary extensively. Some adolescent females reported joining a gang because of family, friends, or a personal reason (eg, experiencing physical or sexual abuse from a loved one). The loss of parental/guardian protection is another risk factor for joining a gang to feel like part of a group.

Case Study 28-2

This 13-year-old female patient presented to the health department stating she needed treatment for sexually transmitted infections (STIs). The patient was concerned that she was exposed to a STI during a recent sexual encounter. During the physical assessment, the nurse asked the patient about tattoos observed on the patient's body. The patient was unwilling to discuss the tattoos or provide additional information regarding her sexual history. Throughout the nurse-patient interaction, the nurse identified other potential indicators of gang affiliation. The nurse understands the intersection of gangs and sexual assault; therefore, the nurse obtained an adverse childhood experience (ACE) score on the patient, resulting in a score of 6. However, the patient denied any concerns for her wellbeing and safety or involvement with gangs. The nurse followed her jurisdictional laws and organizational protocols for mandatory reporting. She also prioritized utilizing screening tools and safety planning measures because she recognized that her patient is an at-risk youth with indicators of possible gang affiliation.

Discussion

The forensic nurse understood that gangs are loosely formed groups that engage in criminal activity and identify with unique symbols and colors that are often displayed as tattoos and/ or branding on gang members. The patient in this case study presented with a high ACE score and multiple risk factors that increase potential gang recruitment. Gangs seek membership from at-risk youth who are commonly vulnerable due to unstable home life to support their criminal activity. Additionally, this patient's high ACE score increased her susceptibility to adverse health outcomes. However, interventions can be initiated to mitigate the long-term effects of trauma. Connecting the patient to resources and support can decrease the patient's risk for adverse health effects associated with a high ACE score.

Summary

Given the prevalence of gang activities, the dynamics of violence and crime impact people who are frequently patients of forensic nurses. Awareness of gang types and their behavioral characteristics will better prepare the health care provider and forensic nurse for the possible escalation of violence in their organization.[12] Forensic nurses should seek education and training on policies addressing organization security, including recognizing the indicators of potential violence.

References

1. US Department of Justice. About violent gangs. Updated April 30, 2021. https:// www.justice.gov/criminal-ocgs/about-violent-gangs

2. Dammers K, Iton AB, Mathis KJ, Speck PM, Nahmias DE. Innovative Tools to Fight Gang Violence. *J Law Med Ethics*. 2007;35(S4):118-119. doi:10.1111/ j.1748-720X.2007.00227.x

3. Garduno LS, Brancale JM. Examining the risk and protective factors of gang involvement among Hispanic youth in Maryland. *J Community Psychol*. 2017;45(6):765–782. doi:10.1002/jcop.21891

4. Nuño LE, Katz CM. Understanding gang joining from a cross classified multilevel perspective. *Deviant Behav*. 2019;40(3):301–325. doi:10.1080/01639625. 2017.1421706

5. Valasik M. Gang violence predictability: using risk terrain modeling to study gang homicides and gang assaults in East Los Angeles. *J Crim Justice*. 2018;58: 10-21. doi:10.1016/j.jcrimjus.2018.06.001

6. Deuchar R. I get more in contact with my soul: gang disengagement, desistance and the role of spirituality. *Youth Justice*. 2019;20(½):113–127.doi:10.1177/ 1473225419889195

7. Carson DC. Examining racial and ethnic variations in reasons for leaving a youth gang. *J Dev Life Course Criminol*. 2018;4(4):449–472. doi:10.1007/s40865-018-0091-z

8. Chakelian A. Freedom has been my word ever since I got out. *New Statesman*. 2020;149(5546):16-17.

9. Densley JA, Pyrooz DC. A signaling perspective on disengagement from gangs. *Justice Quarterly.* 2019;36(1):31-58. doi:10.1080/07418825.2017.1357743

10. National Gang Center. Gang violence protocols for medical facilities. January 16, 2017. https://nationalgangcenter.ojp.gov/insights/34/gang-violence-protocols-for-medical-facilities

11. Clements PC. Gang migration to rural suburban areas: an evolving threat for emergency departments and law enforcement. Evidence Technology Magazine; 2021.

12. Moore CD. Maintaining security when gang members visit your ER. June 13, 2012. https://www.campussafetymagazine.com/hospital/gangs-healthcare-security-preparation-education-are-the-keys/

PRISON VIOLENCE

Anita Hufft, PhD, RN, FAAN

KEY POINTS

1. *Violence in prisons is a health issue which nurses must understand and respond to.*

2. *Sociodemographic and psychological characteristics of inmates are major factors impacting violence in prisons.*

3. *Mentally and physically ill inmates are particularly vulnerable to violence.*

4. *Nurses working in prison settings must be prepared to assess for potential violence and intervene appropriately by collaborating with correctional staff.*

5. *Consistent and frequent training for correctional staff and nurses can be an effective strategy to reduce occurrence and impact of violence on inmates.*

INTRODUCTION

Correctional facilities, prisons, and jails serve to separate criminals from society in order to punish the criminal, protect other members of society, or rehabilitate criminals, so they can return to society as productive members. Among one of the more problematic aspects of prisons is the challenge to provide safety to both inmates and staff. The dangers that exist within prisons often reflect competing interests and factors, which contribute to the violence occurring within these settings. Prison culture is defined, in part, by the behaviors and needs of those individuals and groups who occupy them and who are often characterized by aggression, lack of self-control, and an adversarial relationship with those in whom their care is entrusted.

INCIDENCE AND TYPES OF VIOLENCE IN CORRECTIONAL SETTINGS

The World Health Organization defines violence as "The intentional use of physical force or power, threatened or actual, against oneself, another person, or against a group or community that either results in or has a high likelihood of resulting in injury, death, psychological harm, maldevelopment or deprivation."[1] Prison violence is most commonly considered in terms of inmate-on-inmate assault, sexual assault by inmates or prison staff, excessive violence perpetrated by prison staff, and assault on prison staff by inmates.

Consistently accurate and timely data on violence in prisons and jails are difficult to access and are often not available. It is usually assumed that violence is under-reported, as many statistical databases are dependent upon inmate self-reporting or complete adjudication of the assault or event,[2] and inmates are often reluctant to formally report violence for fear of reprisal. Women are a particularly vulnerable population in prison, composing 7% of the total prison population but 22% of all victims of inmate-on-inmate sexual assault and exploitation and 33% of all victims of staff-on-inmate sexual victimization.[3] Private prisons appear to have more reported violence than public prisons, with estimates of inmate-on-inmate violence 38% higher at private prisons than at public prisons.[3] With respect to violence perpetrated by inmates on health care staff, verbal abuse is more likely to occur than physical abuse and is generally more prevalent among adult male prison populations.

ETIOLOGY OF PRISON VIOLENCE

Factors contributing to prison violence include physical abuse by correctional staff, overcrowding, gang activity, aggressive characteristics among the inmates, a lack of training among correctional staff, and the prison architecture itself. Any policies or actions which mediate the impact of these factors have the potential to decrease the likelihood of prison violence. Some prisoners go into a facility with violent tendencies and poor decision-making abilities. This predisposes them to the use of violence to respond to perceived threats and challenges to their position or role within the hierarchy of the prison community. Overcrowding contributes to prison violence as it disproportionately increases stress in situations when individuals have limited access to personal space and diminished coping skills to address the tension that is presented in such settings.[4] Gang activity and racial tensions are pronounced in prison settings, and overcrowding increases interactions between groups and creates opportunities for confrontations. Inadequate staff training (in both content and frequency) results in problematic staff-inmate interactions, power struggles, and unprofessional responses to challenging inmate behavior. Persons seen as vulnerable or weak are targets for violence among the inmates who are dominant, aggressive, and angry. Those with mental illness, substance abuse disorders, chronic health conditions, and the elderly are more frequently victims of violence or exploitation.

RESPONDING TO VIOLENCE IN PRISON SETTINGS

Nurses working in prisons have a responsibility to see beyond an individual's criminal behavior and background to provide the best possible health care to inmates. The prison population is characterized by higher rates of chronic health problems, infectious diseases, mental health issues, and substance abuse disorders. For many inmates, these conditions are undiagnosed or untreated prior to incarceration. The lack of consistent access to health care among inmates means the nurse is often their first point of contact with the correctional health care system.

Nurses are part of a health care team that must work collaboratively with correctional officers to support the security priorities of the institution. Coordinating timely, compassionate, and evidence-based care within the mandated procedures of the institution is a priority. Additionally, it is necessary to complete a thorough and accurate assessment upon inmates' admission to the institution and throughout their incarceration to identify conditions and characteristics that place them at risk for committing violence, being a victim of violence, or having poor health outcomes.

PREVENTION OF PRISON VIOLENCE

By international law, prisoners have a right to protection against violence.[3] Nurses can promote violence prevention by:

— Supporting therapeutic communication with inmates

— Supporting positive interactions between correctional staff and inmates

— Participating in and supporting violence prevention training for all staff

— Organizing health delivery services, which prioritize provision and respect for inmate health, patient autonomy, privacy of patient records, and honest communication with inmates

Assessment and interpersonal skills are the most important strategies nurses can implement in the prevention of prison violence. Accurate assessments that identify factors related to violence are the foundation for interventions to address inmate needs, reduce risk factors, and promote positive interactions between inmates and staff.

The ability to perform and advocate for the use of aggressive behavior de-escalation by all correctional staff is a key nursing intervention. De-escalation is the first and most effective strategy to respond to potential violence and aggression in health care settings. The aim of de-escalation is to prevent violent behavior, avoid using restraints, reduce patient anger and frustration, maintain inmate and staff safety, and improve interactions. Extensive documentation of factors contributing to aggression in health care settings, along with de-escalation techniques, therapeutic communication, and stress/conflict management, are available for inclusion in professional training. Successful de-escalation promotes inmate and staff feelings of hope, security, and self-acceptance, which form the foundation for an environment in which violence is decreased.[5] Other strategies such as anger management programs can be effective in increasing impulse control and decreasing aggressive problem-solving strategies used by many inmates.

IMPACT OF PRISON VIOLENCE

Prison violence has the potential to negatively impact health, quality of life, and feelings of safety and security among both inmates and staff. Responses to violence in prison include post traumatic stress symptoms and exacerbation of existing mental health problems as well as deterioration of physical health. The higher the incidence of violence in prison, the more likely violence is to occur again, and the negative consequences increase. Witnessing violence can have the same psychologically traumatizing impact as experiencing violence firsthand.[6] Unsafe, violent prison environments are more difficult and expensive to manage, siphoning funding needed for the humane treatment of prisoners. Among staff working in high violence prison settings, there are higher rates of burnout and turnover. General anxiety levels among staff and inmates tend to create and increase negative perceptions of the work environment and dissatisfaction with their work roles.

ETHICAL ISSUES: THE RELATIONSHIP OF CLINICAL DECISION MAKING TO PERCEPTION OF INJUSTICE

Prison settings have restricted patients' access to treatment options and tend to promote a culture that prioritizes security, conformity, and order. Patient autonomy and individualized care are not reflected in prison policies and protocols, which creates professional and ethical challenges for nurses. A perception of substandard treatment due to correctional protocols is one factor impacting distrust between nurses and inmates. Distrust leads to inmates acting out or behaving violently. For instance, intervention options such as pain management are often informed not only by evidence of the clinical efficacy of treatment, but also the potential for diversion to other inmates and fear of misuse and addiction. The health staff is left to make health care judgments based on the prison's protocols and assessment of the individual patient, which are often in conflict with common practice standards.

A careful assessment of patient considerations and needs must be balanced against possible negative outcomes regarding selected health interventions. The consideration of nonmaleficence versus respect for autonomy is a primary source of conflict for ethical decision making in the prison setting. Whenever possible, it is important to prioritize patient autonomy to reduce rationalization of violence as a response to perceived injustice. The nurse needs to consider whether standards of care differ between the community and the correctional setting and if that difference is due to the institution's goals rather than patient welfare.

CASE STUDIES

Case Study 29-1

A prisoner was attacked in the exercise yard. The nurse on duty rushed to the site and was told by one of the other prisoners that the injured man had been stabbed. The correctional officer on duty refused to open the gate to allow the nurse into the exercise yard due to security concerns. The area had not been secured yet, and he was waiting for backup assistance. The nurse observed that the injured prisoner was writhing in pain, and a significant amount of blood appeared to be present.

Discussion

The forensic nurse should consider how the welfare of the injured inmate can be balanced with the welfare of other inmates, correctional staff, and the nurse. Nurses are often the first health care professional to assess and care for inmates. Even with limited access, nurses can and do make a difference in situations such as this.

The nurse has a responsibility to communicate their assessment to correctional staff and administration, even from a distance. The nurse must convey the need for an urgent response in order to provide care for the injured inmate. If the nurse is unable to provide care directly, they may be able to give instructions to a correctional officer who can give immediate care to the inmate until the nurse is admitted. An emergency care bag for these violent settings should always be on hand and include only materials that cannot be used as weapons or for inflicting violence. Nurses need and must demand support and training by the institution in order to cope with constraining circumstances such as these.

SUMMARY

Nurses must be well-informed about the contributing factors of prison violence in order to properly respond. Understanding that the sociodemographic and psychological characteristics of inmates are major factors impacting violence in prisons is critical to constructing strategies for assessment and intervention. Nurses are positioned to assist in the assessment of potential for violence among inmates and in the physical and cultural environment of the prison. Modeling professional caring and critically analyzing the factors impacting violence will allow nurses to effectively collaborate with correctional officers and other staff to initiate appropriate interactions and health interventions with those who are most vulnerable to violence, including mentally and physically disabled inmates. Forensic nurses must pay specific attention to refining their skill in assessing potential violence, and they should advocate for regular training to reduce the occurrence and impact of violence on inmates, correctional staff, and nurses.

REFERENCES

1. Krug EG, Dahlberg LL, Mercy JA, Zwi AB, Lozano R, eds. World report on violence and health: summary. World Health Organization; 2002.

2. Bureau of Prisons. Adjudicated assaults recorded in SENTRY chronological disciplinary records (guilty findings only). Office of Research and Evaluation. Updated September 2020. Accessed September 24, 2021. https://www.bop.gov/about/statistics/statistics_prison_safety.jsp?month=sept&year=2020

3. Modvig J. Violence, sexual abuse and torture in prisons. Accessed October 21, 2021. https://www.euro.who.int/__data/assets/pdf_file/0010/249193/Prisons-and-Health,-4-Violence,-sexual-abuse-and-torture-in-prisons.pdf

4. MacDonald M. Overcrowding and its impact on prison conditions and health. *Int J Prison Health.* 2018;14(2):65-68.

5. The Joint Commission. *De-escalation in health care.* Division of Health Improvement; 2019.

6. Widra E. No escape: the trauma of witnessing violence in prison. Prison Policy Initiative. December 2, 2020. Accessed October 5, 2021. https://www.prisonpolicy.org/blog/2020/12/02/witnessing-prison-violence/

EMERGENCY PREPAREDNESS: NATURAL AND MANMADE DISASTERS

Joyce P. Williams, DNP, MFSA, RN, FAAFS, DF-IAFN, FAAN
David A. Williams, DDS, MS, MPH

KEY POINTS

1. *An all-hazards approach in a disaster maximizes available resources to address the overall scope of emergency preparedness and planning.*

2. *The nurse's primary role in emergency preparedness and the disaster cycle is to provide public health and medical services.*

3. *Individuals and families can exercise disaster preparedness by being informed, gathering knowledge of safety measures, and preparing survival materials.*

INTRODUCTION

Disasters cause injury, death, and economic impact and bring about loss of life and varying levels of mass destruction. Today, disasters are commonly classified into 3 broad categories: natural, manmade, or hybrid.[1] **Natural disasters** are catastrophic events caused by severe weather, global changes, or other nonhuman causes, while **manmade disasters** result directly from human actions. **Hybrid disasters** are caused by a combination of natural events and human actions. Categories of disasters and examples of each are shown in **Table 30-1**.

Table 30-1. Disaster Examples by Category[1]		
NATURAL	MANMADE	HYBRID
Hurricanes/tornados	Stampede	Technical
Earthquake	Transportation/mass transit	Environmental elements
Tsunami/flood/drought	Air disaster	Poor urban planning
Wildfires/bushfires	Pipeline incidents	Pandemics
Extreme heat/cold	Marine/riverine incidents	
	Terrorism/mass shootings	

DISASTER SURVEILLANCE

Changing climates are responsible for more than 9 percent of global deaths each year. Because there are so many variables whereby a disaster may occur, tracking in multiple venues is necessary. Infectious disease outbreaks from emerging viruses spread unknowingly and rapidly. Forensic nurses are key personnel to recognize and report early outbreaks of disease. They also raise awareness of potential hazards and how to address them.

Surveillance constitutes a process of collecting and analyzing data relevant to the detection of changes in health within a community. Syndromic surveillance incorporates nontraditional data to establish a development that may indicate potential threats to a population's health.

Forensic nurses specializing in infection control or epidemiology monitor communities for risk, adverse health events, and recommend ways to decrease hazards.

> "Syndromic surveillance provides public health officials with a timely system for detecting, understanding, and monitoring health events. By tracking symptoms of patients in emergency departments—before a diagnosis is confirmed—public health can detect unusual levels of illness to determine whether a response is warranted. Syndromic data can serve as an early warning system for public health concerns such as flu outbreaks and have been used in responses for opioid overdoses, e-cigarette or vaping product use-associated lung injury, Zika virus infection, and natural disasters."[2]

EMERGENCY PREPAREDNESS RESPONSE

Whenever a disaster happens, the local community experiences impact, and locals are the first to respond. The primary response of the local jurisdiction is to alert the population to impending disaster as soon as possible, and once the disaster has passed, provide the initial response. If the resources to address the incident are insufficient, then the local jurisdiction must declare a local emergency and request assistance from the state government. States have a greater response capacity than the local government; if they have sufficient capacity to meet the needs of the response to the disaster, they initiate state resources to provide the needed services. When state response is sufficient, it is unnecessary to involve the federal government. However, if the disaster exceeds the local and state capacities, then the state's elected officials (eg, governor) requests a federal disaster designation, and if approved, federal resources are accessible (eg, Federal Emergency Management Agency [FEMA]). Forensic nurses are in a unique position to aid in community preparedness because they have the background in patient care as well as the ability to understand the nature of disasters and potential for community response.

ALL HAZARDS APPROACH

An all-hazards approach maximizes available resources to address the overall scope of emergency preparedness and planning, incorporating vulnerabilities and potential threats to the community. Emergency operations centers, as the command center in a community, direct control of and response to carrying out disaster-relief protocols, including short- and long-term preparedness, response, recovery and mitigation. Response models follow the National Incident Management System to coordinate a jurisdiction's overall threat and response to an active situation.

THE DISASTER CYCLE

The federal government defines 4 distinct disaster phases for communities wishing to address disasters proactively. The phases of preparedness, response, recovery, and mitigation are detailed in **Table 30-2**.

NATIONAL RESPONSE FRAMEWORK

The National Response Framework (NRF) guides the national response to all types of disasters and emergencies.[3] The NRF structure helps jurisdictions, citizens, nongovernmental organizations, and businesses develop community plans to stabilize community lifelines and restore services following a disaster. The composition

Table 30-2. Core Competencies of the Disaster Cycle[1]	
PHASES	ACTIVITIES
Preparedness	— Planning, training, and education activities for an event that cannot be mitigated — Individual, local or on a national scale — Includes an environmental scan of the area to determine the types of potential disasters for the area, and estimates of greatest damage
Response	— Occurs immediately in the aftermath of a disaster — During the response phase, business and other operations do not function normally. — Personal safety and well-being in an emergency and the duration of the response phase depends on the level of preparedness, with emphasis on life-threatening and property-threatening activities.
Recovery	— The longest phase, occurring unevenly throughout the affected area with those having the greatest devastation returning to normal more slowly — May be prolonged — Restoration efforts occur concurrently with regular operations and activities in those areas least affected.
Mitigation	— Prevents or reduces the cause, impact, and consequences of disaster — Often happens in response to a previous disaster, with all hazard identification — Ideally occurs prior to event

of the NRF includes 15 Emergency Support Functions (ESFs) and Support Annexes. A specific Federal Cabinet department has primary responsibility for each ESF. In most incidences, registered nurses work under ESF #8, Public Health and Medical Services. ESF #8 includes public health, hospitals, EMS, clinics, and agencies that have involvement in the health section of the emergency response. Another area overseeing registered nurses is ESF #6, Mass Care, Emergency Assistance, Housing, and Human Services, which includes coordination of locations of mass care shelters. **Table 30-2** outlines the phases of the disaster cycle and the steps taken during each phase.

MEDICAL RESPONSE TO DISASTERS
HAZARD VULNERABILITY ANALYSIS
Hospitals endure vulnerabilities after a disaster, and a hazard vulnerability analysis (HVA) is a process for identifying the hospital's highest vulnerabilities to natural and man-made hazards. As leaders, forensic nurses prepare the system for safety to minimize the impact on patients and staff. The HVA also identifies the impact of hazards beyond the hospital and in the community.

HOSPITAL INCIDENT COMMAND SYSTEMS
Forensic nurses can provide guidance and leadership in the hospital's response to disasters. The Incident Command System (ICS) is a standardized approach to the command, control, and coordination of emergency response incident management that is used at the federal, state and local levels. Hospital Incident Command System

(HICS) is a structure specifically designed for hospitals. Within the hospital, the nursing staff provides the greatest number of medical professionals.

CRISIS STANDARDS OF CARE

Providing medical care under catastrophic disaster conditions means the delivery of health care services is likely to change with scarcity of resources. Crisis Standards of Care involve the confluence of ethical, legal, and medical priorities. For instance, equipment running on electricity may need to rely on a generator if a city loses power; when the hospital generator's fuel is exhausted, the equipment ceases to run. In an environment with scarce medical resources, limiting patient morbidity and mortality occurs in a triage environment of collective rather than individual priorities. With the background and knowledge of medicine, and jurisprudence, the forensic nurse can provide input into these difficult decisions.

VOLUNTEERS

Forensic nurses can be active participants working in the community supporting populations in need. In the case of a disaster, volunteers are often needed to assist with other community needs. Volunteers can receive training through FEMA and other sanctioned organizations. Independent Study courses provide the basis for appropriate disaster response and are often required by affiliated disaster response organizations. There are 2 general categories of volunteers – affiliated and unaffiliated.

Affiliated volunteers are members of a recognized volunteer agency. These volunteers have attained specialized skills and have undergone training and certification. They understand agency policies and procedures and their role during disaster response, and they are usually covered by the agency's insurance. Choosing a particular organization reflects individual talents and goals matching actions taken during a disaster. Others choose organizations with sponsorship (eg, religious or fraternal organizations).

Unaffiliated volunteers are individuals not attached to an organization and therefore may or may not have the needed skills or training. They may self-activate or be in groups.

PERSONAL PREPAREDNESS

Personal and family preparedness are essential. Individuals living in a community can exercise disaster preparedness by being informed; gathering knowledge of personal, organizational, and community safety measures; and preparing a disaster kit and other survival materials.[4] The forensic nurse serves as an educator for the community and a model who demonstrates the concept of personal preparedness with a disaster kit and training to share with others. Disaster kits should include 72 hours worth of food and water, medications, batteries, a wireless radio, and chargers. In addition, pet and livestock care materials should be included to provide for their needs when resources are limited during a disaster.

CASE STUDIES

Case Study 30-1

A 120 car train carrying anhydrous ammonia was passing through a small town. The incident occurred ¼ mile from a health care facility, the train collided with a vehicle stalled on the tracks causing it to derail. Twenty train cars came off of the tracks, many of them carrying the anhydrous ammonia, causing leaks.

Discussion

Once the call to emergency personnel was made, the nearby health care facility activated their disaster plan. They began by evaluating the weather conditions and communicating with the emergency response team to determine if it was safe for the team to respond and they also prepared for potential contaminated patients. Upon determining that the team would be safe, the forensic nurses went to the scene to respond to this manmade disaster. Their intervention began with the individuals on the train, those in the vehicle that was struck, and potential victims in the community. These individuals were stabilized and transported by emergency medical services to the nearby health care facility where additional life saving efforts could be enacted.

Once the injured civilians in the area had been safely transported, the forensic nursing staff began implementing recovery efforts in conjunction with emergency response teams and transportation officials. These efforts included containing the leak of anhydrous ammonia, treating those affected by the gas, clearing debris to look for any other injured individuals, and eventually restoring operation of the train. Steps were taken to ensure that any lasting effects of the anhydrous ammonia leak would be mitigated by health care professionals.

Case Study 30-2

An EF-3 tornado tore through a town causing extensive damage to a local warehouse as well as many homes. High winds caused the displacement of more than 250 residents of the town as well as those working in the warehouse at the time of the event. While there was significant warning of the possibility of a tornado and sirens were activated, the warehouse did not have a basement, so staff were left with few options for shelter.

Discussion

In response to this natural disaster, forensic nursing staff at local hospitals were called to enact their response plan. Due to their training in mass disaster response, the local forensic nurses promptly responded to the affected areas to assist injured community members. Due to the extensive property damage, a significant amount of debris blocked many of the injured individuals from nursing staff. In collaboration with the local fire department, the nurses were able to access and transport those trapped within the warehouse for medical treatment. Those with life threatening injuries were treated on site before being transported by emergency medical services to a health care facility for additional treatment.

Recovery efforts lasted several days during which time many community members stayed in a shelter for the displaced run by local emergency services. Forensic nurses had prepared an emergency plan for the community and ensured that the facilities necessary were maintained. Electricity, and waste management systems had been put into place, and food, water, and other necessary supplies were available. Security was maintained at all times. Medical personnel remained on site to facilitate ongoing management for those with health conditions. Housing included age appropriate furnishings for those who were vulnerable or disabled. The emergency preparedness plan set in place ensured that supplies were readily available to all residents by maintaining stores and coordinating deliveries of additional necessary products.

SUMMARY

While mass disasters may cause catastrophic damage, the harmful effects can be mitigated through emergency preparation. All disasters can result in major health crises. Forensic nurses have a responsibility to advise officials on the response to and preparedness for emergencies by providing public health and medical services. Forensic nurses must have plans in place to mitigate the after effects of a mass disaster, especially scarcity of resources. Organizations like the American Red Cross, Salvation Army, and Community Emergency Response Teams can assist in disasters by providing shelter, goods, or services for the community.

REFERENCES

1. National Response Framework, Fourth Edition. Federal Emergency Management Agency. October 28, 2019. https://www.fema.gov/sites/default/files/2020-04/NRF_FINALApproved_2011028.pdf

2. Syndromic Surveillance. Center for Disease Control and Prevention. Updated September 24, 2021. https://www.cdc.gov/nssp/overview.html

3. Emergency Support Function #8 – Public Health and Medical Services Annex. Federal Emergency Management Agency. June 2016. https://www.fema.gov/sites/default/files/2020-07/fema_ESF_8_Public-Health-Medical.pdf

4. Disasters and Emergencies. Ready. Updated November 4, 2021. https://www.ready.gov/be-informed

VI

SPECIAL CRIMES

TECHNOLOGY AND RISK

Elizabeth B. Dowdell, PhD, RN, AFN-C, FAAN
Patricia M. Speck, DNSc, CRNP, FNP-BC, AFN-C, DF-IAFN, FAAFS, DF-AFN, FAAN

KEY POINTS

1. *Trauma is universal, widespread, harmful, and costly to individuals and society at large.*

2. *Technology is growing at an exponential rate, and there are new tools and language that increase risk-taking behavior with both unknown or known persons with or without criminal motives.*

3. *Technology is a useful tool for individuals with nefarious motives, thereby putting all individuals at risk for trauma, which causes negative mental health outcomes.*

4. *Forensic nurses should be familiar with digital natives, screening tools, and the terminology used to communicate with their patients regarding technology.*

INTRODUCTION

Risk-taking by an individual is a pattern of unnecessary engagement in activities or behaviors that are dangerous or highly subject to chance. The risk-taking pattern of behavior is often associated with substance abuse, gambling, high-risk sexual behaviors, and extreme sports.[1,2] Not surprisingly, risk-taking is now also happening in the online world.

The internet is a positive medium for innovation, education, and economic growth around the globe, and for Generation Z, the internet transformed their experience of growing up. Persons born into and raised in a digital world are often called ***digital natives*** as they grew up with digital technology (eg, computers, cell phones, etc.). People born before 1990 are not viewed as digital natives and instead are referred to as ***digital immigrants***. Regardless of status or age, the internet has increasingly become a necessity. Children as young as 18 months old are now introduced to games and educational software through handheld mobile devices (eg, smartphones, tablets). All levels of education are actively using the internet in classrooms and homework assignments, as well as for communication, reports, and social networking. Recently, the COVID-19 pandemic closed many offices and workplaces, creating an era of remote work for millions of adults.[3,4]

ONLINE RISK

Internet risk-taking has grown more common as mobile devices have become part of everyday life, and it frequently has offline consequences. This type of risk behavior is different than the more conventional health risk behaviors of smoking, alcohol use, unsafe sex, and substance abuse.[2,3] Online risk-taking involves a variety of behaviors that tend to cluster together,[2,5,6] and they occur on a variety of websites and social media (**Table 31-1**). Websites often encourage information sharing, and for children and adolescents especially, online risk involves disclosing a wide range of personal information on social media sites, including pictures, names, ages, and locations. Individuals who intend to commit crimes against children often visit these sites because they offer easy access to vulnerable individuals, especially children. From there, those predatory individuals can then entrap and share sexual materials, find like-minded offenders, and maintain some level of anonymity through alias profiles, thereby reducing their risk of detection.[7,8]

Table 31-1. Definitions of High-Risk Online Behaviors[2]

Type of Risk Behavior	Definition of Risk Behavior
Information Sharing	Risky online behavior can be inclusive of more than 1 type of behavior. These behaviors have been found to cluster together, and they include the following: — Sharing personal information (eg, name of school, email address, picture of self) — Corresponding online with an unknown person or later meeting the person offline — Engaging in online initiated harassment (eg, electronic aggression, cyberbullying, posting cruel comments or malicious jokes) — Visiting online sex sites; overriding internet filters or blocks
Social Media	Social media includes different forms of electronic communication that allow the user to create virtual communities and networks. This combination of interactive technologies allows the creation or sharing/exchange of information, ideas, messages, and other forms of expression (eg, pictures and videos).
Cyberbullying	Bullying is a form of unwanted, aggressive behavior involving a real or perceived power imbalance that is repeated or chronic in nature. Cyberbullying is bullying that can occur through any type of digital device and by means of social media, applications (ie, apps), websites, forums, online gaming, or any other online platform where people can view, participate in, or share content.
Self-Exploitation (autopornography)	Autopornography is the creation of explicit or inappropriate pictures of oneself, such as ones that show nudity, sex acts, or simulated sex.
Sexting	Sexting is the electronic distribution of explicit or inappropriate pictures, images, messages, or videos, of oneself or peers, using technology.
Sextortion*	This is a serious crime that occurs primarily online and involves non physical forms of coercion, such as blackmail, to acquire sexual content (eg, photos/videos) of, to obtain money from, or engage in sex with an individual. The perpetrator may also threaten to harm friends or family members by using information they have obtained from the electronic devices.
Cyberstalking	Stalking is a crime of power and control. It is a course of action directed at an individual that causes them to fear for their safety, and it generally involves repeated visual or physical proximity, nonconsensual communication, and verbal, written, or implied threats. Cyberstalking is a form of stalking that includes any course of conduct or action taken by a perpetrator on the internet that leaves the victim with a fear of death or serious bodily injury. It also includes any act that causes, attempts to cause, or would be reasonably expected to cause substantial emotional distress to the victim or the victim's immediate family.
Identity Theft or Identity Fraud	Identity theft and fraud refer to all crimes in which someone wrongfully obtains and uses another individual's personal data in some way that involves fraud or deception, typically for economic gain.

NOTE: In the United States Criminal Code and in many states, there are no "sextortion" offenses; however, the behavior(s) often encompasses multiple federal and state crimes. Dowdell, 2020. Used with permission.

As online connectivity expands, the commission of sexual crimes does as well. The method for online sexual exploitation begins with grooming, live streaming, consuming child sexual abuse materials, and coercing and blackmailing children for sexual purposes. In these cases, the internet acts as a vehicle for targeting and accessing victims. The internet has diminished predatory individuals' need to find victims in person. Instead, they can maintain anonymity and access social media, chat rooms, and other websites from anywhere. Online sexual exploitation often occurs across multiple jurisdictions, with victims and offenders regularly in different states or countries. The intersection of internet use with human sex trafficking of children is significant.[8]

NURSING APPLICATIONS

A public health model delineates the parameters of risk and spells out primary prevention and secondary intervention responses when approaching the problem of technology-based risk. Using the nursing process—a comprehensive assessment of the patient, creating and implementing a treatment plan, and evaluating the intervention—is essential in the creation of an online safety plan. Part of the forensic nursing practice involves routine screening for online risk behaviors and consequences. While it is often time-consuming to ask more assessment questions, the first step in the screening process is to ask every patient about their experiences online and to identify those who report taking risks. The second step in the screening process is for the nurse to then build a rapport with the patient by using what was shared during the assessment or located in the medical history as a foundation for asking specific questions about their risk behavior. Being knowledgeable about online risk behaviors promotes better communication among individuals, families, and other professionals in schools or the community around the serious topic of technology and risk. As practitioners of trauma-informed care, forensic nurses encourage behavior changes regarding the supervision of children to prevent further harm. The forensic nurse should provide supportive suggestions to achieve these changes for both children and the adults in their lives.[9,10] Typical questions to ask parents and their children are located in **Table 31-2**.

Forensic nurses have access to multiple online resources (**Table 31-3**) to help with the care of patients who have been victimized/exploited through online mediums.

Table 31-2. Typical Questions in Screening for Technology Risk[5]

QUESTIONS FOR ALL PATIENTS	QUESTIONS FOR CHILDREN AND ADOLESCENTS
One way to ask about online activity and social media use is to say: "Everyone is spending more time online, and because it affects health and well-being, I ask everyone (patients) about their online life and use of social media and apps."	What device do you use to access the internet (smartphone, tablet, mobile device, laptop, etc.) the most?
During a typical day, how much time do you spend online/on social media sites?	Is your internet access unlimited, or have your parents installed blocks or locks? Do these blocks and locks work?
At what time of day do you use social media?	Do you regularly use FaceTime or another video chat platform to talk with friends, family, or new people?
How many social media and/or online accounts do you have (Instagram, Facebook, Twitter, Tumblr, Snapchat, etc.)?	How important is your internet or online life to you? Use a 1 to 10 scale (1 = not very important, 10 = extremely important). *(continued)*

Table 31-2. Typical Questions in Screening for Technology Risk[5] *(continued)*

QUESTIONS FOR ALL PATIENTS	QUESTIONS FOR CHILDREN AND ADOLESCENTS
Which social media sites and/or apps are your favorite? What makes it/them a favorite?	How would you describe your mood when you are online, offline, at home, and at school?
When you are on and using social media, how do you feel? What is the most common emotion you feel?	Have you ever had a relationship or friendship with someone online? Tell me about them and how you are feeling.
Do you post photos or videos on social media? Can you describe to me the last 2 photos or videos you posted?	If you were to feel uncomfortable or scared from being online, whom would you tell?
Do you have any photos or videos posted that you feel uncomfortable or anxious about?	What device do you use to access the internet (smartphone, tablet, mobile device, laptop, etc.) the most?

© *Dowdell, 2022 Used with permission.*

Table 31-3. Online Resources for Forensic Nurses

National Center for Missing and Exploited Children[11]: Offers information about missing and exploited children. It also helps law enforcement and other agencies. Its toll-free number, 800-THE-LOST or 800-843-5678, is available for reporting 24 hours a day, 7 days a week. The CyberTipline[12] is a reporting mechanism for cases of child sexual exploitation, including child pornography, online enticement of children for sex acts, molestation of children outside the family, sex tourism of children, child prostitution, and unsolicited obscene material sent to a child.

Internet Crimes Against Children Task Force[13]: A national network of 61 coordinated task forces representing more than 3500 federal, state, and local law enforcement and prosecutorial agencies. These agencies are engaged in proactive and reactive investigations, forensic investigations, and criminal prosecutions by helping state and local agencies to develop effective, sustainable responses to online child victimization, including to the online sharing of child sexual abuse images.

The US Postal Inspection Service[14]: A federal law enforcement agency responsible for investigating crimes involving the United States mail, including the prevention of child exploitation by eliminating the distribution of child pornography material. Although pornographic images of children were once solely distributed and traded via mail, the internet has provided a new and more efficient way to continue the victimization of children. Any information regarding child exploitation through the mail or on the internet can be found on their webpage: www.uspis.gov/tips-prevention/child-safety.

US Customs and Border Protection (CBP)[15]: Protects United States borders and also targets cybercrime and the illegal importation/trafficking of child pornography. The CBP tip line for illegal internet activities is 1-800-BE-ALERT. CBP will pay cash awards pursuant to Title 19 of the US Code, Section 1619, for information concerning a violation of customs laws (eg, child exploitation on the internet from different countries or child pornography) if the information leads to the recovery of fines, penalties, or forfeitures.

CASE STUDIES

Case Study 31-1

A 14-year-old female sent her boyfriend a nude picture of herself while she was taking a bath. When they broke up, he shared the picture in a group chat with all of his friends, and then he also posted the picture on his social media page. Other peers at their school saw the picture, and the girl was devastated. She tried to commit suicide and eventually withdrew from school. The boy was charged with distribution of child pornography, and 2 of his friends who had downloaded the photograph were charged with possession of child pornography.

Discussion

Safety is a primary role of all adults. Asking screening questions during routine visits to the school nurse can create an opportunity to increase awareness of the risk-taking behaviors that often plague adolescents, such as sexting and the distribution of revealing images of their underage peers. Having sexual photographs of underage persons on phones, computers, and tablets, whether from social media sites or taken personally, is classified as possession of child pornography. In this case, the boyfriend was the distributor of child pornography, and since his friends re-distributed the image, they also became distributors. Nurses have a responsibility to explain the potential legal ramifications of technology activities and document any interventions taken in their records. School nurses can play a particular role in prevention as they are with vulnerable students throughout the day.

Case Study 31-2

A mother was making dinner for herself and her 9-year-old daughter, who was upstairs in her room. When their dinner was ready, the mother went upstairs and found her daughter with her pants and underwear off, laying in front of her laptop with the webcam on. A voice from the tablet told the girl to spread her labia and to continue touching herself. The mother screamed at the voice and violently shut the laptop. She grabbed the girl and yelled, "get dressed! ... what is wrong with you?!" The mother then called the girl's pediatrician and talked with a nurse, who called the police. The police questioned the child and found out that the girl was on social media playing a game with others when a friend request appeared in her private chat. This "friend" wanted to talk about how much he liked her game character, and he claimed that he was 10 years old. He wanted to learn more about her and asked her to turn the web camera on. Then he asked her to "show and tell," and after several meetings online, she found herself undressing and touching her genitalia for him.

Discussion

Supervision of children is the responsibility of parents and caretakers, especially when technology is involved. In this case, the mother was unprepared and consequently responded in a way to promote shame on her child's actions. The forensic nurse counseled the mother about her response and provided strategies to repair the impact on the child. This included making supportive statements that are appropriate for the child's age, focusing on the child's development and curiosity at this stage in her life. The questions the forensic nurse asked the girl also targeted the child's developmental stage and were trauma-informed. Consequently, the child grew more comfortable during the history portion of her medical-forensic evaluation, eventually saying that she didn't know that what she did was wrong. The child said she was lonely and had been excited that she found a friend online. However, the "friend" turned out to be a 28-year-old male who lived 4 states away from the child and was grooming her. **Grooming** is a characteristic of pedophiles that gradually entices, through positive feedback, the behaviors of exposure for the adult's sexual pleasure. Children rarely understand that this experience is negative because the body's response to self-stimulation feels good, and the sexual intensity is not understood by the child or interpreted as sex. The grooming process makes children an ideal target for continued abuse, as perpetrators can use technology and social media to gain access with a lower risk of arrest than with face-to-face, hands-on abuse.

SUMMARY

Technology permanently changed society, and it is still evolving at an exponential rate. Technology is used to entrap persons, resulting in physical and psychological trauma that leads to negative mental health outcomes. Technology-imposed trauma is universal, widespread, harmful, and costly to individuals and society at large. With new tools and language associated only with technology, there are more risks generationally as the divide grows and the field is rife with persons using technology with nefarious motives. Forensic nurses find it necessary to become familiar with digital natives, as well as the screening tools and terminology needed to communicate with their patients. The resources available to the forensic nurse help to support the patient's understanding of technological risk and provide the nurse with additional methods to screen for risk in patient populations.

REFERENCES

1. American Psychological Association. APA Dictionary of Psychology - Risk Taking. 2020. Accessed January 27, 2022. https://dictionary.apa.org/risk-taking

2. Dowdell E, Noel J. Risk behaviors of high school students who report knowing someone who self-harms. *Issues Ment Health Nurs.* 2020;41(5):415-420. https://doi.org/10.1080/01612840.2019.1663568

3. Cho AN, Dowdell EB. Unintentional gun violence in the home: a survey of pediatric advanced practice nurses' preventive measures. *J Pediatr Health Care.* 2020;34(1):23-29.

4. Parker K, Horowitz JM, Minkin R. *How the Coronavirus Outbreak Has – and Hasn't – Changed the Way Americans Work.* Pew Research Center; 2020.

5. Dowdell EB, Freitas E, Owens A, Greenle MM. School shooters: patterns of adverse childhood experiences, bullying, and social media. *J Pediatr Health Care.* 2022;S0891-5245(21)00290-X. doi:10.1016/j.pedhc.2021.12.004

6. Dowdell EB, Noel J. Having a peer who self-harms: examining risk taking behaviors in high school students. *Issues Ment Health Nurs.* 2020;41(5):415-420.

7. Burgess AW. *Victimology Theories and Applications.* 3rd ed. Jones and Bartlett Learning; 2019.

8. O'Brien JE, Li W. The role of the internet in the grooming, exploitation, and exit of United States domestic minor sex trafficking victims. *J Child Media.* 2020;14(2):187-203.

9. McKenzie KJ, Pierce D, Gunn JM. A systematic review of motivational interviewing in healthcare: the potential of motivational interviewing to address the lifestyle factors relevant to multimorbidity. *J Comorb.* 2015;5:162-174.

10. Dowdell EB, Speck PM. Foundations for trauma informed care in nursing practice. *Am J Nurs.* 2022;122(4):30-38. doi:10.1097/01.NAJ.0000827328.25341.1f

11. National Center for Missing and Exploited Children. https://www.missingkids.org/

12. CyberTipline. National Center for Missing and Exploited Children. https://report.cybertip.org/

13. Internet Crimes Against Children Task Force Program. https://icactaskforce.org/

13. Child Safety. United States Postal Inspection Service. Updated April 2022. https://www.uspis.gov/tips-prevention/child-safety

15. US Customs and Border Protection. Department of Homeland Security. https://www.cbp.gov/

Chapter 32

Offensive Behaviors: Bullying and Sexual Harassment

Steven J. Palazzo, PhD, MN, RN, CNE
Gordon Lee Gillespie, PhD, DNP, RN, FAAN

Key Points

1. *At both the individual and organizational levels, prevention strategies can mitigate the prevalence of bullying and sexual harassment in the workplace.*

2. *Sexual harassment intervention measures can be deployed when identifying cues of escalating harassment behaviors.*

3. *A formal anti-harassment workplace policy is needed to address the prevention and management of bullying and sexual harassment.*

Introduction

There is a high prevalence of unwanted bullying and sexual harassment (ie, sexualized behaviors) toward nurses. Over 40% of nurses experience some form of harassment in the workplace, whether that be verbal, nonverbal, psychological, physical, or sexual violence.[1] While there has been an increased awareness of bullying and sexual harassment toward health care workers, nurses continue to experience offensive and sexually motivated behaviors in the workplace.[1] These behaviors take the form of [2]:

— Unwelcome and unsolicited verbal communication (eg, rude comments, sexually suggestive jokes, intrusive questions, comments about physical appearance)

— Nonverbal communication (eg, hand gestures, staring, and leering)

— Visuals (eg, exposed to explicit material)

— Physical contact of a sexual nature (eg, shoving, touching, fondling, hugging, kissing)

Perpetrators of these types of behavior in the workplace tend to be coworkers, patients, patients' family members, and other visitors.[1] Bullying and sexual harassment in the workplace lead to feelings of humiliation, intimidation, anxiety, depression, sleep disorders, absenteeism, patient safety concerns, and low productivity.[1,3] Furthermore, an omittance or avoidance of patient care is a frequent consequence of sexual harassment when that harassment is perpetrated by a patient. This may lead to an unfavorable outcome for the patient and feelings of shame and inadequacy for the nurse.[4]

In order to mitigate the harmful effects of bullying and sexual harassment in the workplace, it is necessary to develop prevention measures. Two areas of prevention have been identified: the individual and the organization.[5] When feasible, emotional distancing, support from colleagues or bystanders, and mediation by a third party are strategies that work to address the issues at the individual level.[5] To address issues at the organizational level, strategies include establishing policies that encourage discussion and action and removing any tolerance of bullying, sexualized behaviors, and the perpetrators themselves.[5]

CASE STUDIES

Case Study 32-1

During a night shift, this nurse was asked to work in a different unit. Upon arrival, the nurse received a heavier workload assignment than the usual amount given to the nurses of that unit. Two of the nurse's patients were in isolation and required intravenous medications every hour. Each time the nurse passed the central work station, they saw several other nurses sitting and talking there. Because of this, the nurse asked for assistance with their patient workload, but the other nurses laughed and said, "If you can't handle it, then maybe you shouldn't be a nurse." The nurse continued to make efforts to manage their workload but was unable to do so successfully.

During the morning shift change, the other nurses informed the nurse manager that the nurse who floated to their unit was not competent or able to manage a normal patient load. The nurse manager asked the nurse why they could not handle their assignment. The nurse said, "I tried. No one would help me. They gave me too many patients and laughed at me when I asked for help." The nurse manager said, "Well, I have everyone else saying that they offered to help you, and you kept saying that you could do it on your own. I'm really disappointed in your behavior. I do want you to know that I will be informing your own nurse manager about your behaviors. You can go."

Discussion

Bullying behaviors can be enacted by an individual or a group of individuals. The forensic nurse should assess the work environment for signs of bullying, which can be exhibited by assignments that have an imbalance of patient acuity, nurses whispering amongst themselves when coworkers enter and leave the area, and/or nurses reporting that they have been ostracized or bullied. Potential signs of bullying at an organizational level may present as a unit or health system with a high or escalating turnover, absenteeism, and/or an illness rate during a formal evaluation. The forensic nurse should also conduct staff interviews and surveys in order to explore the presence of bullying behaviors, actions attempted to overcome bullying, and responses by management and human resources. Recommendations for preventive actions at the individual and organizational levels include[6]:

— Individual-level prevention and action

  — Informing the employee(s) that their behaviors are negative and are distracting from safe patient care

  — Intervening when witnessing bullying behaviors used by others

  — Reminding coworkers of the expectations for collegiality based on a professional code of ethics

— Organizational-level prevention and action

  — Fostering positive, team-oriented work environments

  — Preventing bullying behaviors through administrative support and resources

  — Educating staff on effective and professional communication

Case Study 32-2

This forensic nurse began employment at a large, urban hospital. A colleague, who was not the nurse's direct report, had become friendly with the nurse over a period of several days. The nurse found their colleague's behavior troubling once it began to involve suggestive comments about their appearance. At first, the nurse dismissed these comments as harmless banter between new colleagues, but their colleague's continued, initiated, and unsolicited banter caused the nurse to become uncomfortable. Despite the nurse's objections, the colleague continued to express a sexualized interest. Days later, the colleague became physical with the nurse by initiating a light touch on the buttocks and by placing their hands on the nurse's shoulders. The nurse confided in a few other colleagues in their unit but was told, "This is how they always behave toward new nurses. Don't worry about it; it's harmless and will pass."

Discussion

In this case, the nurse felt vulnerable because they were new to the organization and other employees seemingly condoned the colleague's sexualized behaviors. The forensic nurse should facilitate an action plan to address the unwanted and uncomfortable behaviors displayed by the colleague. Recommendations for preventive actions at the individual and organizational levels include[5]:

— Individual-level prevention and action

— Establishing clear personal boundaries by using facial expressions and dominant and defensive body language, indicating a discomfort and an intolerance toward the sexualized behavior

— Physically distancing self from the perpetrator

— Confronting directly; saying "stop!" in a clear and strong voice

— Seeking allies, a coalition, or a "show of force" with other colleagues

— Organizational-level prevention and action

— Enacting a robust workplace policy (ie, a signed contract) that formalizes behavioral expectations at the workplace and ensuing consequences for sexual harassment

— Forming a public statement regarding the organization's zero-tolerance policy position on sexual harassment in the workplace

— Establishing an anonymous reporting process that is easy to access

— Mandating training opportunities on de-escalation techniques

— Addressing organizational-level stressors that may contribute to an environment of distress and uncertainty

Case Study 32-3

This team of forensic nurses worked in the emergency department (ED) and encountered a patient who was displaying aggressive sexualized behavior toward them. The patient's behaviors included verbal assaults (ie, offensive, sexualized language) and nonverbal assaults (eg, grabbing at the buttocks and breasts, exposing themselves, blowing kisses). Several times, a new nurse on the team experienced the patient attempting to sexually grab them while using offensive language; therefore, the nurse began withdrawing attempts to care for the patient. Two other experienced nurses in the unit also had encounters with the patient that involved physical and verbal assaults. The team of nurses planned to avoid the patient and only provide the required essential care. They determined what was necessary and arranged a schedule of care for the patient accordingly.

As the day proceeded, care provided to the patient became less frequent, including the assessments that were vital to the protection of the patient from the untoward effects of the injury that placed them in the ED. Over the course of the day, the patient declined and suffered a life-ending cardiac arrest. An investigation ensued and the nurses were found negligent in their care of the patient and were relieved of their positions at the organization.

Discussion

The sexual harassment that was experienced by the nurses resulted in "missed nursing care," therefore reducing the level of quality care and jeopardizing the patient's outcome.[4] This scenario is a common manifestation in EDs where many forensic nurses work.[4] Recommendations for preventive actions at the individual and organizational levels include[5]:

— Individual-level prevention and action

— Identifying your role and responsibilities to the patient as a representative of the organization

— Using direct language and body cues that clearly state boundaries

— Having a coworker present in order to prevent sexualized behaviors

— Organizational-level prevention and action

— Establishing a consultative team to support nurses experiencing sexual harassment

— Developing a campaign that brings awareness to the issue, as well as a patient code of conduct

— Creating a reporting system, including a mechanism to file criminal complaints

— Creating support teams among nurses, management, and security

— Implementing annual and/or monthly training programs

— Administering the MISSCARE (Missed Nursing Care) survey[7] to measure missed nursing care and the reasons for it

— Developing interventions to reduce sexual harassment by patients

Summary

After an incident of workplace bullying or sexual harassment, a nurse may feel shame, guilt, self-blame, embarrassment, and/or ostracization by peers. Because of this, patient outcomes may be jeopardized due to missed nursing care and avoidance. Forensic nurses play an essential role in determining the root causes of workplace bullying and sexual harassment. Forensic nurses also serve as team members who develop strategies in order to prevent and mitigate workplace bullying and sexual harassment incidents, ensuring a better nurse and patient experience in the future.

References

1. Woldegebriel GK, Negarandeh R, Nayen ND, Hasanpour M. Sexual harassment against female nurses: a systematic review. *BMC Nurs.* 2020;19.

2. Shaw E, Hegewisch A, Hess C. Sexual harassment and assault at work: understanding the costs. *Inst Womens Policy Res Publication.* 2018;376.

3. Gender-based violence in global supply chains: resource kit. International Training Centre. Accessed October 25, 2021. https://gbv.itcilo.org/

4. Gabay G, Tikva SS. Sexual harassment of nurses by patients and missed nursing care - a hidden population study. *J Nurs Manag.* 2020;28:1881-1887.

5. Jenner SC, Djermester P, Oertelt-Prigone S. Prevention strategies for sexual harassment in academic medicine: a qualitative study. *J Interpers Violence.* 2020. doi:10.1177/0886260520903130

6. Smith CR, Palazzo SJ, Grubb PL, Gillespie GL. Standing up against workplace bullying behavior: recommendations from newly licensed nurses. *J Nurs Educ Pract.* 2020;10(7):35-45.

7. Kalisch BJ, Williams RA. Development and psychometric testing of a tool to measure missed nursing care. *J Nurs Adm.* 2009;39(5):211-219. doi:10.1097/NNA.0b013e3181a23cf5

Chapter 33

STALKING

Pamela Tabor, DNP, AFN-BC, DF-AFN, DF-IAFN

KEY POINTS

1. *It is essential for forensic nurses to understand what constitutes stalking and recognize that stalking may be an independent crime or may co-occur with other criminal actions.*

2. *Anti-stalking laws exist at both the state and federal levels in the United States; each state and territory, as well as DC, has legislation in place.*

3. *There are tools to assist victims of stalking, such as the computer-based Stalking and Harassment Assessment and Risk Profile (SHARP).*

INTRODUCTION

Stalking is an interpersonal crime that is underscored by a persistent and repeated pattern of unwanted pursuit and harassment. This is a malicious crime that threatens the victim's sense of safety and/or actual safety. It is estimated that 6 to 7.5 million people are stalked annually in the United States. Stalking affects 1 in 6 women and 1 in 17 men at some point during their lifetime.[1]

STALKING BEHAVIOR

There are numerous stalking behaviors, methods, and tactics that induce fear in victims. The widespread use of technology has made it easier for stalkers to act as a constant, invisible intruder and provides limitless opportunities for them to immerse themselves into their victim's life. The 4 categories of stalking behavior are described below (**Table 33-1**).

Table 33-1. Categories of Stalking Behavior[2]		
CATEGORY	DEFINITION	EXAMPLES
Surveillance	Keeping tabs on the victim	Spying; using technology such as a GPS or malware; showing up uninvited; using a third party to harass and spy on victim
Life Invasion	Stalker continually inserts themselves into the victim's life	Phone calls; texting; emailing; spreading damaging gossip; malicious complaints against the victim; sending cards/notes/letters; invading victim's social media; sending unsolicited gifts
Intimidation	The act of inducing fear	Implicit, explicit, and/or third-party threats; forced confrontations; property damage; suicidal threats; threats of harm to victim, their family, or their pets
Interference	Disruption of the victim's life personally, professionally, and/or socially	Initiating spurious legal actions; physical/sexual assault of victim; attacks against third parties; property damage

The most common factors associated with stalking violence include the perpetrator having a close, physical proximity to the victim and disrupting or severing their other personal and intimate relationships. Physical violence is more likely to occur if the stalker and victim had a prior intimate partner relationship.[2] Additional stalking behaviors that may predict physical violence involve the perpetrator loitering outside the victim's home, workplace, or vehicle; threatening physical assault; having a history of abusing partners; vandalizing the victim's home and/or personal property; sending letters to the victim; and scaring the victim enough for them to report being "very frightened." Stalker demographics that significantly increase the risk for violence include a perpetrator who is under the age of 30, has less than a high school diploma, and has a history of substance abuse.[3]

CHARACTERIZING STALKERS

Perpetrators of stalking can be categorized based on the underlying motives for their behavior. There are 4 categories of stalking motivation (**Table 33-2**); however, stalkers may have multiple motives.

Table 33-2. Stalkers' Underlying Motives[4,5]

MOTIVE	CHARACTERISTICS
Simple Obsessional	Most common type of stalker; usually male focusing on ex-wife, ex-lover, or former boss; often feels he was mistreated by the victim; stalking may begin before the relationship ends
Love Obsessional	This type of stalker is a stranger or casual acquaintance; becomes obsessed and begins a pattern of trying to get the attention of the victim; often has celebrities or politicians as the victim
Erotomania	This type of stalker mistakenly believes that the victim is in love with them, and if not for an external barrier, they would be together; may lead the stalker to blame others for standing in the way of the relationship
False Victimization Syndrome	This type of stalker consciously or unconsciously believes that they are the victim and creates a fabricated claim; in these cases, the "supposed victim" is really the stalker; a rare motivation

Another way to categorize a stalker is to determine the relationship between the stalker and their victim (**Table 33-3**).

Table 33-3. Stalker/Victim Relationships[4,5]

RELATIONSHIP TO VICTIM	CHARACTERISTICS
Intimate	Prior relationship exists between the stalker and victim, and the stalker is trying to reestablish that relationship; increased likelihood of prior history of abuse and domestic violence perpetrated by the stalker
Nonintimate	Absolutely no prior relationship, but the stalker focuses on the victim after a brief encounter or by merely observing the victim. Nonintimate stalkers are divided into 2 categories: 1. ***Organized.*** Stalker is methodical and calculating, forming one-way, anonymous communication with the victim. 2. ***Delusional.*** Stalker has a psychological fixation on the victim and falsely believes that there is a relationship or connection with the victim.

STALKING LAWS

Stalking laws in the United States vary between the federal, state, DC, and territory level. The first state to criminalize stalking was California in 1990; as of 2000, all 50 states had anti-stalking laws. There are 3 key elements in anti-stalking laws (**Table 33-4**).

Table 33-4. Key Elements of Stalking Laws[6]

ELEMENT	DEFINITION	CHARACTERISTICS
Actus Reus	The guilty act	Actions and conduct
Mens Rea	The guilty mind	Intent to cause harm and/or fear
Course of Conduct	Pattern of behavior	A pattern-based crime as opposed to an incident-based crime

Stalking is often difficult to prove because fear is subjective. Stalking may include behavior that appears to be benign to others but that holds a special meaning to the victim, causing fear that others may not fully grasp. It can also be difficult to recognize and prosecute stalking because it is an evolving, continual, and progressive crime. Stalking laws serve to criminalize the typically noncriminal behaviors that can appear harmless when considered on an incident-by-incident basis.[6]

STALKING AND INTIMATE PARTNER VIOLENCE

In the context of intimate relationships, stalking is considered to be a specific type of intimate partner violence (IPV). In 21% of intimate relationships in which stalking was reported, the stalking occurs during the time of the relationship; in 36%, the stalking occurs during and after the relationship; and in 43%, the stalking happens after the relationship is terminated.[1,2] With intimate partners, stalkers are also more likely to physically approach the victim, use a weapon, reoffend, initiate insults, display interfering and threatening behaviors, destroy property, follow through on threats, and escalate more quickly.[3]

STALKING AND HEALTH CARE PROVIDERS

Health care workers are at an increased risk of being stalked due to the nature of their work wherein they provide attention, sympathy, and empathy to a stalker. The stalker may then misconstrue these actions as a type of romantic gesture. If the stalker seeks additional time and attention from their health care provider but does not receive it, the stalker may then exhibit delusional thinking, anger, and acts of revenge. Stalking behaviors may also be based on erotomania or a perceived injury or dereliction of duty by the health care provider. These perceptions can lead to incidents of hostility, anger, accusations, threats, and harm.[7]

ASSISTING STALKING VICTIMS

When providing care for victims of stalking, it is important to assure the patient that they are heard and believed. Since stalking is usually covert and difficult to prove, patients should be encouraged to compile and retain corroborating evidence. Corroborating evidence can include, but is not limited to, witnesses to the stalker's tactics, texts, voicemails, computer evidence, pictures, gifts, and any time and/or money that was spent on safety measures. Any victim reports or calls to the police, medical reports (including counseling), requests to be escorted to their car or home, and/or staying at another's house or a hotel should also be noted and receipts retained.[2]

An effective teaching tool for victims of stalking is the Stalking and Harassment Assessment and Risk Profile (SHARP). SHARP is a computer-based program that takes approximately 15 minutes to complete, contains 48 questions, and generates

2 reports. The first report provides a stalking narrative and risk profile, while the second provides information about stalking risks and safety suggestions.[8]

CASE STUDIES

Case Study 33-1

This 24-year-old nurse had been consistently pestered by a former male patient for a few months following his treatment. After encouragement from her coworkers, she went to her hospital's human resources (HR) department and told them about how the former patient would constantly call the front desk asking to speak with her and email her using the contact information provided by the hospital's website. Additionally, he would leave notes on the windshield of her car. In his correspondence he would inform her of what he had observed about her that day; he would talk about who had been with her and what they did, as well as what she was wearing. She also told HR that she had seen him lurking around her home.

Discussion

The nurse and HR utilized the SHARP computer program and then called the police. The nurse had deleted the emails he had sent and had not retained the notes he had written, leaving no physical evidence of his stalking, so the police could not take action until a week later when a GPS tracker was discovered on her car. The police questioned him, and obtained a warrant to search his apartment. There, they found dozens of covert photos of her, binoculars with night vision, and numerous notes written to her that ranged from marriage proposals to a list of various ways to kill her if she did not acquiesce. He was arrested, and a restraining order was obtained until the case could go to trial.

SUMMARY

Stalking is an interpersonal crime that is intrusive, obsessive, harassing, and criminal. For the victim, it evokes fear, loss of control, hopelessness, and can consume their life. Victims may experience anxiety, depression, isolation, drug and alcohol abuse, sleep disturbances, and even suicidal ideation. Trauma-informed forensic nurses should assist these patients by having a working knowledge about stalking, educating patients with tools such as SHARP, and by helping victims create a record of the stalking occurrences and any actions that they have taken to deescalate the situation and protect themselves.

REFERENCES

1. SPARC. Stalking Prevention, Awareness, and Resource Center. Accessed September 2021. https://www.stalkingawareness.org/

2. Connecting the dots: stalking and domestic violence. National Network to End Domestic Violence. February 7, 2020. Accessed 2021. https://nnedv.org/latest_update/connecting-dots-stalking-domestic-violence

3. Rosenfeld B, Harmon R. Factors associated with violence in stalking and obsessional harassment cases. *Criminal Justice Behav.* 2002;29(6):671-691. doi:10.1177/009385402237998

4. Judicial Education Center. Categories of stalking. University of New Mexico. Accessed 2021. http://jec.unm.edu/education/online-training/stalking-tutorial/categories-of-stalking

5. State Stalking Laws. FindLaw. Accessed 2021. https://www.findlaw.com/state/criminal-laws/stalking.html

6. Scott A. Stalking: how perceptions differ from reality and why these differences matter. Goldsmiths University of London. July 15, 2019. Updated June 13, 2021. Accessed 2021. http://research.gold.ac.uk/id/eprint/26591/

7. Bulut S, Usman A, Nazir T. Stalking of healthcare professionals by their clients: the prevalence, motivation, and effect. *Open J Med Psychol.* 2021;10:27-35.

8. The United States Department of Justice. Stalking and harassment assessment and risk profile. Accessed 2021. https://ukcdar.uky.edu/ls/index.php/57925/

Chapter 34

ALCOHOL-ENABLED AND DRUG-FACILITATED CRIMES

Sarah L. Pederson, BSN, RN, AFN-C, SANE-A, SANE-P
Heather Quaile, DNP, WHNP-BC, AFN-C, CSC, IF, FAANP
Jessica M. Volz, DNP, CRNP, FNE A/P, FNP-BC, AFN-C, SANE-A, SANE-P, NE-BC, DM-AFN
Patricia M. Speck, DNSc, CRNP, FNP-BC, AFN-C, DF-IAFN, FAAFS, DF-AFN, FAAN

KEY POINTS

1. *Forensic nurses are prepared for the clinical presentations of alcohol-enabled and drug-facilitated crimes.*

2. *After a suspected alcohol-enabled and/or drug-facilitated crime, the patient's mental health status is always considered prior to gaining consent for the collection of toxicology samples.*

3. *Protection of specimen integrity and adherence to the chain of custody principles are necessary during the collection process and management of toxicology samples.*

4. *The generalist and advanced forensic nurse's interpretation of toxicology results and development of testimony are based on clinical symptom presentations and patient history, not the techniques utilized to analyze the laboratory results.*

INTRODUCTION

Drug and alcohol use is commonly associated with the type of trauma that requires a trauma-informed, person-centered evaluation by a forensic nurse. Forensic nurses should understand the clinical presentations of alcohol-enabled, drug-facilitated, and polysubstance-induced sexual assault. They should also understand their role in identifying and managing toxicology samples collected for potential use in the criminal justice system.

Drug-facilitated sexual assault (DFSA) and alcohol-enabled sexual assault are 2 commonly cited crimes where incapacitation by a substance is a method of choice by criminals.[1] Both DFSA and alcohol-enabled sexual assault require a level of incapacitation that is facilitating the crime of sexual assault. Societal beliefs are that DFSA is the most common type of sexual assault, but in reality, alcohol-enabled sexual assault is far more common.[2] To increase victim vulnerability, perpetrators often employ DFSA methods that include the use of substances to reduce resistance and memory of the event.[3] The methods for alcohol-enabled and drug-facilitated sexual assault at large include the voluntary and involuntary consumption of alcohol or drugs or polydrug use, either in isolation or in combination with each other.[1]

Perpetrators of sexual violence target vulnerabilities in individuals as a way of identifying victims that they intend to rape. Common targets for DFSA include adolescents engaging in risk-taking behaviors, dependent children and adults, and other vulnerable persons. Perpetrators also have a predictable method of isolating their victims. They may weaponize drugs and alcohol against victims in 1 of 3 ways[1]:

1. The patient voluntarily ingests a drug or alcohol; the incapacitating effects create an opportunity for a sexual assault crime to take place.

2. The patient involuntarily ingests a drug that the perpetrator provided.

3. The patient voluntarily ingests a drug believing that the drug is another. The perpetrator's intent is to render the victim incapacitated by knowing the effects of the actual drug that they gave the victim. The defense is that the victim took the drug; the ploy is that the drug was not properly represented.

Other examples of drug-facilitated and alcohol-enabled crimes include driving under the influence, homicide, poisoning, occupational exposure, physical assault, drug-endangered children, and human trafficking.

The forensic nurse is aware of patient presentations following suspected drug-facilitated and alcohol-enabled crimes, often recommending or ordering toxicology testing for them. Forensic nurses obtain consent and conduct their examination using trauma-informed, person-centered techniques to assess the capacity of consent for testing. Suspicious symptoms often include loss of memory with or without unexplained injury, reported voluntary or involuntary ingestion of a substance, and signs and symptoms of impairment (**Figure 34-1**).

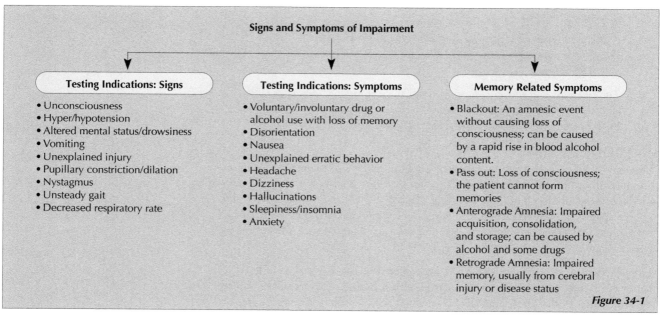

Figure 34-1. Signs, Symptoms, and Memory Related Symptoms of Impairment. Pederson S, Volz J, Quaile H, Speck P. 2021. Used with permission.

The testing capacity for toxicology samples varies between jurisdictions. In suspected cases of drug-facilitated or alcohol-enabled crimes, the forensic nurse should obtain additional information from the patient to determine the type of biological sample to be collected.[4] Blood and urine are the most commonly tested specimens in the living patient. In the deceased patient, autopsy findings should include any identified drugs that may provide information relevant to the death investigation. **Figure 34-2** outlines the common drugs and the recommended time frame for sample collection, as well as their potential biological sources, that should be obtained regardless of whether the victim is living or deceased.

The forensic nurse is trained in procedures for management of evidence, including the processes of identification, collection, packaging, and storage, while maintaining

Drug- and Alcohol- Facilitated SA Specimen Collection Timeframe

Blood: May be collected within approximately 24 hours after the ingestion, or if clinically symptomatic
Urine: May be collected within approximately 120 hours after the ingestion

Postmortem Toxicology Specimens	**Living Person Biological Specimens**	**Commonly Used Drugs** (Approximate detection time in urine)
• Blood	• Amniotic fluid	• Cocaine
• Bile	• Blood	• Diazepam
• Brain	• Breast milk	• Lysergic Acid Diethylamide (LSD)
• Gastric contents	• Hair	• Methadone
• Hair	• Nails	• Methamphetamine
• Heart (blood)	• Urine	• Methaqualone
• Kidneys	• Saliva	• Phencyclidine (PCP)
• Liver	• Sweat	• Phenobarbital
• Lung		• Propoxyphene
• Vitreous humor		• Tetrahydrocannabinol

Figure 34-2

Figure 34-2. Common drugs used, time frame recommendations for sample collection, and potential biological sources. Pederson S, Volz J, Quaile H, Speck P. 2021. Used with permission.

the principles of chain of custody. The chain of custody begins with the patient who presents with evidence on their body. The forensic nurse then identifies and implements processes for the collection and management of the sample, creating a chronologic paper trail that follows the evidence when transferred to the proceeding professional.[5]

When drugs are a method used in a crime, prosecution is exceptionally challenging. However, when a forensic nurse protects aspects of specimen collection and adheres to management and chain of custody principles, successful prosecution is more likely. Frequently, detection of a substance is a significant obstacle.[6] Often, drug metabolization occurs quickly, and any delay in seeking medical care will increase the likelihood of rapid metabolite excretion. Other prosecuting limitations are tests that screen for specific drug groups, not individual types of drugs. In many parts of the country, testing limitations are the tests for basic toxicology panels conducted in emergency departments or state crime laboratories.[5] Without a biochemistry background, the forensic nurse cannot interpret the toxicology results. Rather, the forensic nurse monitors health outcomes from toxicity, documents symptoms from a multitude of body systems, and refers patients when necessary. Furthermore, a forensic nurse's testimony reflects only clinical symptom presentations, patient history, and interventional tests and treatments, not the forensic or toxicology laboratory techniques used to analyze samples provided from the forensic nursing practices.

CASE STUDIES

Case Study 34-1

This 19-year-old female college student presented to a sexual assault center. The patient stated that she was at an off-campus party the night before and drank a beer that was given to her by a male acquaintance. After that, she recalled experiencing only a few hazy memories, including what seemed to be a man on top of her having penetrative sex. The patient woke up the next morning with a bad headache, not wearing underwear, and with vaginal pain. She looked for her underwear on the ground, but she could not locate them. She then called her roommate to come pick her up and told her roommate that she believed she was sexually assaulted the night prior.

Discussion

In this case study, the patient was given the drug during the evening, when her body's natural inclination was to rest. Patients often do not remember the assault itself but wake up the next morning knowing that something is wrong. While some perpetrators physically force or threaten victims to engage in a sexual act, there has been increasing awareness around DFSA crimes. Some of the most common places where alcohol and DFSA crimes occur are clubs, bars, and college campuses. In fact, drug or alcohol-related sexual assaults on college campuses are more frequent than forcible sexual assaults. However, it is not uncommon for a DFSA to occur during a casual date or other interaction. During the forensic examination and data collection, the forensic nurse must preserve evidence and maintain the chain of custody. The forensic nurse has a relationship with the toxicology laboratory and is responsible for knowing their requirements for collection, packaging, labeling, storage, handling, transportation, and delivery of specimens. Furthermore, policies help each facility for the storage of these samples when patients are undecided about reporting.

SUMMARY

Whether voluntary or involuntary, drugs and alcohol use are common methods for increasing vulnerability in targeted persons. Drug-facilitated and alcohol-enabled crime presentations vary widely, but forensic nurses have trauma-informed, patient-centered education and skilled practices to successfully care for patients in various settings with various presentations within the context of their state license.

When testing specimens, determining the type to collect for testing and preserving them in a comprehensive management plan is necessary to ensure the test's success. Lastly, an essential part of the forensic nurse's role in the clinical setting is to understand the experiences of their patients.

REFERENCES

1. Krebs CP, Lindquist CH, Warner TD, Fisher BS, Martin SL. College women's experiences with physically forced, alcohol- or other drug-enabled, and drug-facilitated sexual assault before and since entering college. *J Am Coll Health.* 2009;57(6):639-647. doi:10.3200/JACH.57.6.639-64

2. Faugno D, Speck PM, Spencer MJ, Giardino AP. *Sexual Assault Quick Reference.* 2nd ed. STM Learning, Inc.; 2016.

3. Hammer RM, Moynihan B, Pagliaro EM. *Forensic Nursing: A Handbook for Practice.* 2nd ed. Jones & Bartlett Learning; 2013.

4. Lynch VA, Duval JB. *Forensic Nursing Science.* 2nd ed. Elsevier-Mosby; 2011.

5. US Department of Justice, Office on Violence Against Women. A national protocol for sexual assault medical forensic examinations: adults/adolescents. April 2013. https://www.justice.gov/ovw/file/846856/download

6. Research Triangle Institute. Continuing education and training: drug-facilitated sexual assault topics. https://www.rti.org/brochures/continuing-education-and-training-drug-facilitated-sexual-assault-topics

Sexual Violence

Christine Foote-Lucero, MSN, RN, CEN, SANE-A, SANE-P, AFN-C
Loretta Tsu, MA, BSN, RN, SANE-A, SCRN

Key Points

1. *Sexual assault is any sexual contact or act performed by one person on another without consent.*

2. *Forensic nurses should understand the best practice for treatment of patients affected by sexual violence.*

3. *During a medical forensic examination (MFE), a patient's medical, emotional, and forensic needs should be met through thorough examination, treatment, testing, intervention, and documentation.*

Introduction

Sexual violence can have profound and lasting effects on patients of all ages and genders. *Sexual assault* (SA) is any sexual contact or act performed by one person on another without consent, involving force, threat of force, refusal of consent, or the inability to provide consent.[1] SA encompasses many types of sexual contact, including rape, attempted rape, unwanted sexual touching, forced sexual activities, and attempts to force someone into sexual activity. SA is pervasive, with 20% of women and 3% of men in the United States experiencing completed or attempted rape during their lifetime.[2] More than 50% of SA cases involve an intimate partner, and about 40% involve an acquaintance, so only a minority of cases involve a stranger. In addition, the prevalence of false reporting is low at about 2%.[2] Reported SA cases only represent a fraction of those committed, as only 10% to 15% of all SAs are reported to law enforcement given that those who know their assailant are less likely to report.[1] SA can involve alcohol and drugs, with alcohol being the most common substance.

Role of the Sexual Assault Nurse Examiner

All health care team members who respond to patients affected by sexual violence must provide trauma- and violence-informed care. Sexual violence can have short- and long-term health consequences, and responding clinicians are uniquely positioned to help mitigate them. The role of the sexual assault nurse examiner (SANE) is to conduct a MFE while providing patient-centered care. This process can validate a patient's concerns, mitigate trauma, provide safety, and promote healing. The SANE should simultaneously address the medical, emotional, and forensic needs of the patient. Medical needs include treatment of injuries and evaluation for sexually transmitted infections (STIs) and pregnancy. Emotional needs include acute crisis intervention, advocacy referral, and appropriate follow-up counseling. Forensic needs include thorough documentation of the patient's history and physical findings, proper collection and handling of evidence, and eventual presentation of findings and conclusions in court.[3]

History

Once the patient consents to the MFE, a history should first be documented. It should include the patient's exact statements, quoted directly, to ensure accuracy and avoid misinterpretation. It should focus on the precise details of the assault for the purposes of medical diagnosis and treatment, including considerations for bodily and anogenital injury; assessment for risk of pregnancy and STIs; evaluation of each specimen's evidentiary value; determination of any loss of consciousness or memory; and evaluation of the use of weapons, force, restraints, or threats. The history should be obtained in a sensitive and supportive manner, starting with open-ended questions. Any support persons at the bedside should refrain from interrupting or asking leading or suggestive questions.[1]

PHYSICAL AND ANOGENITAL EXAMINATION WITH EVIDENCE COLLECTION

A thorough head-to-toe examination with a detailed anogenital examination should be performed on all patients with their consent. The clinician should carefully note from the history what body parts could be a potential source of DNA transfer so that these areas can be swabbed, in addition to where injuries may be located. The clinician should record injuries carefully using objective terminology and the patient's subjective symptoms. Supplemental photodocumentation is necessary to support written documentation.

On female patients (**Figure 35-1**), the detailed anogenital examination should begin with a gross visual inspection of the outer labia majora, followed by separation of the labia majora to evaluate the labia minora. Then labial traction is performed to visualize the vestibule, including the mucosal area within the labia, such as the clitoris and surrounding area, urethra and periurethral tissue, hymen, posterior fourchette, and fossa navicularis. Each structure should be assessed and photographed with a binocular microscope (ie, a colposcope) at varying magnifications. Once external genital evidence collection is complete, the clinician should proceed with inspection of the anus, perianal folds, and perineum. Evidence from this area should be collected before speculum insertion, as consideration must be given to the natural gravitational flow

Figure 35-1. The genital structures of the adult female.

Figure 35-2. The genital structures of the adult male.

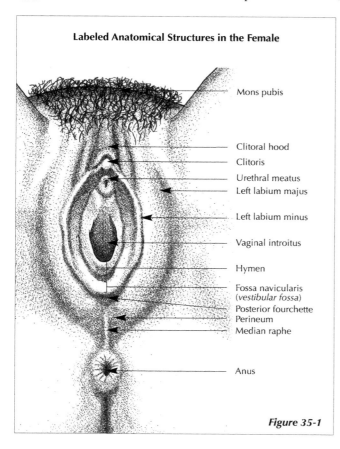

Labeled Anatomical Structures in the Female

Mons pubis

Clitoral hood
Clitoris
Urethral meatus
Left labium majus

Left labium minus

Vaginal introitus

Hymen

Fossa navicularis
(*vestibular fossa*)
Posterior fourchette
Perineum
Median raphe

Anus

Figure 35-1

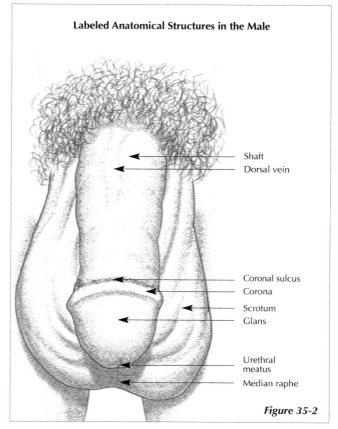

Labeled Anatomical Structures in the Male

Shaft
Dorsal vein

Coronal sulcus
Corona

Scrotum
Glans

Urethral
meatus
Median raphe

Figure 35-2

of secretions from the vaginal vault to the anal folds.[4] Then, the clinician inserts the speculum to assess and perform evidence collection from the vagina and cervix. The clinician should also consider the collection of STI swabs. After all evidence collection, the final step is a detailed assessment of the hymen in the estrogenized patient, including using a large cotton-tipped swab or a foley catheter.

On male patients (**Figure 35-2**), the detailed anogenital examination should begin with careful inspection of the scrotum and the penis, including the shaft and glans. If the patient is not circumcised, the foreskin should also be thoroughly retracted for a comprehensive examination. As with female patients, each structure should be assessed and photographed, and evidence should be collected per protocol. Once external genital assessment and evidence collection are completed, the clinician should inspect the anus, anal folds, and perineum, followed by additional evidence collection. **Figures 35-3** and **35-4** show possible examination positions for patients.

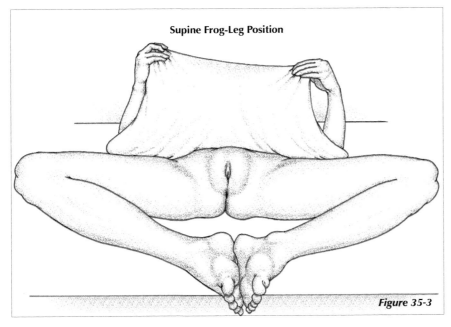

Supine Frog-Leg Position

Figure 35-3

Figure 35-3. Genital examination of the female in the supine frog-leg position.

Prone Knee-Chest Position

Figure 35-4

Figure 35-4. Prone knee chest position affords an optimal view of the posterior hymen, vestibule, and vagina in prepubescent female patients, and perineal and anal view in both male and female patients. The patient should be assisted to a prone position, with head and torso flush with the exam table. The knees are placed about 18 inches apart and should remain on the exam table at approximately a 90-degree angle, while the buttocks are raised.

DRUG-FACILITATED SEXUAL ASSAULT

Drug-facilitated sexual assault (DFSA) includes any SA involving the use of drugs and/or alcohol that renders the patient unable to consciously give or deny consent. Patients may report a degree of intoxication inconsistent with the quantity of drugs and/or alcohol they report voluntarily ingesting. The patient may also report amnesia, loss of consciousness, confusion, dizziness, blurred vision, drowsiness, nausea, and/or vomiting. Immediate action must be taken to preserve blood and/or urine specimens due to the rapid metabolism of most substances.[4]

CASE STUDY

Case Study 35-1

This 23-year-old female, presented to the emergency department (ED) complaining of vaginal and anal pain and was concerned she had been sexually assaulted. She told the triage nurse that she went to a club with friends the previous night but did not remember the night's events after drinking 1 to 2 alcoholic beverages, even though she regularly drank that amount socially and had never had this type of response. She awoke 8 hours later in her friend's apartment. Her underwear was missing, her skirt was on backwards, and her bra was on the floor. She reported vomiting prior to her arrival to the ED and felt lightheaded and weak. The ED triage nurse escorted her to an ED treatment room and consulted the forensic nurse examiner (FNE).

The FNE responded to the patient's room; introduced themselves; and explained their role, the MFE, reporting options, medications, and evidence collection. The FNE reviewed applicable consents and paperwork with the patient and obtained the patient's signature. The FNE discussed pregnancy risk and emergency contraception as well as prophylactic care for STIs. After the FNE provided education on the risks, benefits, and possible side effects of all medications, the patient agreed to take STI medications but decided against emergency contraception because she had an intrauterine device (IUD). The FNE knew that DFSA specimens are time-sensitive, so blood and urine specimens were collected first.

After obtaining a thorough history of what the patient could remember, the FNE collected oral swabs so she could have food and beverages with the medications. She agreed to have her clothing collected for evidence and disrobed over a drop cloth. The FNE assisted her into a gown and then collected the clothing and drop cloth. Each item of clothing was photographed and then placed into its own paper bag, sealed, and labeled. Next, the FNE performed a thorough head-to-toe examination, uncovering only the body parts needed for assessment, and then covered them again to maintain the patient's modesty and privacy. The FNE documented and photographed bruising to the upper arms, erythema to the inner thighs, and abrasions to the knees. The FNE collected evidence from the patient's body, such as her neck, breasts, and fingernails. The examination continued with a detailed anogenital examination using a colposcope for visualization and evidence collection. The FNE explained each step to her and proceeded only with her consent. The FNE noted injuries such as lacerations to 6 o'clock of the posterior fourchette and 3 o'clock of the anus. The FNE then proceeded with speculum insertion to assess the vagina and cervix. Evidence was collected, and photographs were obtained. Upon speculum removal, the hymen was then thoroughly evaluated with the use of a foley catheter balloon.

Once the examination was complete, the FNE and the patient discussed safety planning and crisis interventions. The FNE provided her with appropriate patient education, referrals for medical and psychological care, and community resources. After obtaining a set of vital signs, she was discharged home with a family member.

Discussion

During the patient's examination, she reported drinking alcohol, which is the most common substance used for DFSA. Still, DFSA can also include benzodiazepines, opioids, muscle relaxers, over-the-counter sleep aids, and street drugs like ecstasy, cocaine, ketamine, and GHB (ie, the "date rape" drug). Early preservation of blood and urine for evidence collection can help with detection of substances used to facilitate DFSA.

Her injuries were consistent with common extragenital trauma, such as bruises, abrasions, or erythema to the thigh, upper arm, face, or neck.[1] Although genital injury findings are not commonly found, the most common location for injury in women is the posterior fourchette. Other anatomical locations include the labia minora, hymen, fossa navicularis, vulva, vagina, perineum, and cervix. Anal lacerations, swelling, and bruising are also markers for nonconsensual sexual intercourse and should increase the suspicion for lack of consent.[5]

SUMMARY

Sexual violence is prevalent, and its physical impact on patients can include genital and nongenital trauma as well as contraction of STIs, general health risks, pregnancy, substance abuse, and sexual dysfunction. The psychological impact can last for years and typically includes depression, anxiety, fear, posttraumatic stress disorder, self-blame, and shame. An MFE provides an opportunity for the forensic nurse to mitigate many of the short- and long-term effects of sexual violence. Some of the most important aspects of the MFE include addressing these medical and psychological needs, as well as restoring the patient's sense of control, validating the patient's concerns, providing safety, and promoting healing.

REFERENCES

1. Bates CK. Evaluation and management of adult and adolescent sexual assault victims. UpToDate. Updated July 29, 2021. Accessed January 11, 2022. https://www.uptodate.com/contents/evaluation-and-management-of-adult-and-adolescent-sexual-assault-victims

2. Statistics. National Sexual Violence Resource Center. Accessed January 11, 2022. https://www.nsvrc.org/statistics

3. *Evaluation and Management of the Sexually Assaulted or Sexually Abused Patient.* American College of Emergency Physicians; 2013. https://icesaht.org/wp-content/uploads/2016/06/Sexual-Assault-e-book-1.pdf

4. Ferrell J, Caruso C. Sexual Assault Evidence Recovery. In: Lynch VA, Duval JB, eds. *Forensic Nursing Science.* 2nd ed. Mosby, Inc.; 2011:144-154.

5. Sommers MS, Fargo JD. Discriminating between consensual intercourse and sexual assault: genital-anal injury pattern in females. *J Forensic Leg Med.* 2021;79. doi:10.1016/j.jflm.2021.102138

NONFATAL STRANGULATION

Valerie Sievers, MSN, RN, CNS, AFN-C, SANE-A, SANE-P, DF-AFN

Diana K. Faugno, MSN, RN, CPN, AFN-C, SANE-A, SANE-P, FAAFS, DF-IAFN, DF-AFN

Jessica M. Volz, DNP, CRNP, FNE A/P, FNP-BC, AFN-C, NE-BC, SANE-A, SANE-P, DM-AFN

Patricia M. Speck, DNSc, CRNP, FNP-BC, AFN-C, DF-IAFN, FAAFS, DF-AFN, FAAN

"Domestic violence offenders do not strangle their partners to kill them. They strangle them to let them know they can kill them — any time they wish!"

— *Casey Gwinn, JD Alliance for HOPE International*

KEY POINTS

1. *Strangulation is widely known to be associated with domestic violence (DV), family violence, and intimate partner violence (IPV), and it can be lethal.*

2. *Strangulation is often unrecognized as there can be no obvious signs of physical injury.*

3. *Patients who present with a description of strangulation need a health care professional with a high index of suspicion for potentially urgent and emergent critical injuries to the neck and head.*

4. *A trauma-informed approach to patients affected by strangulation is a key component to completing a comprehensive evaluation.*

INTRODUCTION

As early as the 1990s, violence against women was widely recognized as a health concern.[1] In the past 17 years, recognition of nonfatal strangulation within the context of DV or IPV has received greater attention. This is largely in response to a seminal study that helped shape understanding about strangulation, law enforcement responses, health care practice, legislation, and research.[2-4] The San Diego study[3] of 300 victims of nonfatal strangulation identified that the majority of persons reporting strangulation lacked significant visible injuries. Researchers found that 50% of the victims had no visible injuries, and 35% of the victims had injuries too minor to photograph. Additionally, many of these victims did not receive a referral for an evaluation in an emergency department (ED).[2] Early studies increased awareness of nonfatal strangulation as a life-threatening serious injury, creating an impetus for legislation and the development of best medical practices related to clinical evaluation and treatment.[3-5]

THE STRANGULATION ACT

Strangulation is often referred to as choking, throttling, or suffocating by patients experiencing the external application of pressure to the neck, which results in alteration of consciousness after the interruption of blood flow. **Strangulation** is a common and lethal form of DV[3-6] with negative physical and psychological outcomes, often a result of "reduced blood flow to or from the brain via the external compression of blood vessels in the neck."[6] There are 2 methods of strangulation described in **Table 36-1**. Studies in the 1940s[7] found that in adult males, 4 pounds (1.8 kg) of pressure or less can obstruct the jugular veins and 5 to 11 pounds (2.3 kg to 5 kg) can occlude the carotid arteries. There are no specific studies that focus on the amount of pressure required for strangulation in women or children, but due to size and structural differences, the amount of pressure necessary is believed to be lower.

Table 36-1. Methods, Characteristics, and Descriptions of Strangulation[6]	
METHODS	CHARACTERISTICS AND DESCRIPTIONS
Manual strangulation	— Hands or other body parts applied to the victim's neck
	— Most common form of strangulation between 2 or more persons
Ligature strangulation	— Object applied to the victim's neck
	— More commonly used in suicide hangings

Nonfatal strangulation is more common than realized and is known to impact victims of DV, human trafficking, sexual assault, child abuse, and elder abuse. Up to 68% of all high-risk DV victims experience repeated strangulation that goes unreported.[2,8] The risk of being killed increases 7- to 10-fold after experiencing a singular incident of strangulation.[5,9] If a person is lucky enough to survive strangulation, the anoxic or traumatic brain injury increases the chance of long-term consequences from strokes and global dementias.[2,9] Therefore, early recognition, detection, and intervention are key to survival.

ANATOMY OF THE NECK

The neck is comprised of subcutaneous fat, muscle, cartilage, bone, vessels, nerves, lymph nodes, and salivary glands. The anterior and anterolateral neck are underlying structures that are especially vulnerable to the intentional and external pressure from strangulation. These structures include the hyoid bone, larynx, trachea, jugular veins, and carotid arteries. The vertebral arteries are located on the lateral side of the neck. The importance of the neck structure is best understood in terms of the role of the individual structure and their relationships with the cardiovascular and respiratory systems. The anatomy and features in strangulation are identified in **Figure 36-1** with descriptions featured in **Table 36-2**.

Figure 36-1. Vital neck structures. (Illustration courtesy of Yesenia Aceves and the Training Institute on Strangulation Prevention.)

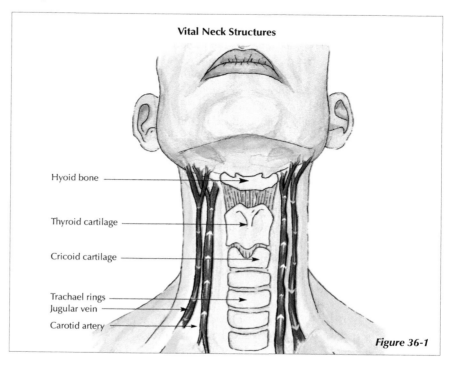

Vital Neck Structures

Hyoid bone

Thyroid cartilage

Cricoid cartilage

Trachael rings
Jugular vein
Carotid artery

Figure 36-1

Table 36-2. Names and Descriptions of Neck Features[6]

NECK ANATOMY	DESCRIPTION
Carotid Arteries	Originates from the aortic arch at the top of the heart
	Located on the left and right sides of the neck
	Protected by neck muscles
	Lies slightly deeper and medial to the jugular veins
	Carries approximately 80% of the oxygenated, nutrient-rich blood from the heart to the head and brain
	Pressure inside the carotid arteries exerts the force required not only to deliver oxygenated blood but to diffuse oxygen throughout the brain tissues
Jugular Veins	Vessels located on the left and right sides of the anterior neck
	Located more external and lateral to the carotid arteries
	Returns the majority of CO_2 gases in deoxygenated blood from the brain and head back to the heart and lungs where the CO_2 gases are exhaled as waste
Vertebral Arteries	Originates from the subclavian arteries
	The primary blood supply to the upper spinal cord, brainstem, cerebellum, and the posterior circulation of the brain
	Carries 15% to 20% of the brain's blood supply
Trachea	A hollow tube located along the body's midline that connects the larynx to the 2 main bronchi of the lungs
	Incomplete, highly elastic, C-shaped cartilage rings located anteriorly along the tracheal wall
	Primary function is supporting air flow to and from the lungs
Hyoid Bone	A horseshoe-shaped bone located at the base of the mandible and above the larynx
	Free-floating (ie, not connected to any other bone in the body)
	Main function is supporting a wide range of tongue, pharyngeal, and laryngeal movements, including swallowing
	Fracture of the hyoid bone leads to difficulty swallowing (ie, dysphagia), painful swallowing (ie, odynophagia), and pain on neck rotation

ASSESSMENT AND EVALUATION

When there is suspicion of strangulation, physical abuse, sexual assault, human trafficking, or DV, establishing a safe environment is essential in applying the first principle of trauma-informed care.[10] For more information on trauma-informed care, please see chapter 5. With cases of strangulation in particular, the provider's approach affects the patient's response. They must recognize that a patient may not think of strangulation as injury, especially with multiple ongoing episodes of violence and abuse. Patients may use the term "choking" or describe a history that includes attempted smothering. The history from the patient should be documented in quotes, using their exact words.

It is best to use language that is culturally humble and inclusive, to be nonjudgmental, and to ask developmentally appropriate and open-ended questions.[11,12] Often, patients do not understand the technical language used by the health care provider, so it is important to ask questions that reflect the patient's level of understanding. Asking the patient to describe symptoms and the circumstances for those symptoms is also necessary. Suggested approaches[10,11] for following trauma-informed care principles include:

— A brief introduction of the nurse and their role: "My name is Jane Doe, and I'm your nurse today."

— Ask about their preferences: "What would you like me to call you?" *and/or* "May I have permission to talk to you about your neck and breathing symptoms?"

— Make a statement of an observation, ask permission to continue the conversation, and talk about symptoms *after* the patient grants permission: "You sound hoarse, may I ask you about your symptoms?" *or* "Did something happen that hurt your neck or throat?" *or*

"Did anything happen that made you feel like it was hard to breathe?"

Trauma-informed care is person-centered, and questions such as these are part of changing nursing practices to ensure patients feel comfortable and secure throughout their examination.[11]

Physical Assessment and Documentation

The physical assessment includes a thorough head-to-toe physical assessment and a focused evaluation. There are several standardized tools for health care professionals to use during the medical-forensic examination. A sample standardized assessment tool can be seen in **Figure 36-2.** The *Strangulation Documentation Tool*[12] guides the health care professional through documenting a comprehensive history and detailed documentation of all injuries. In addition to diagrams of injuries, photodocumentation provides a record of the patient's injuries and condition at the time of the examination. Most patients with a clear history of strangulation do not have any visible injury at the time of the medical forensic examination.[13] However, there are a variety of symptoms patients may describe or exhibit after experiencing strangulation that imply certain injuries.

Common symptoms and injuries following strangulation include the following[6,12,13]:

— Breathing changes (ie, difficulty breathing or hyperventilation)

— Vision changes (ie, blurred vision, 'spots' in the visual field)

— Voice changes (ie, a raspy or hoarse voice)

— Hearing changes (ie, 'ringing in the ears,' loss of hearing)

— Difficulty swallowing or speaking

— Coughing

— Confusion (ie, memory loss or a history of loss of consciousness)

— Bladder or bowel incontinence

— Bruises and abrasions to the face, neck, chest, ears, arms, shoulders, and hands

— Scratches to the face and neck (from attempts to remove hands or ligature from the neck)

Victim Name _____ Date of Birth _____ Case #_____ Report # _____

LEFT EYE - OUTER EYELID/UPPER AND LOWER CONJUNCTIVA/SCLERA

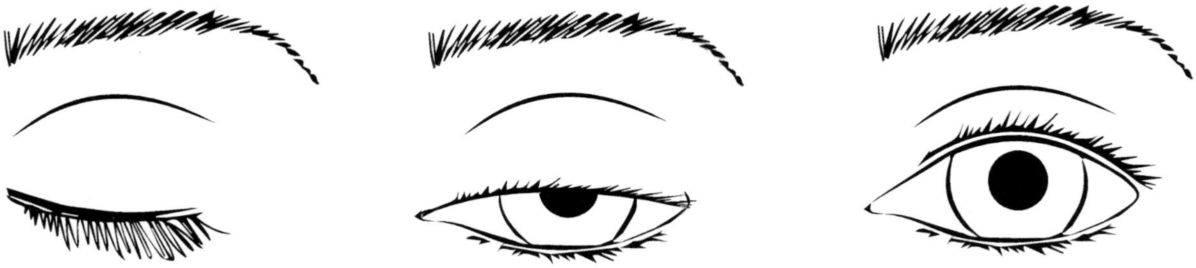

RIGHT EYE - SCLERA/UPPER AND LOWER CONJUNCTIVA/OUTER LID

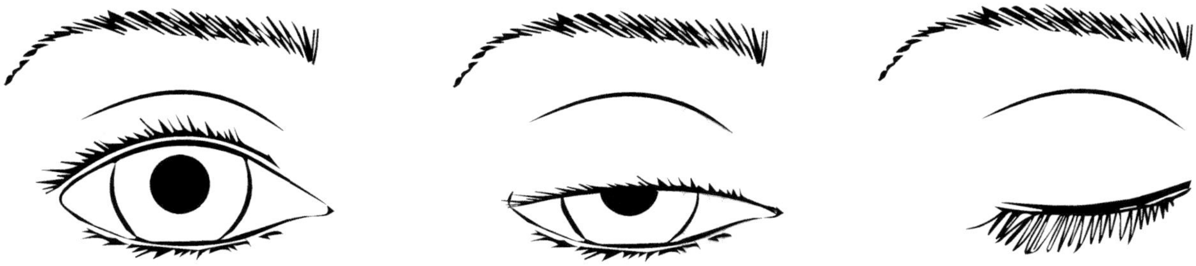

MOUTH - PALATE/TONGUE/FRENULUMS/INNER AND OUTER LIPS

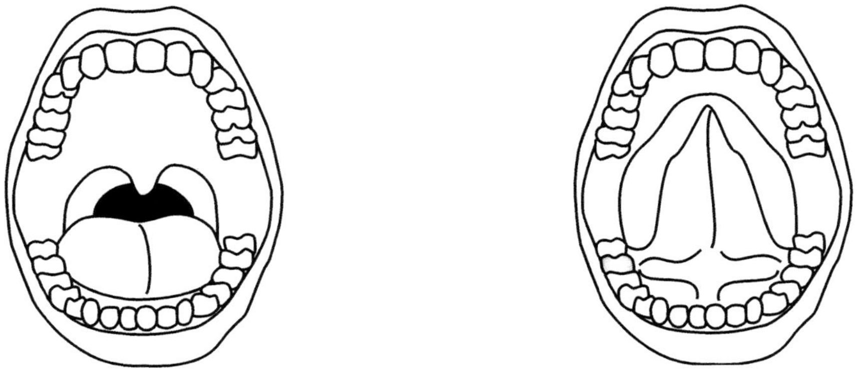

Forensic Nurse Examiner Name/Signature _____

Courtesy of Sally Sturgeon, DNP, RN, SANE-A, AFN-BC.

Figure 36-2

Figure 36-2. *Sturgeon's SAVEcD Tool - Strangulation Assessment for Victims with Evidence Collection and Documentation*

— Subconjunctival hemorrhages

— Petechial hemorrhages (eyes, eye lids, face, ears, neck, scalp, mouth, palate, uvula)

— Pain, discomfort, areas of tenderness

— Traumatic alopecia

EVIDENCE COLLECTION

When making decisions about evidence collection, the forensic nurse should be guided by the patient's history and any physical evidence identified during the medical forensic examination. In cases of strangulation, evidence includes both physical samples and the patient's history of the event.

To secure evidence in a trauma-informed manner, the nurse should initially ask the patient for permission to question them (eg, May I ask about the events leading to your visit here?). With the patient's consent, the nurse may then ask the following questions[10-12]:

— Do you know when the strangulation event occurred?

— Are you wearing the same clothes you had on during the strangulation, or have you changed your clothing since then?

— Have you bathed or showered since the strangulation?

— Was there a struggle? Did you scratch or injure the person who strangled you?

The evidence necessary following a strangulation includes the patient's DNA standards (buccal swabs); clothing; and swabs (trace evidence) of any scratches, abrasions, or bruises on the face, neck, and/or chest, which may yield DNA from the strangler. Collection of any physical evidence must follow evidence management guidelines and the chain of custody.[6] For more information on evidence collection, see chapter 11.

TREATMENT

Following a thorough evaluation, treatment for the strangulation should be completed. Effective care always involves a trauma-informed team approach and can include neurologists, neurosurgeons, ED personnel, and ear, nose, and throat specialists. A consensus of physicians and nurses developed the Recommendations for Medical/ Radiographic Evaluation of Acute Adult, Non-Fatal Strangulation, an evaluation and treatment algorithm (**Figure 36-3**).[14] The most desirable radiographic study for assessing vascular injury to the neck vessels is a computed tomography angiogram (CTA). The imaging in a CTA helps radiologists visualize vessels to detect any vascular injury that potentially puts patients at risk for stroke and obstruction.[12,14] Soft tissue swelling also puts patients at risk for airway obstruction.[9] Providers should follow up with patients for 1 year if they experienced neurological changes during strangulation, or longer, with referral to specialists, if there was anoxic traumatic brain injury.[13]

DISCHARGE AND SAFETY PLANNING

Throughout the entire patient encounter, the forensic nurse plans for safety both during and after the encounter and discharge. Essential elements of effective discharge planning include risk assessment, identification of relevant options, and assistance with implementation.[15] For persons who experienced strangulation as part of DV, the Johns Hopkins Danger Assessment-5 [12,16] should be used to self-assess for risk of homicide.

RECOMMENDATIONS FOR THE **MEDICAL/RADIOGRAPHIC EVALUATION** OF ACUTE ADULT/ADOLESCENT, **NON/NEAR FATAL STRANGULATION**

v10.31.22

Prepared by **Bill Smock, MD; Bill Green, MD; and Sally Sturgeon, DNP, SANE-A**

Endorsed by the **National Medical Advisory Committee:**
Cathy Baldwin, MD; Ralph Riviello, MD; Sean Dugan, MD; Steve Stapczynski, MD; Ellen Tailiaferro, MD; Michael Weaver, MD

GOALS:
1. Evaluate for acute medical conditions requiring immediate management/stabilization
2. Evaluate carotid and vertebral arteries for injuries (dissection/thrombosis)
3. Evaluate airway structures and other bony/cartilaginous/soft tissue neck structures

STRANGULATION PATIENT PRESENTS TO THE EMERGENCY DEPARTMENT

HISTORY (ANY of the following; current **OR** assault related and now resolved)

1. Loss of consciousness
2. Visual changes: "spots," "flashing lights," "tunnel vision"
3. History of altered mental status: "dizzy," "confused," "lightheaded," "loss of memory," "any loss of awareness"
4. Breathing changes: "I couldn't breathe," "difficulty breathing"
5. Incontinence (bladder or bowel)
6. Neurologic symptoms: seizure-like activity, stroke-like symptoms, headache, tinnitus, decreased hearing, focal numbness, amnesia
7. Ligature mark or neck contusion
8. Neck tenderness or pain/sore throat/pain with swallowing
9. Change in voice: unable to speak, hoarse or raspy voice

PHYSICAL EXAM (ANY Abnormality)

1. Functional assessment of breathing, swallowing, and voice
2. Thorough examination of neck, eyes, TMs, oral mucosa, nose, airway, upper torso for: tenderness, swelling, bruising, abrasions, crepitance, bruit
3. Venous congestion/petechial hemorrhages/scleral hemorrhages
4. Ligature mark = HIGH RISK
5. Tenderness of airway structures/carotid arteries = HIGH RISK
6. Mental status/complete neurologic exam

CONSIDER ADMINISTRATION OF ONE 325MG ASPIRIN IF THERE IS ANY DELAY IN OBTAINING A RADIOGRAPHIC STUDY

RECOMMENDED RADIOGRAPHIC STUDIES TO RULE OUT LIFE-THREATENING INJURIES* (including delayed presentations of up to 1 year)

1. CT Angio of carotid/vertebral arteries (GOLD STANDARD for evaluation of vessels and bony/cartilaginous structures, less sensitive for soft tissue trauma) or
2. MRA of carotid/vertebral arteries
3. Carotid Doppler Ultrasound (NOT RECOMMENDED - Unable to adequately evaluate vertebral arteries or proximal internal carotid arteries)
4. Plain Radiographs (NOT RECOMMENDED - Unable to evaluate vascular and soft-tissue structures)
5. Consider fiberoptic direct laryngoscopy to evaluate possible larygeal injury or airway compromise

POSITIVE RESULTS

1. Consult Neurology/Neurosurgery/Trauma Surgery for admission
2. Consider ENT consult for laryngeal trauma or dysphonia
3. Perform a lethality assessment per institutional policy

NEGATIVE RESULTS

Discharge home with detailed instructions, including a lethality assessment, and to return to ED if: neurological signs/symptoms, dyspnea, dysphonia or odynophagia develops or worsens

IF THE CTA IS NEGATIVE, CONSIDER OBSERVATION OF NEAR-FATAL STRANGULATION PATIENT IF THE AIRWAY IS OF CONCERN. OBSERVATION HAS NO ROLE IN RULING OUT A VASCULAR INJURY.

Graphic Design by Yesenia Aceves

*References on page 2

Reprinted with permission from Training Institute on Strangulation Prevention.

Figure 36-3

Figure 36-3. Recommendations for the Medical/Radiographic Evaluation of Acute Adult, Non-Fatal Strangulation

CASE STUDIES

Case Study 36-1

This female patient, met her boyfriend in college. He was very attentive and demanded all of her time when she was not in class. She loved the attention and progressively became more isolated from her friends; by her senior year, she was only going to work and to school. The boyfriend became increasingly possessive of her, looking at her bills, checking her email, and monitoring her texts. When the patient turned 22- years- old, he talked her into moving in with him. The night she moved into his place, she arrived in the ED with law enforcement. Their neighbors had called the police because the yelling and threats coming from the couple's home were so loud that they were afraid for the girl's safety. When law enforcement arrived, they saw that she was injured, so he boyfriend was arrested.

In the ED, the patient told the triage nurse that her boyfriend got home from work and immediately accused her of talking to another man. The patient explained to the nurse that the man in question was just someone from school. She said, "I didn't know what he was talking about!" She then reported that when he heard the denial, he grabbed her phone and started looking through her texts. The patient said,

> I was climbing on him trying to get my phone back and yelling at him. He saw other guys' names from my classes and work, and he got really mad and pushed me down on the couch. I was sitting up, and he was pushing my head back until I was hanging over the back of the couch, and then he 'choked' me.

When asked to describe the choking, she stated, "He had his 2 hands around my neck and was squeezing so hard… He was calling me a whore." She then reported that she could not breathe, and she "was trying to talk, and it came out in squeaks without words." She stated, "He was choking me for a long time, and then he started laughing." When he let go, the patient said she was crying and trying to catch a breath. She turned away from him on the couch and held her neck. She said her boyfriend then "bear hugged" her from behind and "started biting me, and I started screaming." A neighbor rang the doorbell multiple times and yelled that he had called the cops. She said, "When he heard that, he got up, got my purse and jacket, opened the door, and told me to get out." She explained that he punched her in the face, pushed her out the door, and locked it behind her. The police arrived shortly after. When asked about her neck injuries and the bite marks, she told the patrol officer that they were from "having sex." She told the triage nurse, "I didn't want to get him in trouble." The patrol officer had noticed that she was coughing and holding her neck, so he encouraged her to be seen in the ED. She was transported by ambulance to the ED and was later discharged after being medically cleared. She left the hospital, declining a medical forensic examination and the care of the forensic nurse.

The patient's symptoms worsened 2 days later. She called the patrol officer, who then brought her to see the forensic nurse. When asked about the symptoms she experienced following the fight, she said that she was now coughing and "clearing her throat a lot," her back and neck were sore, and her voice was raspy. During the examination, the forensic nurse observed irregular bruising on both sides of her neck, linear abrasions on her neck and chest, the bruising and swelling of her lips, and self-inflicted bite marks on her tongue. she stated that she did not remember biting her tongue, but "all I could think about then was that I couldn't breathe and didn't feel pain." She stated that she was sure she "didn't pass out because I was staring at him the whole time while he was choking me, and that's why he was laughing at me. He said my eyes were bugging out!" The forensic nurse also noted multiple double-arched bite marks on her posterior neck and back. She told the forensic nurse that she reached out to her older sister, who had taken her in and was helping her to "get over him."

Later, the forensic nurse heard that the patient had moved back with the boyfriend. He had appeared in court, but the patient dropped the charges and did not appear for her scheduled follow-up appointment with the advocate and forensic nurse.

Discussion

This case is complex, presenting the forensic nurse with a scenario to analyze the biology of trauma and healing, the psychological conflicts that occur in DV relationships, and the social risk that occurs when data predicts mortality (eg, increased risk of homicide when strangulation is used in DV). The forensic nurse has basic nursing knowledge about the assessment of hypoxic and anoxic brain injury and the subsequent neurological outcomes. With how the patient answered the forensic nurse's questions, the nurse was able to evaluate the demeanor of the patient to inform the documentation.

In this case, the patient had multiple patterned injuries, with some evidence of underlying structural injury to the larynx. This included a hoarse voice, poor memory of how injuries occurred (eg, tongue), and fear of worsening outcomes. If the patient had completed the medical forensic examination instead of leaving the ED as soon as she was cleared, the generalist forensic nurse would have consulted with an advanced practice provider who could complete the medical work-up, including contrast imaging of the neck. Finally, the patient needed a referral to a primary health care provider to follow the healing process and to screen for potential serious sequelae, including mental health outcomes.

In addition, the follow-up facility needs to partner with community agencies serving DV victims/survivors and their children. Frequently, forensic health care clinics or family justice centers are found in urban areas, while rural agencies are sparse. Regardless, it is incumbent on the forensic nurse to identify and refer patients to the agencies that serve those affected by interpersonal violence and crime.

SUMMARY

Strangulation is often unrecognized, but it is still a pervasive method used by aggressors, especially in populations that are affected by intimate partner and interpersonal violence. Health care professionals and the interprofessional team have the skills and responsibility to identify strangulation and intervene using a trauma-informed approach. Health care providers must counsel strangulation victims about the complications and lethality of their experience and provide resources for self-assessment, safety planning, and healing after discharge, specifically to prevent a future fatality.

REFERENCES

1. Violence Against Women. American Nurses Association. Accessed December 20, 2021. https://www.nursingworld.org/practice-policy/nursing-excellence/official-position-statements/id/violence-against-women/

2. Sorenson SB, Joshi M, Sivitz E. A systematic review of the epidemiology of nonfatal strangulation, a human rights and health concern. *Am J Public Health*. 2014;104(11):e54-e61. doi:10.2105/AJPH.2014.302191

3. Strack GB, McClane GE, Hawley D. A review of 300 attempted strangulation cases. Part I: criminal legal issues. *J Emerg Med*. 2001;21(3):303-9. doi:10.1016/s0736-4679(01)00399-7

4. McClane GE, Strack GB, Hawley D. A review of 300 attempted strangulation cases. Part II: clinical evaluation of the surviving victim. *J Emerg Med*. 2001;21(3):311-5. doi:10.1016/s0736-4679(01)00400-0

5. Hawley DA, McClane GE, Strack GB. A review of 300 attempted strangulation cases. Part III: injuries in fatal cases. *J Emerg Med*. 2001;21(3)317-22. doi:10.1016/s0736-4679(01)00401-2

6. Faugno DK, Sievers V, Shores M, Smock W, Speck PM. *Domestic Violence and Nonfatal Strangulation Assessment*. STM Learning, Inc.; 2020.

7. Rossen R, Kabat H, Anderson JP. Acute arrest of cerebral circulation in man. *Arch Neurol Psychiatry*. 1943;50(5):510–528.

8. Pritchard AJ, Reckdenwald A, Nordham C. Nonfatal strangulation as part of domestic violence: a review of research. *Trauma Violence Abuse*. 2017;18(4):407-424.

9. Rosen T, LoFaso VM, Bloemen EM, et al. Identifying injury patterns associated with physical elder abuse: analysis of legally adjudicated cases. *Ann Emerg Med*. 2020;76(3):266-276. doi:10.1016/j.annemergmed.2020.03.020

10. SAMHSA's Concept of Trauma and Guidance for a Trauma-Informed Approach. Substance Abuse and Mental Health Services Administration. 2014. Accessed December 20, 2021. https://scholarworks.boisestate.edu/cgi/viewcontent.cgi?article=1006&context=covid

11. Dowdell EB, Speck PM. Foundations for trauma-informed care in nursing practice. *Am J Nurs.* 2022;122(3).

12. Faugno D, Trujillo A, Bachmeier B, Speck PM. *Manual Nonfatal Strangulation Assessment.* STM Learning, Inc.; 2017.

13. Matusz EC, Schaffer JT, Bachmeier BA, et al. Evaluation of nonfatal strangulation in alert adults. *Ann Emerg Med.* 2020;75(3):329-338. doi:10.1016/j.annemergmed.2019.07.018

14. Smock W, Sturgeon S. Recommendations for the medical-radiographic evaluation of acute adult, non-fatal strangulation. Family Justice Center. 2019. https://www.familyjusticecenter.org/wp-content/uploads/2019/04/Recommendations-for-Medical-Radiological-Eval-of-Non-Fatal-Strangulation-v4.9.19.pdf

15. Davies J. *Victim Defined Safety Planning: A Summary.* Greater Hartford Legal Aid; 2017.

16. Messing JT, Campbell JC, Snider C. Validation and adaptation of the danger assessment-5: A brief intimate partner violence risk assessment. *J Adv Nurs.* 2017;73(12):3220-3230. doi:10.1111/jan.13459

Traumatic Brain Injury

Sean P. Dugan, MD, FAAP, SAFE
Jessica M. Volz, DNP, CRNP, FNE A/P, FNP-BC, AFN-C, NE-BC, SANE-A, SANE-P, DM-AFN

Key Points

1. *Traumatic brain injury (TBI) is an event following an anoxic injury; it is not a syndrome.*

2. *TBI is an alteration in the normal function of the brain as a result of external forces (eg, blow to the head, shaking, strangulation, other intentional anoxic events).*

3. *TBI is a common injury seen in sexual and domestic assault (ie, intimate partner violence [IPV]).*

4. *It is best practice to screen for TBI in all patients with suspected neck, head, and/or brain injury following a sexual or domestic assault.*

5. *A thorough neurological examination is part of the medical forensic evaluation when there is suspicion of neck, head, and/or brain injury.*

Introduction

TBI is defined as an alteration in the normal function of the brain caused by external forces. Previous definitions sought to limit the scope of this diagnosis by framing it as a blow to the head, shaking, blast wave, or penetration. Modern definitions, however, have included hypoxic (ie, decreased oxygen) and anoxic (ie, no oxygen) brain injuries. While researchers acknowledge that the mechanisms of injury for TBI may be different, such as a blow to the head versus strangulation, the neurological sequelae of both manifest with similar symptoms.[1]

Epidemiology and History

Recent epidemiological studies identified strangulation as a lethality indicator in domestic violence events. In the United States, 1 in 3 women experience domestic violence at some point during their lifetime. Up to 92% of those women report experiencing trauma to the head and nearly half report experiencing strangulation.[1] Strangulation is also reported in 12% of all sexual assaults. TBI is reported by 75% of those who experience IPV. Of those, 50% report repetitive TBI.[2] The Centers for Disease Control and Prevention report that in 2014, TBI was diagnosed at approximately 2.9 million emergency department (ED) visits, hospitalizations, and autopsies. Furthermore, in 2018, TBI resulted in 223 050 hospitalizations; in 2019, there were 60 611 deaths.[3] Consequently, TBI is a leading cause of disability in the United States.

Research into the neurological sequelae of strangulation, often in the form of memory problems, dates back to the late 1800s. Women who report having been strangled perform worse on assessments of long-term and working memory compared to women without the experience of strangulation.[4] The proposed cause of these memory problems are hypoxic and anoxic brain injuries as a result of the strangulation event. These injuries deny oxygen to brain cells, thereby killing them in the areas of the brain that are most sensitive to oxygen deprivation, which are the hippocampus and the 3rd and 5th layers of the neocortex where memory formation occurs.

Publications, even dating back to the 1940s, show that oxygen deprivation of approximately 5 to 10 seconds—with complete occlusion of the carotid arteries, vertebral arteries, and jugular veins—causes a loss of consciousness (LOC), which is when anoxic brain injury begins. The rate of anoxic cellular brain death is approximately 32 000 neurons per second. Since each neuron forms up to 10 000 connections with neighboring cells (called synapses), approximately 230 million synapses are lost with each second of anoxia.[5]

SYMPTOMOLOGY

General awareness about the dangers of strangulation has increased over the last decade due to growing epidemiological literature, case studies, and pressures from domestic violence health care providers and nurses. In response, the American Academy of Neurology released a position statement regarding the dangers of strangulation, stating[6]:

> The medical literature and the cumulative experience of neurologists clearly indicate that restricting cerebral blood flow or oxygen delivery, *even briefly*, can cause permanent injury to the brain, including stroke, cognitive impairment, and even death. Unconsciousness resulting from such maneuvers is a manifestation of catastrophic global brain dysfunction.

Manifestations of TBI symptoms are often delayed, appearing hours, days, or even weeks later. Symptoms include neurological manifestations such as new onset epilepsy, chronic dizziness (ie, vertigo), frequent headaches, sleep disruptions, new onset decline in vision and hearing acuity, focal numbness and tingling, and difficulty remembering the time around the event and/or difficulty forming new memories since the event.[1,2,4] Understanding neuronal cellular death provides a foundation for assessment and documentation by forensic nurses who, once suspicious of the hypoxic or anoxic event, refer the patient for mitigation of medical outcomes with trauma-informed intervention and management.

TRAUMATIC BRAIN INJURY SCREENING

To assist in documentation, a structured evaluation of sexual or domestic assault in a medical forensic evaluation is necessary. Forms that screen for TBI, such as the Cal OES 2-502 Strangulation and Head Injury Addendums,[7] assist in structured evaluation. Since short-term memory is affected immediately, the individual who experienced strangulation to the point of unconsciousness may not remember losing consciousness, and when asked, might deny LOC. Using a logical sequence of questions, demonstrated on the Cal OES 2-502 Strangulation and Head Injury Addendum,[7] all aspects of screening occur. Additionally, a structured evaluation form listing specific, evidence-based symptoms can be helpful. Symptoms leading to LOC include inability to breathe, vision and hearing changes, feelings of dizziness, lightheadedness, or fainting. After an initial screening, patients are asked directly whether there was LOC during their assault. If the patient denies LOC, the provider's questions should become targeted to address the possibility of a gap in memory. It may be helpful to ask the patient, "From the start of the event you just described to the end of the strangulation, when all of the pressure was gone from your neck, do you remember every single moment or is there a gap in your memory?" Being silent and allowing ample time for the patient to respond gives them enough time to replay the memory in their mind. If the patient discloses a gap in memory, then this symptom represents the onset of brain anoxia, thereby indicating TBI. Hypoxia and subsequent anoxia reveals the level of intentional injury and potential health sequelae.

NEUROLOGICAL EVALUATION

Because neurological examinations are part of the basic training of a registered nurse, forensic nurses are aware of this type of evaluation and likely have improved skills in this area. A review of the location and function of each cranial nerve may help the forensic nurse in categorizing the symptoms that follow a strangulation event. Grouping cranial nerves into 3 categories assists in the examination by forensic nurses (**Figure 37-1**).

Figure 37-1. *Grouping of Cranial Nerves into Senses, Eye Movement, and Facial Sensation and Movement*

Grouping of Cranial Nerves

Senses
- CN I-Olfactory
  Smell
- CN II-Optic
  Sight
- CN VIII-Vestibulocochlear
  Hearing
- CN IX-Glossopharyngeal
  Taste

Eye Movement
- CN III-Oculomotor
  Most Eye Movement
- CN IV-Trochlear
  Eye Abduction* and Intorsion
- CN VI-Abducens
  Eye Abduction*

*Eye Abduction: Look towards your ear. Eye Adduction: Look towards your nose.

Facial Sensation/Movement
- CN V-Trigeminal
  Facial Sensation, Chewing
- CN VII-Facial
  Facial Expression (Smile)
- CN X-Vagus
  Palatal Elevation with saying "Ahh"
- CN XI-Accessory
  Shoulder Shrug
- CN XII-Hypoglossal
  Tongue Protrusion

Figure 37-1

Easily assessed components of the cranial nerve examination include the following groups:

— ***The senses:*** Have there been any changes to the patient's smell, sight, hearing, or taste?

— ***Eye movement:*** Are the patient's extraocular movements intact?

— ***Facial sensation and movement:*** Test the patient's facial sensation, have them chew/bite down, smile, stick their tongue out, say "ahh," swallow, and shrug their shoulders.

Once the cranial nerve examination is completed, the forensic nurse then proceeds through the rest of the neurological examination which includes testing the deep tendon reflexes, strength, proprioception (ie, Romberg sign), upper extremity coordination (finger to nose), and gait. All of these neurological examination techniques are part of the basic registered nursing training.

CASE STUDIES

Case Study 37-1

This 16-year-old girl was brought to the ED by law enforcement for care by a forensic nurse with specialized training in sexual assault response. The girl appeared tired and had a difficult time recalling the order of events that had occurred. The patient disclosed that pressure was applied to her neck during the sexual assault. The forensic nurse then used the Strangulation Addendum of the Cal OES 2-502[7] to screen the patient for injuries to the neck, head, and brain. The patient disclosed that after pressure was applied to her neck, she was unable to breathe and experienced blurred vision, a ringing sensation in her ears, dizziness, lightheadedness, feeling faint, and disorientation. She denied LOC, but after being asked to replay the memory, she disclosed that there was a gap in memory between the onset of the hypoxic symptoms and the end of the strangulation. She also said that she did not remember the perpetrator letting go and that she felt disoriented and dizzy for several minutes afterwards. The physical examination revealed that the patient had a raspy voice and significant neck tenderness, but otherwise there were no visible bruises to her neck. During the neurological examination, she reported feeling dizzy during the Romberg testing. The forensic nurse examiner worked with the medical team who ordered a computed tomography angiogram of the patient's neck and provided education, treatment, and referral for the TBI.

Discussion

The forensic nurse in this case was able to screen the patient for strangulation and TBI, gathering significant information. The forensic nurse was careful to follow a logical sequence of questions to determine that a gap in memory was present despite the patient initially denying LOC. Missing detailed elements of the TBI event could have resulted in missed diagnosis of TBI by the medical team. The forensic nurse conducted a thorough neurological examination, which demonstrated dizziness during Romberg testing and an unsteady gait. She reported her findings to the medical team members, who were able to provide the appropriate diagnostic evaluation, treatment, and referral.

Case Study 37-2

This 45-year-old female presented with a neighbor to the ED for multiple bruises to her head and face, and she was having difficulty answering questions. The nurse used trauma-informed care principles, thereby allowing the patient to disclose that her husband of 13 years had hit her in the head on numerous occasions. The forensic nurse was then called to assess the patient. After obtaining consent, the forensic nurse conducted a domestic assault forensic medical examination, guided by the Head Injury Addendum of the Cal OES 2-502.[7] The patient denied strangulation but disclosed multiple blows to her head and face. Several of the blows caused her to "see stars," and the final blow resulted in LOC. She had multiple gaps in memory including before, during, and after the assault. The neighbor described how the patient walked over to her house and told her about the assault; however, the patient had no memory of this conversation and did not remember how she got to the ED. On physical examination, the patient had numerous tender and swollen bruises on her face; several other areas were numb to soft touch. The patient screened positive for multiple TBIs, and the forensic nurse made the appropriate referral to the medical team for evaluation and treatment of her head and brain injuries.

Discussion

It is common for patients who experience IPV to present to the ED with injuries. In this case, the medical staff was able to involve the forensic nurse who utilized a domestic violence medical forensic examination form that includes a screening for head injury and TBI to guide the assessment. The forensic nurse was able to screen this patient appropriately. The nurse also conducted a thorough neurological examination and discovered areas of numbness. As a result, the patient was referred to the medical team for additional medical evaluation and treatment.

SUMMARY

TBI is not a syndrome. It is an intentional event with a specific mechanism of injury resulting in brain cell injury and/or death and subsequent neurological symptoms. Forensic nurses, familiar with the resources available to screen for neck, head, and brain injuries, develop skilled capacity in the performance of a thorough neurological examination. Following a sexual assault or domestic violence assessment, the standard is to include a structured neurologic assessment with patients who have disclosed or who are suspected of having injury to the neck, head, or brain. The sequence of the questions and examination uses a structured approach to provide the best opportunity for a patient to recall the events that occurred throughout the intentional injury, specifically if there is LOC or a gap in memory. The employment of trauma-informed principles (see chapter 5), promotion of safety, and using silence as a reflective tool all help to give voice to the victim.

REFERENCES

1. Campbell J, Anderson J, McFadgion A, et al. The effects of intimate partner violence and probable traumatic brain injury on central nervous system symptoms. *J Womens Health*. 2018;27:(6)761-767. doi:10.1089/jwh.2016.6311

2. Valera E. Increasing our understanding of an overlooked public health epidemic: traumatic brain injuries in women subjected to intimate partner violence. *J Womens Health*. 2018;27;(6):735-737. doi:10.1089/jwh.2017.6838

3. Centers for Disease Control and Prevention. Traumatic brain injury and concussion. 2021. Accessed January 11, 2022. https://www.cdc.gov/traumatic braininjury/index.html

4. Valera E, Daugherty J, Scott O, Berenbaum H. Strangulation as an acquired brain injury in intimate-partner violence and its relationship to cognitive and psychological functioning: a preliminary study. *J Head Trauma Rehabil.* 2022;37:15-23.

5. Desai S, Rocha M, Jovin T, Jadhav A. High variability in neuronal loss: time is brain, requantified. *Stroke.* 2019;50:34-37.

6. American Academy of Neurology. AAN position statement on the use of neck restraints in law enforcement. 2021. Accessed January 11, 2022. https://www.aan.com/advocacy/use-of-neck-restraints-position-statement

7, California Clinical Forensic Medical Training Center. State of California governor's office of emergency services forensic medical report domestic violence examination Cal OES 2-502 form. 2022. Accessed January 11, 2022. https://www.ccfmtc.org/forensic-medical-examination-forms/

Military Sexual Assault and Violence

Teresa Devitt-Lynch, MSN, RN, AFN-C, AFN-BC, SANE-A
Andrea B. Ward-Wiley, MS, BSN, RN, SANE-A, GFN-C

Key Points

1. *Incidences of sexual assault in the military are grossly underreported.*

2. *Barriers, or perceived barriers, to reporting in the military are different from those of civilians who are sexually assaulted due to the military's culture and structure.*

3. *Military culture is one of distinct and unifying practices, traditions, language, and guiding principles that influence the perception and response to sexual and physical violence.*

Introduction

As within the general population, sexual assault knows no gender in the military. Both male and female service members, their family members, and federal civilian employees are affected by sexual violence. The Department of Defense (DOD) produces an annual report on sexual assault in the military. The 2020 report[1] reflected 7816 reports of sexual assault. These numbers are believed to be an underrepresentation, as most sexual assaults go unreported. The estimated number of sexual assaults in 2019 was approximately 20 500.[1]

Barriers to Reporting and Seeking Health Care

Like any survivor of abuse, military members are often reluctant to make an official report or seek care. There are many unique barriers (real and perceived) to reporting and receiving care when one serves in the military. Military culture and structure affect both the incidence of sexual assault and the barriers to reporting sexual assault. Negative use of military culture and structure affects both individuals and the military unit as a whole, which could ultimately impact national security.

Confidentiality Breaches

Many cases of sexual assault will occur within small, tight-knit commands. Victims may be worried that if they report or seek care, everyone in their command will know they were sexually assaulted. This is due to the fact that commands will work, train, eat, shower, and sleep in close quarters together with few days off. There is constant connection not only with those who may learn about the assault and pass judgment but also with their assailant.

Unhealthy or Non-Supportive Command Climates

There are military commands that have unhealthy or non-supporting environments, much like any workplace. However, the military member cannot simply resign from their job like a civilian employee can, and transferring from one command to another can be difficult or impossible depending on the nature of the assignment. The military work environment can include harassment, hazing, or retaliation, creating a physically unsafe or unaddressed environment. Commanders and lower ranking military personnel alike can, at times, consider those types of assault like hazing and bullying to be the norm, so members can be wary of reporting sexual assault or seeking care.

RETALIATION FROM LEADERSHIP OR PEERS

A victim may worry that if they report their sexual assault—especially if it was committed by someone in their command—their Command might take the side of the assailant and retaliate against them in terms of assignments given, duties assigned, or promotions denied. The victim may also fear that peers will ostracize them. These fears are some of the perceived barriers for reporting, as ostracization and retaliation do not always occur, but there is still a dependency on the goodwill and respect of leadership due to the military's power dynamics.

PUNISHMENT FOR COLLATERAL OFFENSES

In cases of sexual assault, drugs and/or alcohol may be in play. Underage alcohol consumption and recreational drug use are both illegal while serving in the military; however, a member may choose to underage drink or use drugs. Those members that do participate in alcohol and drug use may worry that they could be punished for those offenses if they report that they were sexually assaulted while under the influence.

MILITARY CULTURE AND FORENSIC NURSING

Cultural competency in forensic nursing facilitates an effective therapeutic relationship through respectful patient care and contributes to positive health care outcomes.[2,3] As such, the military culture needs to be taken into account when caring for service members, as they will require different care than civilian patients. Behaviors, beliefs, and values of current service members, veterans, family members, and civil defense employees are shaped through their military service experiences and influence the perception and interpretation of violence and help-seeking behavior.[4]

The DOD is composed of 3 service departments and 5 branches of service, as indicated in **Figure 38-1**.

Figure 38-1. *Department of Defense Organizational Structure*

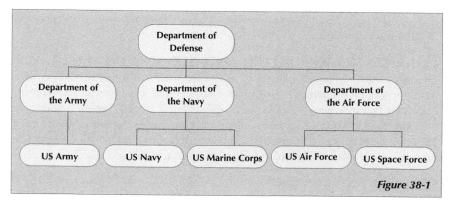

While each corps is a subculture of the military and follows its own set of values, they are all grounded in the Warrior Ethos, sometimes referred to as the Military Ethos. The Warrior Ethos outlines the fundamental principles of military culture and includes selflessness, loyalty, stoicism, moral code, and excellence. In alignment with the Warrior Ethos, military culture is centered on structure, organization, and clear delineation of leader and subordinate roles. For instance, unlike within civilian cultures, military leaders are responsible for the personal and professional actions and wellbeing of subordinates at all times. Additionally, soldiers, airmen, sailors, and marines must prioritize the accomplishment of their mission and command cohesiveness.[3-5]

Indoctrination into the military culture and the Warrior Ethos begins with the initial training called basic training or boot camp, in which civilian individualism is deconstructed and the military principles of obedience, discipline, self-sacrifice, comradery, and courage are introduced with continual reinforcement and conformity throughout service members' careers.[5]

While the Warrior Ethos makes strong soldiers, sailors, marines, and airmen, it also creates vulnerabilities that can make reporting and seeking care difficult, as shown in **Table 38-1**.[4,6] Culturally competent care for military sexual violence victims and suspects is dependent upon the forensic nurse's understanding that the Warrior Ethos and military culture have significant influence over the military members' recognition and interpretation of sexual violence, help-seeking behaviors, and health care engagement. It is also reliant upon the forensic nurse's ability to identify the extent to which patients identify with the Warrior Ethos and degree of enculturation.[4] This is done through research and understanding of the military culture and how it affects patients.[3,4] Understanding the influence of military culture upon health-related behaviors helps the forensic nurse appropriately interact with military patients and create an appropriate treatment plan to reach optimal health outcomes.

Table 38-1. Warrior Ethos Military Strengths and Weaknesses in Help-Seeking Behavior Related to Sexual Violence[2-4, 6]

Strength to service	Ethos category	Vulnerability to help-seeking
Commitment to mission accomplishment and protecting comrades	Loyalty	Reporting sexual violence would be equivalent to "whistle-blowing" and betraying the loyalty of comrades and superiors; no longer viewed as team player; fear of retaliation
Placing the welfare of others above one's own	Selflessness	Not seeking help for sexual violence because personal health is not a priority and absence from unit would impact the workload of fellow servicemen
Following an internal "right" versus "wrong" moral compass	Moral code	Feeling of betrayal when the assailant is a fellow service member who violated the moral code
Toughness and ability to endure hardships without complaint	Stoicism	Not acknowledging significant symptoms and suffering related to sexual violence; need to maintain courage and strength and not display weakness
Becoming the best and most effective professional possible	Excellence	Self-blame and shame related to "allowing" the sexual violence to happen

CASE STUDIES

Case Study 38-1

An active-duty sailor, was stationed on the USS Carl Vinson. His ship pulled into port in San Diego, and the ship members were granted liberty in town. The sailor, who was only 18 years old, found a bar with his friend that would serve them alcohol despite them being underage. While using the restroom, the sailor was bombarded by 2 other males and was sexually assaulted. He returned to the ship to sleep and did not tell anyone what happened to him until the next morning, when his friend saw a bruise on his back while he was changing clothes. After telling his friend what happened, the sailor reluctantly decided to go to a nearby civilian ED to be seen because of the pain he was experiencing and for evaluation for possible sexually transmitted infections. After talking with the forensic nurse, the sailor consented to a sexual assault forensic examination but declined to report the crime to law enforcement. During the examination, he expressed self-blame and frequently commented that he should not have been drinking and should have fought off the attackers. He also declined the 2 days of leave the forensic nurse offered him because that would cause the other sailors in his unit to "pick up his slack."

Discussion

Having an understanding of the military culture and Warrior Ethos, the forensic nurse was able to identify the cultural influences in the sailor's emotional and psychological reaction to the trauma. She relayed this information to him and reaffirmed that the violent trauma he experienced was neither his fault nor a reflection on his level of masculinity. She also informed him this trauma did not have to impact his capabilities of fulfilling his military duties, and his feelings were normal. She also provided the advocate, who had little experience in supporting military victims, with some information and tips on supporting the sailor.

SUMMARY

To develop cultural competence when caring for military patients, forensic nurses must identify and evaluate their own beliefs and seek educational sources to understand military culture. Forensic nurses must identify and evaluate their own beliefs, biases, and experiences with military service members, veterans, family members, and culture through self-reflection. Agreement with military culture or supporting the military's mission and operations is not required to establish a therapeutic relationship with military patients. It is imperative, however, that negative beliefs and biases toward the military or its functions are identified and self-mitigated so as to not interfere with the provision of comprehensive and compassionate care.[3,4] Forensic nurses must also understand that both the structure and culture of the military influence the incidence of sexual assault and may create barriers to reporting an assault.

REFERENCES

1. Annual Report on Sexual Assault in the Military. Department of Defense. March 15, 2021. Accessed October 14, 2021. https://www.sapr.mil/sites/default/files/DOD_Annual_Report_on_Sexual_Assault_in_the_Military_FY2020.pdf

2. Research on Interpersonal Victimization in the Military. Center for Victim Research. Accessed October 14, 2021. https://ncvc.dspacedirect.org/bitstream/id/2659/CVR%20Annotated%20Bibliography_Interpersonal%20Victimization%20in%20the%20Military.pdf

3. Sanghera N. Developing military cultural competency to better serve those who have served us. The Journal of the Association of Schools and Colleges of Optometry: Optometric Education. 2017. Accessed October 10, 2021. https://journal.opted.org/article/developing-military-cultural-competency-to-better-servethose-who-have-served-us/

4. Westphal RJ, Convoy SP. Military culture implications for mental health and nursing care. *Online J Issues Nurs.* 2015;20(1). doi:10.3912/OJIN.Vol20No01Man04

5. Redmond SA, Wilcox SL, Campbell S, et al. A brief introduction to the military workplace culture. *Military Culture.* 2015;50(1):9-20. doi:10.3233/WOR-141987

6. Bourke J. Military sexual trauma: Gender, military cultures and the medicalization of abuse in contemporary America. *J War Cult Stud.* 2021. doi:10.1080/17526272.2021.1884785

Chapter 39

Military Service and Forensic Nursing Response to Violence

Victoria A. Franz, DNP, APRN, FNP-C, AFN-BC, SANE-A, SANE-P, SAMFE
Shelli A. Larkin, MSN, WHNP-BC, NE-BC, SANE-A
Patricia M. Speck, DNSc, CRNP, FNP-BC, AFN-C, DF-IAFN, FAAFS, DF-AFN, FAAN

Key Points

1. *Military members face challenges in receiving care without consequence.*

2. *The Department of Defense (DOD)'s Sexual Assault Prevention and Response (SAPR) program provides resources for military members.*

3. *There are 2 reporting options for military members – restricted and unrestricted.*

4. *The DOD offers centralized training for forensic nurses who maintain clinical competencies by participating in continuing education on an annual basis.*

5. *The DOD standardized Evidence Recovery Kits, medical forensic examinations, and comprehensive documentation.*

Introduction

In response to the Tailhook scandal in 1991, when 83 women and 7 men accused US Navy and Marine Corps officers of improper and indecent conduct or sexual assault, the DOD reviewed their process for treatment and care of victims of sexual assault in the military.[1] The former Secretary of Defense Donald H. Rumsfeld directed Dr. David S. C. Chu, the former Under Secretary of Defense for Personnel and Readiness, to review the DOD's process,[2] and the DOD quickly assembled the Care for Victims of Sexual Assault Task Force. The task force was charged with evaluating the current response to sexual assault and subsequently produced the *2004 Task Force Report on Care for Victims of Sexual Assault*.[3] Drs. Cynthia Ferguson, Linda Ledray, and Patricia Speck, forensic nurses with military service backgrounds, received invitations to participate in stakeholder groups, representing each branch of the health care task force. Following a comprehensive review with stakeholder input, the task force released a series of recommendations.[3]

One of these recommendations emphasized the need to establish a single point of accountability for sexual assault policy within the DOD, which led to the creation of Joint Task Force for Sexual Assault Prevention and Response. The task force focused its initial efforts on developing a new DOD-wide sexual assault policy that incorporated recommendations set forth in the *Task Force Report on Care for Victims of Sexual Assault*. The Ronald W. Reagan National Defense Authorization Act for Fiscal Year 2005 (PL108-375) mandated a policy by January 1, 2005.[2] In January 2005, the DOD presented Congress with a comprehensive policy on prevention and response to sexual assault.[4] The policy provided a foundation for the DOD to improve prevention of sexual assault, significantly enhance support to reporting and non-reporting victims, and increase accountability.

The current SAPR policies and procedures established more than 1200 sexual assault response coordinators, chaplains, lawyers, and law enforcement officials as first responders at all major installations, training more than 1 million service members.[4] The overarching elements of SAPR efforts became permanent with the approval of DOD Directive 6495.01, the "Sexual Assault Prevention and Response Policy," in October 2005. The SAPR Office now serves as the DOD's single point of authority for sexual assault policy and provides oversight to ensure that each branch of the military service's programs complies with DOD policy.[4] Healthcare for military members of all branches, their family members, and other Tricare beneficiaries falls under the Defense health Agency (DHA). The DHA recently established the Forensic Healthcare Program (FHP) under Health Affairs. The FHP provides oversight of forensic health care, to include care provided to patients with a disclosure of sexual assault. This care may be rendered directly within the military treatment facility (MTF) or through agreements called memorandums of understanding (MOUs), with community resources, surrounding US Armed Forces installations. The medical professionals, forensic nurses, and other forensic examiners, responding to the medical needs of victims of abuse are under the umbrella of the DHA.[4]

MILITARY RESPONSE TO VIOLENCE

The military response to sexual abuse is patient-centered, trauma-informed, and gender-neutral, and it emphasizes a culture of safety.[5,6-8] Affording victims autonomy and control over the process of reporting and having advocates available 24/7 is necessary to provide resources to those affiliated with the military.[9] Under the DOD's SAPR procedures, service members and their adult family members have 2 reporting options for sexual assault – *restricted* and *unrestricted*.[4-9] A ***restricted report*** allows the victim to receive medical, behavioral, and advocacy support, while not reporting to law enforcement or to their military unit or command. An ***unrestricted report*** includes notifications to law enforcement or to their military unit or command.[4-9]

By congressional mandate and DOD policies, sexual assault medical forensic examiners (SAMFE) may be registered nurses, advanced practice registered nurses, physician assistants, or physicians, and they are trained at a 2-week standardized course at the US Army Medical Center of Excellence. Both SAMFEs and forensic health examiners (FHE) are required to have standardized training, maintain annual clinical competencies, and complete annual abuse/trauma-related continuing education in order to maintain credentials within the MTF.[6-10,20] The SAMFE course meets education eligibility for nurses trained as sexual assault nurse examiners to seek certification with the International Association of Forensic Nursing as an Adult/Adolescent Sexual Assault Nurse Examiner.[11,12] These practices have been derived from the American Association of Colleges of Nursing's *Essentials*[15] and Forensic Nursing Certification Board (FNCB) Forensic Nursing Core Competencies.[13]

After the disclosure of physical or sexual abuse, FHPs perform all aspects of trauma-informed care for patients, which include the acute assault medical forensic examination and follow-up primary medical care. Forensic health care within the MTFs is carried out by specially trained FHE/SAMFEs.[6-9,12,14,20] In accordance with guidance from the DHA, those performing acute medical forensic evaluations for adolescent/adults (post-puberty and above) after a sexual assault have up to 168 hours to collect a Physical Evidence Recovery Kit (PERK). For prepubescent children, they have up to 72 hours for collection.[14,16] Kits collected within a MTF are standardized across the globe, and they are sent to be analyzed at the Defense Forensic Science Center (ie, the DOD's major crime lab, also known as the US Army Criminal Investigation Laboratory [USACIL]). When DNA allele detection reaches the threshold for the Combined DNA Index System (CODIS), forensic scientists enter the profile. The USACIL analyzes DOD and non-DOD kits in cooperation with other jurisdictional

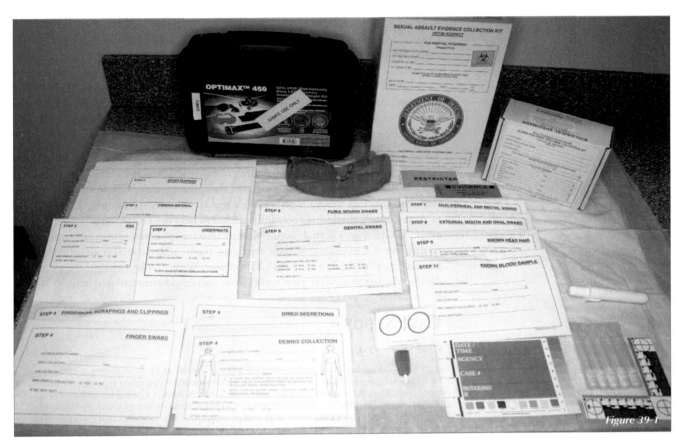

crime labs. **Figure 39-1** shows various evidence collection and documentation tools that may be utilized by a forensic nurse at the MTF.

Figure 39-1. Examples of various evidence collection tools including a sexual assault evidence collection kit, blood and urine specimen collection kit, and step-by-step guide with diagrams for evidence collection and photodocumentation.

PERSON-CENTERED ADVOCACY

In the event that an abused patient is an intimate partner or child of a military member, the military offers medical care that includes access to interpersonal violence and nonfatal strangulation medical forensic evaluations as well as additional Family Advocacy Program resources.[9] A restricted reporting option is unavailable for pediatric patients with a disclosure of or suspected assault/abuse.[9] All health care providers within the MTF, including FHEs and SAMFEs, are mandatory reporters.[9]

When a military service member or TRICARE (ie, the military health care program) beneficiary is the victim, and forensic health care is not readily available within the MTF, the military procedures allow collection at MOU facilities following local policies and procedures.[6-8,20] Within the MTF, documentation for sexual assault across all branches of the military is currently accomplished using a standardized DOD form.[10] The DD2911 is a comprehensive form, used by FHE/SAMFEs and community MOU forensic nurses in the documentation of the patient's medical history, presenting illness or injury (eg, from the assault), and assault-related details. These details guide the physical evaluation and sample collection. Accurate and objective documentation of findings and injuries should follow. The encounter record (DD2911) is retained for 50 years,[6-8] and restricted kits are stored for a minimum of 10 years after collection.[9]

Medical forensic health care within the MTF for either restricted or unrestricted reports ensures patient choice. It includes options for injury evaluation and treatment, specialized referrals, the collection of forensic samples,[4] emergency contraception, immunizations, and testing and prophylaxis for sexually transmitted infections (STIs).[17]

Special Circumstances for Military Members

Often, alcohol and drugs are used to create vulnerability in victims of sexual assault.[1,5,18] If alcohol-enabled or drug-facilitated sexual assault (DFSA) is suspected or reported, regardless of unrestricted or restricted reporting, and with the patient's permission, the FHE/SAMFE collects a DFSA kit within 96 hours.[6-8] The DFSA kit processing occurs at the Dover Air Force Base Armed Forces Medical Examiner System's toxicology lab. Toxicology testing includes over 200 potential metabolites of over-the-counter drugs, prescription medications, illegal substances, and others.[6-8]

Trauma-informed approaches to facilitate post-event recovery are standard in established episodic and ongoing behavioral and medical health care and are present in specialized forensic health care programs and primary care.[2,5] To better support victims, the CATCH Program gives people making a restricted report the opportunity to anonymously disclose suspect information to help the DOD identify serial offenders. CATCH allows sexual assault victims (service members and adult dependents) to discover if the suspect in their restricted report may have also assaulted another person (eg, a "match" in the CATCH website). With that knowledge, the victim can decide whether to convert their report from restricted to unrestricted in order to initiate an investigation of the suspect.[19]

Case Study

Case Study 39-1

A 21-year-old soldier presented to the MTF with a "friend" at 11 PM reporting sexual assault by fellow soldiers while at a hotel party. The victim advocate discussed reporting options with the victim. She chose an unrestricted report, and the US Army Criminal Investigation Division (CID) was notified. The soldier consented to a medical forensic examination performed by the SAMFE, which included toxicology and photography. She was concerned about collateral misconduct as she admitted that she had been drinking, and they were not supposed to be off base. She recalled being vaginally assaulted by 5 different persons, and she also reported anal penetration and no use of condoms. She had a pre-existing contusion to her left shin as a result of a fall during physical training. Her first pap smear was 5 weeks before the assault. She had no pregnancy history, was not currently in any relationship(s), and was sexually active with 1 past partner before she joined the military. Her last menstrual period was 2 weeks prior to arrival. She took oral contraceptive pills "for acne" but "may have missed a few days during her recent field exercise." She reported no other medical history.

The SAMFE collected all samples per protocol and patient history including urine and blood for toxicology. Medical laboratory testing included general blood work and testing for STIs. The patient accepted STI and HIV prophylaxis as well as emergency contraception. She was up to date on her immunizations. She denied both suicidal and homicidal ideation. The victim advocate arranged temporary housing in different barracks from her classmates, and she accepted a referral to behavioral health. Sixteen weeks later, CID sat down with her to advise her on the results of the forensic analysis of the specimens in her PERK. Seven DNA profiles were identified from the vaginal, cervical, and anal samples, including her female "battle buddy" and a male classmate, the same "friend" who drove her to the emergency room the night she was seen by the SAMFE. Four years later, all 7 identified perpetrators received non-judicial punishments and dishonorable discharges from the military. One, upon discharge from the military, was picked up by a state bureau of investigation due to a CODIS hit for involvement in additional sexual crimes. The victim, still in recovery, is now married and continues to receive services for Military Sexual Trauma through her local Veterans Affairs hospital.

Discussion

Forensic nurses should consider the unique barriers that the patient overcame to report her sexual assault. In this case, the unique factors assisted in the forensic nurse's decisions related to evidence, resulting in high DNA recovery from her medical forensic examination in the evidence collection kit. There were a number of factors recognized by the forensic nurse that led to the patient having a drug-facilitated toxicology kit collected, being offered emergency contraception during her medical forensic examination, and being a candidate for HIV post-exposure prophylaxis.

Summary

Forensic nurses caring for members of the Armed Services and their families are in a unique situation to facilitate collaboration with community partners. The forensic nurse should be cognizant that sexual assault in the military is complex and related to the diverse and transient environment of service members and their families. The specialized training afforded by FHE/SAMFEs prepares the forensic nurse to treat these patients in a trauma-informed, comprehensive, and compassionate manner cohesive to the military culture.[4-8]

REFERENCES

1. Ogden J. Institutions in Crisis: Tailhook '91 and the US Navy. The Kenan Institute for Ethics at Duke University. 2009. https://kenan.ethics.duke.edu/wp-content/uploads/2018/01/TailhookUSNavy_Case2015.pdf

2. United States Department of Defense Sexual Assault Prevention and Response. Mission & History. https://www.sapr.mil/mission-history

3. Embrey EP, Arnold KA, Bingham C, et al. Task Force Report on Care for Victims of Sexual Assault. April 2004. https://www.sapr.mil/public/docs/reports/task-force-report-for-care-of-victims-of-sa-2004.pdf

4. Department of Defense Directive 6495.01: Sexual Assault Prevention and Response (SAPR) Program. January 23, 2012. Updated November 10, 2021. https://www.esd.whs.mil/Portals/54/Documents/DD/issuances/dodd/649501p.pdf

5. Marino MA, Wolgast KA, Speck PM, Kenny DJ, Moriarty H. American Academy of Nursing Policy Brief: Military sexual trauma. *Nursing Outlook*. 2019; 69:486-491.

6. Department of Defense Instruction 6495.02, Volume 1: Sexual Assault Prevention and Response: Program Procedures. March 28, 2013. Updated November 10, 2021. https://www.esd.whs.mil/Portals/54/Documents/DD/issuances/dodi/649502_vol1.PDF?ver=cgGWF8znmrSsFAimctzJFQ%3d%3d

7. Department of Defense Instruction 6495.02, Volume 2: Sexual Assault Prevention and Response: Education and Training. March 28, 2013. Updated April 9, 2021. https://www.esd.whs.mil/Portals/54/Documents/DD/issuances/dodi/649502_vol2p.PDF?ver=x0Y2PHlLAnffN3xcghUPbg%3d%3d

8. Department of Defense Instruction 6495.02, Volume 3: Sexual Assault Prevention and Response: Retaliation Response for Adult Sexual Assault Cases. June 24, 2022 Updated November 10, 2021. https://www.esd.whs.mil/Portals/54/Documents/DD/issuances/dodi/649502_vol3.PDF

9. Department of Defense. Instructions 6400.01: Family Advocacy Program. May 1, 2019. https://www.esd.whs.mil/Portals/54/Documents/DD/issuances/dodi/640001p.pdf

10. Department of Defense. Form 2911: Sexual Assault Forensic Examination Report. 2005. Updated September 1, 2015. https://www.sapr.mil/public/docs/miscellaneous/toolkit/dd2911__Sept_2015.pdf

11. US Department of Justice, Office on Violence Against Women. National Training Standards for Sexual Assault Medical Forensic Examiners. August 1, 2018. https://www.ojp.gov/pdffiles1/ovw/241903.pdf

12. Lechner M, Britton-Susino S, Daiber D, et al. *Sexual Assault Nurse Examiners Education Guidelines*. International Association of Forensic Nurses; 2018.

13. Giddnes J, Bartels J, McCurren C, et al. *The Essentials: Core Competencies for Professional Nursing Education AACN*. American Association of Colleges of Nursing; 2021.

14. US Department of Justice, Office on Violence Against Women. A National Protocol for Sexual Assault Medical Forensic Examinations: Adults/Adolescents. April 1, 2013. https://www.justice.gov/ovw/file/846856/download

15. *Forensic Nursing Core Competencies for Generalist and Advanced Forensic Nursing Practice.* 1st ed. Forensic Nursing Certification Board; 2021:1-60.

16. US Department of Justice, Office on Violence Against Women. A National Protocol for Sexual Assault Medical Forensic Examinations: Pediatric. April 2016. https://www.justice.gov/ovw/file/846856/download

17. Centers for Disease Control and Prevention. STI Treatment Guidelines. Sexual Assault and Abuse and STIs: Adolescents and Adults. 2021. https://www.cdc.gov/std/treatment-guidelines/sexual-assault.htm

18. US Department of Defense Sexual Assault Prevention and Response. Catch a Serial Offender (CATCH) Program. August 2019. Accessed October 1, 2021. https://www.sapr.mil/CATCH

19. Krebs CP, Lindquist CH, Warner TD, Fisher BS, Martin SL. College women's experiences with physically forced, alcohol- or other drug-enabled, and drug-facilitated sexual assault before and since entering college. *J Am Coll Health.* 2009;57(6):639-647. doi:10.3200/JACH.57.6.639-649

20. Department of Defense Instruction 6310.09: Healthcare Management for Patients Associated with a Sexual Assault. May 7,2019. https://www.esd.whs.mil/ Portals/54/Documents/DD/issuances/dodi/631009p.pdf?ver=2019-05-07-104626-470

CAMPUS SEXUAL ASSAULT

Josie Doss, PhD, RNC-OB, AFN-C, SANE-A
Shantee Henry, DNP, RN, SANE-A

KEY POINTS

1. *Sexual violence is pervasive on college campuses but remains largely unreported.*

2. *Persons experiencing sexual assault on college campuses are at an increased risk for depression, anxiety, post traumatic stress disorder (PTSD), and unsuccessful academic endeavors due to the increased likelihood of continued interaction with the perpetrator.*

3. *Institutional reporting and disciplinary processes are required by the federal Title IX Educational Amendments of 1972 (Title IX).*

4. *The Jeanne Clery Disclosure of Campus Security Policy and Campus Crime Statistics Act (Clery Act) is a federal mandate that requires institutions of higher education to disclose information about crime on campuses.*

INTRODUCTION

College students, primarily female students between the ages of 18 and 24, are at an increased risk for sexual violence both on and off campus.[1] In 2019, the Association of American Universities report[2] indicated that the overall rate of non-consensual sexual contact (ie, penetration, attempted penetration, sexual touching, or inability to consent) on college campuses is 13%. The report further indicates that rates for women (20.4%) and those who identify as transgender, nonbinary, gender questioning, lesbian, bisexual, or gay (20.3%) are 4 times higher than the rates for men (5.1%). The majority of these assaults are believed to occur during the first or second semester of college and the latter part of the calendar year[2,3] and are often committed by individuals known to the survivor.[1]

Alcohol and drug use are factors contributing to sexual violence,[4] with 75% to 80% of student victims reporting that they consumed alcohol prior to the event.[2] Approximately 66% of these victims reported offender alcohol consumption prior to the event. For the 3.7% of women who reported non-consensual penetration, 11.8% suspected another substance was given to them without their knowledge prior to the incident.[2]

Campus sexual assault is widely under-reported.[1] Approximately 1 in 5 female college student victims report their assault to law enforcement.[5] Drug-facilitated sexual assault reporting is even lower. Survivors surveyed in the report provided a number of reasons for not reporting: they could "handle it themselves," the incident was not serious enough to merit a report, embarrassment, lack of proof, confusion about what happened, uncertainty about what constitutes assault, fear of retaliation, lack of knowledge about how to report, and/or fear of how the criminal justice system would treat them.[1,2] Despite college resource availability, only 29.5% of women and 17.8% of men who reported non-consensual penetration contacted a campus-based program or resource.[2]

People who experience sexual violence face an increased risk of behavioral or emotional consequences including depression, anxiety, and PTSD.[2] Small college campus communities almost guarantee the victim will see the accused in classes, the dorm, the cafeteria, or at other campus events, making it harder to recover. Survivors often experience academic consequences that include decreased class attendance, difficulty concentrating, and difficulty going to work. These symptoms are often more prevalent among members of the LGBTQ+ community, who should be given additional referrals to address their specific needs in recovery.[2]

LEGISLATION

There are 2 significant federal legislations governing treatment of sexual assault victims and the accused on campuses. Title IX of the Educational Amendment Act of 1972 and the Jeanne Clery Disclosure of Campus Security Policy and Campus Crime Statistics Act guide institutional response to incidents of dating violence, domestic violence, sexual assault, and stalking.

TITLE IX

Title IX guarantees equal access to education for all and consequently prohibits discrimination on the basis of sex in educational institutions receiving federal financial assistance.[6] Title IX requires that colleges receiving federal funding have policies and procedures to combat gender-based sexual violence and harassment. These schools also must respond to survivors' needs in order to ensure equal access to education.[6]

Students, faculty, or staff who experience any form of sexual harassment or violence have the ability to file a formal complaint with the Title IX office located on their campus. All college employees, including faculty, staff, and administrators, are mandated reporters and are required to report any disclosures of sexual assault to the college's Title IX office, where victims are provided with written information on available resources, including counseling, legal assistance, and other on and off campus services. The Title IX office will also advise the victim on their right to file criminal charges. The US Department of Education's Office for Civil Rights is responsible for investigating when schools fail to follow up on a complaint or to protect the victim.[6]

CLERY ACT

Enacted in 1990, the Clery Act requires both public and private colleges and universities that participate in federal student aid programs to report campus crime data, support victims of violence, and publicly outline the policies and procedures in place to improve campus safety with initial and ongoing prevention and awareness education.[7] Under the Clery Act, institutions accepting federal funding must create and disseminate an annual security report (ASR) to employees and students detailing initiatives to improve campus safety. ASR data includes criminal offenses (eg, homicide, murder, sexual assault, robbery, aggravated assault, burglary, motor vehicle theft, and arson), gender offenses (eg, domestic violence, dating violence, and stalking), hate crimes (eg, larceny-theft; simple assault; intimidation; and destruction, damage, or vandalism of property), and any arrests and referrals for disciplinary action (eg, weapons law, drug abuse, and liquor law violations).

RESPONSE TO CRIME ON CAMPUS

Violence on campus is treated in a manner similar to other environments. If the person feels they are in immediate danger, they should call 911 as soon as possible. After the event, victims may choose to report, and when they do, many campuses have sexual assault centers, campus police, and campus health centers to respond. If sexual assault services are not available on campus, campus services will refer survivors to community resources.

The forensic nurse's role on or in collaboration with campuses is often as a Sexual Assault Nurse Examiner (SANE). The forensic nurse responding to a case of sexual assault has subspecialty education and follows standards of practice and care. A few of the forensic nurse's tasks include completing a medical and nursing evaluation for injury (physical, psychological, and emotional) and collecting, storing, and transporting forensic evidence to law enforcement. The forensic nurse who is also a faculty member has the opportunity to work with campus officials to support administrative activities, plan employee and student educational events about campus sexual assault, and prepare resources for students and employees alike. Advanced practice nurse faculty, such as those in the fields of family health, psych-mental health, and women's health, often expand their practices on campuses by developing and implementing campus health services to support the long-term recovery of survivors.

CASE STUDIES

Case Study 40-1

An 18-year-old cisgender female college freshman met her friends at a local bar to celebrate fall midterms. They were drinking and having fun when a classmate from her biology class asked them to join him at a house party. They agreed, and she rode there with her classmate. The classmate said he had to stop at his dorm room to get a jacket. While there, he offered her a glass of water, which she drank. After a few minutes, she started feeling dizzy and weak. The guy started kissing her and fondling her breasts. She tried to push him off, but she was very weak. She sporadically remembers him penetrating her vaginally and anally. After, he left her in the dorm alone, and she called a friend to pick her up. She reported the sexual assault to campus police the next day. They responded by asking her to not report the incident to police and initiated an internal investigation. During this time, the accused remained on campus and appeared in their common classes with her. The victim experienced nightmares, panic attacks, and had difficulty sleeping and concentrating. She then found herself on academic probation and decided it was too hard to continue seeing the accused, so she dropped out of school at the end of the spring semester.

Discussion

This student presented with several risk factors for campus sexual assault. She was an 18-year-old female undergraduate who, after a night of drinking, was in the company of a male who had also been drinking. In this case, she went to his dorm room and was offered a drink that she accepted. Unknown to her was the additional substance that made her dizzy, weak, and unable to fight off the advances of the assailant. She reported the incident to campus police, who should have known the requirements of Title IX and the Clery Act. They should have facilitated her report to local police when she requested, as the community's resources included SANE evaluation and community assistance. Failure to protect the victim following the assault likely contributed to the behavioral and emotional consequences she experienced and her subsequent withdrawal from the university.

SUMMARY

Sexual violence is pervasive on college campuses, but reporting is limited. Risk factors include being a freshman or sophomore undergraduate student between the ages of 18 and 24 and being a sexual or gender minority. Any student who experiences sexual violence and remains on campus is likely to encounter their assailant through various campus events, including classes, cafeteria dining, and dorm living. The revictimization associated with these encounters triggers anxiety reactions and increases the rates of behavioral and emotional problems, which may result in academic struggles and failure. Title IX provides student victims with access to resources and support following an incident. Forensic nurses may be responsible for providing forensic medical examinations as a SANE, counseling students about the services available to them, or educating the campus community about risk factors, prevention, and reporting requirements. The forensic nurse has leadership competencies that are useful for the development and implementation of these campus-based services.

REFERENCES
1. Krebs CP, Lindquist CH, Warner TD, Fisher BS, Martin SL. College women's experiences with physically forced, alcohol- or other drug-enabled, and drug-facilitated sexual assault before and since entering college. *J Am Coll Health.* 2009;57(6):639-647. doi:10.3200/JACH.57.6.639-649

2. Cantor D, Fisher B, Chibnall S, et al. Report on the AAU Campus Climate Survey on Sexual Assault and Sexual Misconduct. The Association of American Universities. Updated October 20, 2017. Accessed December 15, 2021. https://www.aau.edu/sites/default/files/AAU-Files/Key-Issues/Campus-Safety/AAU-Campus-Climate-Survey-FINAL-10-20-17.pdf

3. Kimble M, Neacsiu AD, Flack WF Jr, Horner J. Risk of unwanted sex for college women: evidence for a red zone. *J Am Coll Health*. 2008;57(3):331-8. doi:10.3200/jach.57.3.331-338

4. Centers for Disease Control and Prevention. Sexual Violence. Updated February 5, 2021. Accessed December 15, 2021. https://www.cdc.gov/violenceprevention/sexualviolence/index.html

5. Sinozich S, Langton L. Rape and Sexual Victimization Among College-Aged Females, 1995-2013. US Department of Justice. December 2014. Accessed December 15, 2021. https://bjs.ojp.gov/content/pub/pdf/rsavcaf9513.pdf

6. Office of Civil Rights Headquarters. Title IX of the Education Amendments of 1972. US Department of Health & Human Services. Accessed December 15, 2021. https://www.hhs.gov/civil-rights/for-individuals/sex-discrimination/title-ix-education-amendments/index.html

7. Clery Center: At the heart of campus safety. The Jeanne Clery Act. Updated January 3, 2017. Accessed December 15, 2021. https://clerycenter.org/policy/the-clery-act/

WORKPLACE VIOLENCE

Gordon Lee Gillespie, PhD, DNP, RN, FAAN
Steven J. Palazzo, PhD, MN, RN, CNE

KEY POINTS

1. *A security walkaround, completed by a forensic nurse, can aid in identifying additional and necessary security interventions for the prevention of workplace violence.*

2. *Workplace violence prevention interventions can be deployed upon identifying cues of escalating aggressive behaviors.*

3. *To address the prevention and management of workplace violence by intimate partners, a formal policy should be in place.*

INTRODUCTION

In the categories of health care and social assistance, approximately 1 out of every 50 nonfatal occupational injuries or illnesses that required days off from work were due to workplace violence.[1] The causality of these incidents included simple assaults, aggravated assaults, robberies, and rape/sexual assaults. Furthermore, in 2019, there were a reported 20 890 intentional injuries in the United States, of which the following was found to be accounted for: pain (5210); bruises and contusions (4070); sprains, strains, and tears (3430); and fractures (990).[1] The long-term consequences of workplace violence victimization include burnout, absenteeism, presenteeism, substance abuse, chronic illness, posttraumatic stress disorder (PTSD), physical or sensory disability, and change of employers.

There are 4 categories of workplace violence based on the relationship of the aggressor to the worker[2]:

1. *Criminal-intent workplace violence* (eg, Stephen Paddock shooting into the crowd of the Route 91 Harvest Music Festival in Las Vegas, Nevada, injuring both spectators and festival workers)

2. *Customer/client workplace violence* (eg, a male patient running through a nursing station at St. John's Hospital in Minnesota, hitting nurses with a metal pole)

3. *Coworker workplace violence* (eg, opposing members of the United States Congress making derogatory comments about other Congress members). *Note: this type of workplace violence is addressed in chapter 32 of this book.*

4. *Personal relationship workplace violence* (eg, an estranged husband going to his wife's workplace and shooting and killing her while she was working)

CARE OF WORKPLACE VIOLENCE VICTIMS

After an incident of workplace violence, employees may experience embarrassment or humiliation from being victimized in front of their coworkers, guilt for not being able to prevent the violence, and anger against the aggressor or coworkers who they may have perceived as failing to intervene. The forensic nurse's initial step is to assess the employee for physically life-threatening injuries and any other wounds. This assessment will include documenting the injuries sustained, taking photographic evidence, and documenting the worker's self-reported symptoms and history of the event. Treatment plans will vary based on the severity and type of injuries incurred. Treatment may also warrant mental health counseling and a referral to their employer's employee assistance program.[3,4] Evaluation may initially focus on pain management for physical injuries and an acceptance of their referral to an employee assistance program. Long-term evaluation can include evaluating for symptoms of PTSD and/or changes in the worker's performance.

During the care of a victimized employee, the forensic nurse can demonstrate trauma-informed care by promoting the employee's safety. For many employees, their aggressor might be receiving treatment in the same department (eg, emergency department [ED]); therefore, it is important for the employee to be physically separated from them. The forensic nurse may also discuss the incident and evaluate the victim's perception of the trauma in order to better understand their perspective and experience.[4] In addition, the forensic nurse can help the worker identify coping strategies that will reflect the worker's strength and resilience.

CASE STUDIES

Case Study 41-1

In a relatively small suburban hospital, this man entered the lobby of the ED during the night shift, asking to see a patient. The lobby clerk asked for the patient's name and stated that he would need to check with the patient's nurse before letting the man into the treatment area. The man pushed the clerk aside, burst through the unlocked door and into the treatment area, and then ran past the nursing station, rushing through the back door into the main hospital. After security completed an extensive search of the hospital, they discovered that the wallets and purses for 3 patients and 1 laboratory technician were missing, presumably taken by the man. The ED staff described him as being 30 to 50 years of age, White or Hispanic, weighing between 120 to 190 pounds, and being between 5'6" and 6'1" tall with red or brown hair.

Discussion

In this case, access to the ED treatment area, and subsequently the main hospital, was unfettered. Physical security measures are an important component for the prevention of criminal-intent workplace violence. The forensic nurse can facilitate a security walkaround of the ED and other hospital wings with representatives from administration, patient services, security, and risk management.[5] The purpose of the security walkaround is to identify actual and potential security risks.[3] During the security walkaround, the forensic nurse should interview staff about past events of workplace violence and solicit strategies that they believe could have prevented the events.[3]

Recommendations for this case include locking all access points into the ED, installing closed circuit televisions (CCTV), providing radios in order to directly contact security when needed, and having a procedure for a hospital-wide security lockdown.[3-5] Restricting access into the ED would prevent unauthorized persons from entering the treatment area. CCTV enables early intervention by allowing security or ED clerks to witness the lobby altercation as it is taking place. In addition, the CCTV would provide a more accurate description of the offender. Radios allow for the clerk or other ED staff to directly contact security, therefore reducing the response time, which can be particularly prolonged during night shift. A hospital-wide security lockdown limits the ability of the perpetrator to move within the hospital without being detected.

Case Study 41-2

At an inpatient psychiatric unit, this social worker was leading a group counseling session. During the session, a client with a history of intermittent explosive disorder and chronic substance abuse stood up and paced behind their chair while running their hands through their hair repeatedly. The social worker asked, "Are you able to sit back down with the group, or do you want to return to your room for a break?" The client immediately began cursing, kicked a chair, walked over to the social worker, and then began punching them while they tried to get away. Another client in the focus group ran to get help from other staff members.

Discussion

In this case, the forensic nurse can train psychiatric staff on the behavioral cues for pending workplace violence. These cues include staring, changes in tone and volume of speech, anxiety symptoms, mumbling or incomprehensible speech, and pacing.[5] In addition, a prior history of mental health diseases and disorders further increases the risk for becoming violent.[5] As symptoms escalate, staff should request assistance or, at minimum, be immediately available should an event continue to escalate towards violence. The forensic nurse can also recommend that staff wear locator/alarm devices that can be activated in the event of an emergency. Locator devices provide an additional safety measure by routinely identifying the location of all staff members and can send help if a staff member is found to be in an unexpected location.

During a root cause analysis of the event, the advanced-practice forensic nurse would explore the client's pharmacologic treatment regimen and adherence. It may be discovered that the client's regimen is not adequately preventing substance abuse withdrawal symptoms. Based on the client's history of intermittent explosive disorder, it would have been warranted to have a second staff member co-facilitate the group therapy session.[3] Additionally, an advanced forensic nurse should select patient chairs that are heavily weighted, thereby preventing patients from picking them up and using them as projectiles.[5] Decorative wall pictures should also be permanently mounted so that they cannot be used as a weapon during an altercation.[3,5]

Case Study 41-3

This home health care aide in a rural community was assigned to visit 3 homes per shift, where they were required to provide hygiene care, a light cleaning of the patients' living rooms and bedrooms, and a respite for the patients' spouses. Several times during the past 2 weeks, the aide's ex-spouse followed them in a separate vehicle while travelling between home health care visits. During one visit, the ex-spouse entered the home of the aide's patient and accused the aide of having a sexual affair. The patient called 911, but the ex-spouse left before a deputy sheriff could arrive. During the aide's last work day at her third home visit, the ex-spouse pulled into the patient's driveway behind the aide, and they began arguing. The ex-spouse then punched the aide, pulled them into the vehicle, and handcuffed them to the inside door handle of the backseat. The ex-spouse quickly drove away. The aide has not since returned to work, and coworkers have not yet been able to get in contact with them. The employer notified the sheriff's office after 3 days of missed work.

Discussion

In this case, the forensic nurse can evaluate the home health care agency's policy for managing reports of personal relationship violence.[2] Although the violence was enacted by an ex-spouse, these acts represent workplace violence because the aide was on duty at the time of both events.[2] The forensic nurse should verify or recommend the addition of policy aspects for employees to report instances of threatening or violent behaviors from current or former partners. Employers can monitor their home health care staff's location through GPS trackers, or the employee can contact the employer's office, noting the times that they arrive and depart from a home site.[2,3] This would allow the employer or police to trace the last known location of a missing employee. Self-defense and de-escalation training could also be beneficial, as it protects the employee from aggressors both inside and outside of patient residences.[2-4] In addition, the use of personal alarms that trigger a response by local law enforcement to the scene of a violent encounter could be implemented. The forensic nurse can also educate employees on the known personal relationship workplace violence risks and tips for mitigating them. Those tips include watching for familiar vehicles when traveling between home health care sites and remaining in their vehicle until they have surveyed their surroundings and deemed it presumably safe to enter a residence (this should also be done when leaving a residence before walking back to their vehicle).

SUMMARY

Incidents of workplace violence can originate from persons with no business relationship to health care, patients and clients, and past or current personal partners of workers. The violence experienced by employees while at work can impact their physical and mental well-being. Forensic nurses are situated to assist the health care and social assistance sector in exploring the root causes of workplace violence as well as recommending strategies to victimized workers and health systems for the prevention of further workplace violence.

REFERENCES

1.   Injuries, illnesses, and fatalities. US Bureau of Labor Statistics. Accessed August 8, 2021. https://www.bls.gov/iif/

2. Small TF, Gillespie GL, Kean EB, Hutton S. Workplace violence interventions used by home healthcare workers: an integrative review. *Home Healthcare Now.* 2020;38(4):193-201.

3. Guidelines for preventing workplace violence for healthcare and social service workers (OSHA Pub. No. 3148-06R). US Department of Labor; Occupational Safety and Health Administration. 2016. https://www.osha.gov/sites/default/files/publications/osha3148.pdf

4. Gillespie GL, Fisher B, Kennebeck S, et al. Leveraging a public health framework and community advisory board to innovate workplace violence intervention strategies. *Adv Emerg Nurs J.* 2019;41(4):357-371.

5. Gillespie GL, Palazzo SJ. Violence should not be part of the job: universal violence precautions in acute care. *Am Nurse J.* 2021;16(3):18-22.

Chapter 42

Forensic Nurses on a SWAT Team: Care Under Fire

Deborah Pierce, RN, BSN, CEN, ATCN, TNCC, TECC, TPATC
Jeremy Ackerman, MD, PhD, FACEP

Key Points

1. The provision of medical support for a law enforcement Special Weapons and Tactics (SWAT) team requires specialized training so the forensic nurse is able to effectively meet the demands of "care under fire."

2. The planning and preparation for each mission is essential for overcoming the challenges of caring for injured individuals during an active tactical situation.

3. Field care of an injured person with potential ongoing threats is unique due to limited resources and security concerns, unlike care rendered in a hospital.

Introduction

Providing medical support for a law enforcement SWAT team is a uniquely challenging and fulfilling role for a forensic nurse. The assessment, treatment, and transportation of acutely injured persons during tactical SWAT operations is frequently filled by nurses and other advanced health care providers who are trained to respond under fire. Nurses' roles within a SWAT team vary from contractors to employees to volunteers. Forensic nurses work under the supervision of and in collaboration with a physician or medical director. Where there is independent, advanced nurse practice, other collaborators often consist of additional advanced practice providers, including physicians. Nurses working with SWAT teams may function in a health care provider role exclusively; may be deputized in a limited law enforcement role; or be fully trained and a duly sworn law enforcement officer. In contrast to hospital-based care, providing care in the field relies only on the equipment carried in, much like a medic in the military war theater. Due to the nature of tactical engagements in the United States, there is a heavy emphasis on management of penetrating trauma, primarily gunshot wounds. A forensic nurse in this role is primarily responsible for care of injured until traditional emergency medical services (EMS) is available on scene, which includes officers but also bystanders and suspects, as conditions permit. SWAT acts to preserve evidence, but the medical SWAT role focuses on preservation of life, and rarely involves evidence collection. Once the scene is secure, investigators, crime scene personnel, and patrol officers secure and lead management of the scene.

SWAT teams often have a paramedic who joins the team when they are called out on a mission. While less commonly used, a forensic nurse's training and scope of practice enhances a team's medical response capabilities, beyond the paramedic's role. Caring for injured persons, often police officers, under tactical conditions is uniquely different from hospital or clinic care because the environments are hostile, unsecured, and inherently dangerous. Tactical training and careful planning are required to assure medical care is delivered safely. Specialized training is necessary to understand and anticipate tactical movements and concerns of the SWAT team. A forensic nurse working in an evolving high-stress setting needs specific training to re-focus critical response skills and adapt to delivering lifesaving treatment while under fire. Depending on the needs and interests of the law enforcement agency, nurses may be eligible to complete additional training to be sworn in as an armed law enforcement officer.

TRAINING

Nurses, specifically forensic nurses, who want to master the medical SWAT response role need additional training. Advanced education in emergency procedures with certification is essential. Forensic nurses with dual or triple certifications in emergency nursing, forensics, advanced critical care, trauma care, transport nursing, and weapons safety are ideal candidates for the role. Once the basic education and certification is accomplished, completing a National Association of Emergency Medical Technician (NAEMT), Tactical Emergency Casualty Care (TECC), or Tactical Combat Casualty Care (TCCC) course,[1] is essential to refocus existing knowledge to this care setting.

Beyond medical training, training in law enforcement, tactics, and weapons handling is essential. Additional challenges in providing emergent care during the SWAT response include working in a dangerous environment and handling and removing the layers of armor, gear, and weapons. Basic knowledge of weapons handling and use requires proficiency and is an acquired skill, which will be required for any nurse wanting to become a sworn officer. The combination of these skills is critical for the forensic nurse to successfully serve the medical SWAT response team and safely handle weapons that officers or the public are carrying.

FIELD CARE

In the past, officers injured on a scene received little care until they were transported to a hospital by an ambulance that was staged nearby or in a police vehicle. Programs like Stop the Bleed[2] training give bystanders the ability to recognize life-threatening bleeding and intervene effectively. Trainings for TECC and TCCC improve officer awareness of early interventions and save lives. The awareness of a method to save lives, combined with limited availability of EMS resources on active scenes, led to increased emphasis on self-rendered, buddy-rendered, and on-the-scene medical-asset-rendered care. Most of the critical treatment steps are within the advanced forensic nurse's scope of practice collaborative agreements, when necessary, and in the generalist forensic nurse's scope of practice with physician-approved standing orders.

In the traditional nursing care plan, following the "ABCs" of nursing (ie, airway, breathing, circulation)[3] is the standard approach to trauma. Current data from both military and civilian casualty care show that ABCs are not the most effective way to prioritize care immediately following injury.[4] Instead, the MARCH[5] acronym is used (ie, massive hemorrhage, airway, respiration, circulation, head and hypothermia) with an initial focus on bleeding control, maintaining an airway, and respiration. The MARCH method is evidence based and can be delivered with limited resources in the field. The MARCH approach is summarized in **Table 42-1**.

Table 42-1. MARCH Approach to Trauma[5]	
ACRONYM MEANING	DESCRIPTION
Massive Hemorrhage	— The initial approach to bleeding control under fire
Airway	— Basic airway concerns are rapidly addressed after hemorrhage control has been established, but in some cases they may be addressed simultaneously

(continued)

Table 42-1. MARCH Approach to Trauma[5] *(continued)*	
ACRONYM MEANING	DESCRIPTION
Respiration	— Traditional assessment and support of breathing — Emphasis placed on assessment and intervention for tension pneumothorax
Circulation	— Refers to assessment and treatment for shock, necessary to restore adequate circulation
Hypothermia	— A key part of the "trauma triad of death" — Note, in military training, "H" may also stand for head injury and should be recognized if present

MISSION PREPARATION

Mission preparation requires meticulous planning, and careful consideration is needed to select supplies and equipment for a SWAT mission. This includes selection and preparation of medical equipment, planning for inherently dangerous situations, and working with environmental hazards by assessing weight and size constraints. For the medical SWAT response, appropriate body armor and ballistic helmets are recommended on the peripheral scene even if the expectation is that the medical response team will not be entering the primary zone of danger. There are several pieces of equipment that are necessary for the environment, but flashlights and trauma scissors are critically useful on the scene. Tactical teams frequently use tear gas and flashbang devices; therefore, eye and ear protection, as well as a gas mask, are important. Depending on the team and the nurse's role within that team, the nurse may be assigned additional equipment such as night-vision goggles, a tactical radio, and weapons.

Each officer is equipped with 2 tourniquets that are easily accessible on their duty belt or on their body armor (ie, 1 for them and 1 for a fellow officer, if needed). They also carry an individual first aid kit (IFAK) that contains the initial medical supplies to be used on any officer with life-threatening injuries. The contents of the IFAK and more advanced kits carried by medical staff (eg, rapid kit) or stored in vehicles (eg, advanced kit) are summarized in **Table 42-2**.

Table 42-2. Medical SWAT Mission Kit Contents*		
INDIVIDUAL FIRST AID KIT (IFAK) FOR EACH OFFICER	RAPID KIT (SMALL PROVIDER KIT)	ADVANCED KIT
— Combat tourniquets (2)	— Duplicates of IFAK	— Duplicates of rapid kit
— Combat bandages	— Nasopharyngeal airway device	— Warming blankets
— Clot promoting bandage	— Oral airway device	— Intravenous (IV) kits and fluids
— Chest seal	— Supraglottic airway device	— Eye care
— Thoracostomy needle	— Collapsible bag valve mask (BVM)	— Burn care
	— Malleable splints	— Minor wound closure

*A limited supply of medications may be carried, depending on standing orders, but few medications improve the likelihood of survival after traumatic injury.

Finally, planners create a medical risk assessment and response plan immediately before each mission. On every mission, there is an assessment of known risks, unplanned potential risks, and the possible barriers to providing care. This discussion includes factors like weather conditions, traffic, pedestrian safety, transportation logistics, and the medical response in the event of multiple casualties.

CURRENT ISSUES

Traditionally, EMS can only enter the scene when it is deemed safe. Therefore, rapid transport of an injured officer to a hospital can be problematic. Scene safety must be assured before paramedics approach, resulting in long delays if the threats persist. For this reason, the injured may be transported in a law enforcement vehicle. The transport vehicle and its route should be planned ahead of time. SWAT teams may have access to additional resources like armored vehicles and helicopters, which can aid rescue and evacuation efforts. Experience demonstrates that effective deployment of these resources requires significant planning and training. Because there is wide variability in geography, equipment available to teams, and typical encounters, each team must plan their own specific strategies and training to have viable options to facilitate and complete evacuations.

TRAUMA-INFORMED CARE

Trauma-informed care has 6 principles familiar to forensic nurses: safety; trustworthiness and transparency; peer support; collaboration and mutuality; empowerment and choice; and sensitivity to cultural, historical, and gender issues. In any stressful circumstance, nurses forge trust bonds with the team members, unique to the tactical setting. The medical staff must trust that the officers maintain their safety, and the officers must trust that if they get injured, the medical staff will render quality care and focus on their survival. Co-training is a critical time to acquire skills and create these trusting relationships that are necessary for survival on a mission. Two key principles learned during this training are collaboration and mutuality. On a mission, the nurse has a previously forged relationship with the potential patient (eg, an officer), and the mutual agreement on potential care rendered is made long before the trauma itself happens. The trust forged in this collaboration positions the nurse in this role to attend to both the physical and emotional concerns of officers and their families.

CASE STUDIES

Case Study 42-1

This SWAT team was called out on a mission at 2:00 AM to a hostage situation with 2 armed men holding a family at gunpoint. The team's nurse performed a threat assessment, noting the high risk of violence and darkness. They checked their own helmet, armor, and light sources, and ensured that the medical kits for caring for multiple casualties were complete and packed. On arrival at the briefing point, the commander designated an evacuation vehicle where the nurse stayed, and he also advised that the helicopter would be available to the team. A landing zone was designated for transfer of an injured officer requiring rapid transport to the hospital. Use of tear gas was only going to be deployed if there was active gunfire to avoid exposing the children in the home.

During the mission, an officer was struck in the thigh by gunfire from the home. He immediately put a tourniquet on his leg. He then realized he could not stand up because his injury rendered his leg too unstable to move, but he was able to provide information and cover the house with his firearm. The team deployed tear gas into the house, and the officer continued to support the team from the ground. In the face of tear gas, the suspects rapidly surrendered. This allowed 2 officers to carry the injured officer to the designated vehicle. The nurse was prepared to receive the injured officer in the evacuation vehicle and had already notified the local trauma center that there was an injured officer coming to their facility by improvised air transport. Upon receiving the patient, they performed a rapid assessment and implemented Stop the Bleed measures by performing needed interventions. The officer was taken to the helicopter where the patient and nurse were secured according to the transport plan, and the officer was delivered to the hospital with minimal blood loss.

Discussion

Anticipation is a key element for a SWAT nurse. In this instance, there were quite a few things that the nurse knew they must anticipate. They prepared for restricted visibility due to darkness by making sure their flashlight was completely charged and placed on their vest. They made sure that they had medical supplies readily available to treat anticipated gunshot wounds, and because they knew there was potential for tear gas deployment, they took their gas mask with them. A safety plan and equipment to aid secure transport in the helicopter were in place.

The officer was trained and prepared to render immediate care to himself. This allowed him to quickly apply a tourniquet himself and resume providing aid to the team from a seated position on the ground. His safe rescue on scene, transportation to the rescue vehicle, transfer to the helicopter, and transport on the helicopter were the collective result of training of all team members and the pilot.

On arrival to the vehicle, the nurse performed the 5 stages of the nursing process—assessment, diagnosis, planning, implementation, and evaluation—in conjunction with the MARCH algorithm. They performed interventions as needed as consent to be treated had been established long before this incident, and the officer trusted the nurse because of their ongoing relationship as team members. If during transport he expressed his discomfort from the tourniquet, the nurse would reassure him and get verbal consent to leave it in place, thereby maintaining mutuality. As in other areas of nursing, communication is important in this setting, as trauma creates significant vagal nerve activation. In this case, the team communicated to the nurse, transport officer, and driver that a man was down, which allowed everyone to adequately prepare. Communication to the local trauma center was vital, as they had to assure that the helipad was clear and ready for landing and prepare for the patient.

Flight poses additional barriers to patient assessment and communication. The barriers of verbal communication in a loud helicopter were anticipated, as was the potential for safety issues. If, for instance, the officer signaled to the nurse that he was anxious due to his fear of heights, the nurse would use available equipment to reassure him and present a calm countenance to help allay his fears. As a nurse, they also understand that anxiety can be a sign of an acute physical condition, such as shock or pulmonary embolism.[6] In this case, they would reassess the symptom of anxiety as physical compromise.

When care of the patient is relinquished to the nurses at the trauma center on arrival, it would be appropriate for the SWAT nurse to stay with them for moral support as a team member until other support persons become available or they go into surgery. This nurse followed up by visiting the officer in the hospital the next day, providing updates and emotional support for other concerned teammates and supporting the officer's wife by helping her with arrangements for equipment and supplies that would be needed when he got home.

Summary

SWAT teams, by nature, are called into hazardous environments where there is great potential for injury and limited resources for treatment. Unlike hospital nursing where vitals are the first assessment, the goal of the medical SWAT response is to identify the source of the immediate threat to life (in most cases, gunshot wounds), treat the issue with aggressive use of tourniquets and wound packing, assure a patient's airway is open, and transport the patient as soon as possible. Measuring blood pressure and noting an exact pulse are not the priority, as these measurements are determined by the amount of blood loss. The focus of the medical SWAT responder must be shifted toward controlling the hemorrhage first and assessing blood loss second. The medical SWAT responder must perform ongoing assessment of mentation and level of consciousness, coupled with airway assessment and management, which are all good predictors of measured vital signs but are more clearly associated with interventions. Medical personnel without law enforcement certification and advanced tactical training will usually be in a nearby location and will not be entering the dangerous environment. It is therefore important that officers on a SWAT team receive continuous and ongoing education and training to be able to administer lifesaving care to themselves and each other as a first line of care. Finally, the forensic nurse medical SWAT responder who accompanies the patient to the hospital trains to assure that extra gear and weapons are removed safely from the officer, to be able to effectively assess wounds, and to maintain safety for all involved. Working on a medical SWAT response team provides an emerging job opportunity for the forensic nurse with the proper knowledge, skills, and training.

REFERENCES

1. National Association of Emergency Medical Technicians (NAEMT). *TECC: Tactical Emergency Casualty Care.* 2nd Ed. Jones & Bartlett Learning; 2019.

2. Surgeons ACo. Stop The Bleed. Published 2019. Accessed 2021. http://stopthebleed.org.

3. Phillp J, Humphreys M, Ewens B. *Nursing Emergency Medical Patients.* Wiley-Blackwell; 2010.

4. Puryear B, Roarty J, Knight C. *EMS Tactical Combat Casualty Care.* StatPearls Publishing; 2021.

5. Gerecht R. Trauma's Lethal Triad of Hypothermia, Acidosis & Coagulopathy Create a Deadly Cycle for Trauma Patients. *JEMS.* 2014;39(4):56-60.

6. Urden LD, Stacy KM, Lough ME. *Critical Care Nursing: Diagnosis and Management.* 7th Ed. Elsevier Health Sciences; 2013.

ASSESSMENT

SINGLE BEST ANSWER MULTIPLE CHOICE

1. The document that influenced Forensic Nursing Core Competencies is:

   A. FNCB Core Competencies

   B. AACN Essentials

   C. ANA Nursing Code of Ethics

   D. IAFN Scope and Standards of Practice

2. The following is NOT a key element in forensic nurse core concepts:

   A. Knowledge attainment

   B. Technology management

   C. Lifelong learning

   D. Independence

3. The concepts defining relationships in nursing are:

   A. Nurse, crime, victim, and legal system

   B. Nurse, patient, environment, and health

   C. Patient, perpetrator, and legal system

   D. Patient, nurse, crime, and health

4. When stressed, a person can expect:

   A. Pupil dilation

   B. Reduced heart rate

   C. Reduced digestion

   D. Increased micturition

5. A key component of compassion fatigue is the stress resulting from:

   A. High workload every shift with COVID-19

   B. Adequate Staffing for the shift

   C. Minimal overtime

   D. Working with patients who have experienced traumatic events

6. Which of the following are Mindfulness Based Stress Reduction (MBSR) techniques that nurses might use to decrease burnout and stress?

    A. Singing

    B. Working extra hours

    C. Journaling and/or poetry writing

    D. Open discussion of stress with colleagues

7. When a provider ignores the lived experience of trauma's association with a patient's health, the explicit bias is:

    A. Overconfidence bias

    B. Adversarial bias

    C. Aggregate bias

    D. Confirmation bias

8. Where a person is born, grows, lives, and works are examples of:

    A. Social determinants of health

    B. Health disparities

    C. Adverse childhood experiences

    D. Millennium goals

9. When patients receive information that requires intentional partnering and equal treatment of all persons, the trauma informed care principle is:

    A. Safety

    B. Mutuality and collaboration

    C. Empowerment and choice

    D. Cultural, historical and gender issues

10. Variability in healing is associated with

    A. Age, location, and chronic illness

    B. Denying moisture over the wound

    C. Stiches to near the separate edges

11. Funding for forensic nursing was hampered by:

    A. Domestic violence response programs

    B. Forensic nurses and their programs

    C. Psyche-MH diversion programs

    D. Hospital systems

12. Criminology is the study of:

    A. Criminals and their behavior

    B. Criminals and the criminal justice system

    C. Victims and their responses

    D. Victims and the criminal justice system

13. Victimology is the study of:

    A. Criminals and the criminal justice system

    B. Criminals and their behavior

    C. Victims and their responses

    D. Victims and the criminal justice system

14. The stage of healing characterized by heat and redness is:

    A. Hemostasis

    B. Inflammatory

    C. Proliferative

    D. Maturation

15. Wound descriptions include:

    A. Labeling of entrance and exit

    B. Shape, body location, and size, being as subjective as possible

    C. Type and caliber of weapon

    D. Shape, body location, and size, being as objective as possible

16. The best way to package clothing evidence is:

    A. Place each item in its own plastic bag.

    B. Place all items in a paper bag.

    C. Place each item in its own paper bag.

    D. Please all items in a plastic bag.

17. Violence against NA/AI women includes all EXCEPT:

    A. Lack of access to services

    B. Lack of trust in institutional services

    C. Reduced incarceration

    D. Increased incarceration

18. Which of the following is not a barrier to conducting suspect examinations:

    A. Lack of knowledge

    B. Lack of training

    C. Lack of funding

    D. Lack of personnel

19. What are the steps in the Disaster Cycle?

    A. Preparedness, Response, Recovery, and Mitigation

    B. Prevention, Response, Recovery, and Mitigation

    C. Preparedness, Response, Recovery, and Completion

    D. Preparedness, Prevention, Recovery, and Mitigation

20. The recommendation of personal preparedness includes:

    A. Prepare, prevent, recover, and mitigate

    B. Be informed, make a plan, get a disaster kit

    C. Notify local, state, and federal agencies of situation

    Prepare your organization's response to disaster

21. All of the following are true of trauma EXCEPT:

    A. Individuals who experience trauma may experience anxiety if there is a lack of trauma resolution

    B. Children who experience trauma are less susceptible to substance abuse

    C. Individuals who experience trauma are susceptible to PTSD

22. Establishment of best practices in forensic nursing is the charge of

    A. NIST

    B. FNCB

    C. OSAC

    D. AAFS

23. Chain of custody is:

    A. A logarithmic accounting of evidence handling

    B. A method for safety with prisoners

    C. A method for victims to track their evidence

    D. An animal restraint

24. A forensic nurse testifies to what the patient says when there is a:

    A. Justice mission exception

    B. Direct knowledge exception for medical treatment

    C. Hearsay exception for medical diagnosis

    D. Nursing advocacy exception

25. A forensic nurse can release a record to law enforcement under this law exception:

    A. TVPA

    B. SAFER

    C. ADA

    D. HIPAA

26. The Office of Management and Budget (OMB) categorizes minority groups into (choose the best answer):

    A. Social, economic, and educational groups

    B. Ethnic and racial groups

    C. Ethnic, racial, and gender groups

    D. Gender and racial groups

27. The responsibility of the forensic nurse when providing testimony in a criminal trial is to:

    A. Demonstrate prosecutorial bias

    B. Educate the jury

    C. Support the elements of investigation

    D. Testify using technical language

28. In a criminal trial, the person who qualifies or declares that a witness can testify as an expert based on credentials and expertise is the:

    A. Attorney for the government

    B. Jury

    C. Attorney for the Defendant

    D. Judge

29. Jurisdictional maze between federal and tribal authorities means:

    A. An increase in the prosecution rates on tribal crimes

    B. A reduction in prosecution with tribal land crime

    C. Federal prosecution is primary with sex crimes

    D. Tribal jurisdiction is for NA/AI only

30. Without the availability of a forensic nursing telehealth program, this patient faced the following 2 major barriers to accessing expert forensic nursing care:

    A. Lack of internet access and lack of internet safety measures

    B. Living in a remote area and limited hours at the clinic

    C. Living in a remote area and living in a community without access to forensic nurses

    D. Not wanting to call the police and fear of retaliation

31. Which of the following is not true of photographic documentation?

    A. Obtain verbal and written consent before taking photographs

    B. Take photos at a 90° angle

    C. Ensure photographs and documentation contain the same information

    D. Do not wear gloves if your hands will be in the photograph

32. Like most patients who have utilized telehealth forensic nursing services, the patient in this case scenario reported:

    A. Feeling re-traumatized

    B. Feeling geographically isolated

    C. The physician seemed inept

    D. Feeling cared for and was glad to be able to access expert care

33. Where does violence against adolescents and adults primarily occur?

    A. At school

    B. At work

    C. At home

    D. At public events

34. Adverse childhood experiences are:

    A. Common and children are able to overcome without intervention

    B. Common and children experience long-lasting health impact and early death

    C. Uncommon and families are often used to mitigate the health outcomes

    D. Uncommon and children overcome the impact with healthy living and support

35. Who must a nurse contact should they suspect child abuse?

    A. The nurse manager

    B. The attending doctor

    C. Child Protective Services

    D. The child's guardians

36. Research on violence against elders has shown:

    A. Few elders are vulnerable to abuse

    B. Family members are never abusers of the elderly

    C. Violence against elders is pervasive across all socioeconomic levels

37. Deliberate injury in the elderly may be difficult to detect due to:

    A. Polypharmacy and co-morbid conditions

    B. Bruises look the same to all medical providers

    C. Deliberate injury only occurs with emotional abuse

38. The Social Determinant of Health related to where you live is

    A. Education attainment and inequality

    B. Receiving optimal health care

    C. Neighborhood and built environment

    D. Social work context

39. To be protected by the Americans with Disabilities Act (ADA), a person must have a disability, which is defined by the ADA as a physical or mental impairment that substantially limits _____ or more major life activities.

    A. Three

    B. Five

    C. One

    D. Two

40. Barriers to reporting sex crimes and interpersonal violence in LGBTQIA+ populations include all EXCEPT:

    A. Services serving cisgender individuals only

    B. Heterocentric services

    C. Trans male in heterocentric agencies

    D. Absence of criminal justice advocacy

41. How does heteronormativity frame the health care response to LGBTQIA+ people who have experienced sex crimes? Select all that apply:

    A. It provides a baseline standard of care for patients regardless of gender or sexual orientation

    B. Much medical research is focused on heterosexual cisgender individuals

    C. Many states do not require health care providers to take training courses on caring for LGBTQIA+ patients

    D. As the dominant social culture, heteronormative beliefs may inform health care provider's actions

    E. Providers may have personal biases against LGBTQIA+ patients

42. Stating "Heather has Tourette's syndrome" is an example of using:

    A. Identity first language

    B. Disability first language

    C. Person first language

    D. Medical-legal terminology

43. Smuggling is the:

    A. Transportation of persons into countries legally

    B. Exploitation of people who cross international borders

    C. Sheltering and feeding those who cross international borders legally

    D. Illegal transportation/harboring of persons across international borders

44. Human trafficking includes the acts listed below EXCEPT:

    A. Commercial sex

    B. Labor in agriculture

    C. Elder abuse

    D. Child soldiers

45. Wrap around services are necessary for:

    A. Elopement

    B. Recovery

    C. Truancy reversal

    D. Standard of living

46. Gang classification generally includes:

    A. Ten or more members and linkage to a name that is not recognized by anyone else to keep their gang identity private.

    B. Independent identity and public recognition by others that they are a criminal gang.

    C. Three or more members, shared identity, and the purpose is to engage in criminal activity.

    D. Maintaining an anonymous identity to engage in criminal activity without getting caught.

47. Identify the 3 violent gang types:

    A. Organized Criminal Gangs, Street Gangs, International Gangs

    B. Organized Criminal Gangs, Prison Gangs, Foreign-born Gangs

    C. Motorcycle Gangs, Prison Gangs, Street Gangs

    D. Motorcycle Gangs, Organized Criminal Gangs, Prison Gangs

48. Inmates who are at highest risk for victimization in prison settings include:

    A. Inmates who are guilty of violent offenses

    B. Inmates who have lower levels of education

    C. Members of gangs

    D. Inmates with chronic illnesses, substance abuse disorders, mental illness and the elderly

MULTIPLE CORRECT ANSWER MULTIPLE CHOICE

1. Factors that can directly impact family dynamics and risk for violence include:

    A. Financial and/or housing instability

    B. Substance use disorders

    C. Education level

    D. Adverse childhood experiences

2. Which are components of a nursing forensic examination?

    A. Focused assessment

    B. Review of system interview.

    C. Photography and body diagrams

    D. Detailed injury assessment

    E. Collection of forensic evidence

3. Which ways can the forensic nurse help a someone who has experienced dating violence?

    A. Obtain a medical and forensic history using trauma-informed principles

    B. Provide a detailed head-to-toe assessment to determine the extent of injuries

    C. Identify and collect potential evidence that is on the body and clothing

4. When documenting injuries in medical-legal cases, the nurse should use which of the types:

    A. Written narrative

    B. Diagrams

    C. Photographs

5. Arrest the perpetrator Responses to prison violence such as post-traumatic stress symptoms and exacerbation of existing mental health and physical health problems are experienced primarily by:

    A. Inmates who are victims of violence from other inmates

    B. Health staff who are the victims of inmate violence

    C. Inmates and staff who witness violence

    D. Staff who do not witness violence

6. With whom do forensic nurses consult for scientific identification of remains?

    A. Forensic odontology

    B. Forensic engineer

    C. Forensic anthropology

    D. Forensic epidemiologist

7. Which community resources may be helpful in to a college student recovering from sexual assault?

    A. Rape crisis center

    B. Trauma recovery program

    C. College counseling services

    D. Crime victim compensation program

TRUE OR FALSE

1. The age of a child at the time of trauma influences their ability to process trauma.

    — True

    — False

2. SANE is available 24/7?

    — True

    — False

3. A male cannot be raped by a female.

    — True

    — False

4. Intentionally damaging a family member's property is an act of domestic violence.

    — True

    — False

5. The damaging effects of family violence can span generations

    — True

    — False

6. Inmates are not at a higher risk for sexual victimization because there are always guards around.

    — True

    — False

7. All states in the US have specific protocols related to suspect examinations.

    — True

    — False

8. One tactic of coercive emotional and psychological abuse is cruelty and violence toward household pets.

    — True

    — False

ANSWER KEY

SINGLE BEST ANSWER MULTIPLE CHOICE

1. B	13. D	25. D	37. A
2. D	14. B	26. B	38. C
3. B	15. D	27. B	39. C
4. C	16. C	28. D	40. D
5. D	17. C	29. B	41. B, C, D, E
6. C	18. D	30. C	42. C
7. C	19. A	31. D	43. D
8. A	20. D	32. D	44. C
9. B	21. B	33. C	45 B
10. A	22. C	34. B	46. C
11. A	23. A	35. C	47. C
12. B	24. C	36. C	48. D

MULTIPLE CORRECT ANSWER MULTIPLE CHOICE

1. A, B, C, D

2. C, D, E

3. A, B, C

4. A, B, C

5. A, B, C

6. A, C

7. A, B, C, D

TRUE OR FALSE

1. True		6. False
2. True		7. False
3. False		8. True
4. True		
5. True		